Sensors for Physiological Monitoring and Digital Health

Sensors for Physiological Monitoring and Digital Health

Guest Editors

Ganesh R. Naik
Elena Pirogova
Margaret Lech

MDPI

Basel • Beijing • Wuhan • Barcelona • Belgrade • Novi Sad • Cluj • Manchester

Guest Editors
Ganesh R. Naik
College of Medicine and Public Health
Flinders University
Adelaide
Australia

Elena Pirogova
School of Engineering
RMIT University
Melbourne
Australia

Margaret Lech
School of Engineering
RMIT University
Melbourne
Australia

Editorial Office
MDPI AG
Grosspeteranlage 5
4052 Basel, Switzerland

This is a reprint of the Special Issue, published open access by the journal *Sensors* (ISSN 1424-8220), freely accessible at: https://www.mdpi.com/journal/sensors/special_issues/W1YX1019R9.

For citation purposes, cite each article independently as indicated on the article page online and as indicated below:

Lastname, A.A.; Lastname, B.B. Article Title. *Journal Name* **Year**, *Volume Number*, Page Range.

ISBN 978-3-7258-5359-5 (Hbk)
ISBN 978-3-7258-5360-1 (PDF)
https://doi.org/10.3390/books978-3-7258-5360-1

Contents

About the Editors

Ganesh R. Naik

Ganesh R. Naik is a highly respected figure in biomedical engineering and signal processing. Ranked in the top 2% of global researchers by Stanford University, he earned his PhD from RMIT University in 2009. Currently a senior academic at Torrens University Australia, Dr. Naik is a prolific mid-career researcher. He has edited 16 books and authored more than 150 papers in peer-reviewed journals and conferences. His expertise is widely recognized, as he serves as an associate editor for several major publications, including *IEEE ACCESS* and *Frontiers in Neurorobotics*. Dr. Naik has been awarded numerous prestigious fellowships throughout his career, including a Baden–Württemberg Scholarship from Germany, a BridgeTech industry fellowship from the Australian government, and an international fellowship from the Royal Academy of Engineering UK in 2025. Before his current position, Dr. Naik held significant research roles. He was a research theme co-lead at the Adelaide Institute for Sleep Health at Flinders University from 2020 to 2023. Prior to that, he was a Postdoctoral Research Fellow at Western Sydney University, where he led the data analysis for a major sleep project and developed algorithms for wearable sleep technology. His postdoctoral career also included a Chancellor's Postdoctoral Research Fellowship at the University of Technology Sydney from 2013 to 2017.

Elena Pirogova

Elena Pirogova is a Professor of Biomedical Engineering. She graduated with a Doctor of Philosophy (PhD) in Biomedical Engineering from the Department of Electrical and Computer Systems Engineering, Monash University, Australia, in 2002. Prof. Pirogova currently works in the School of Engineering, STEM College, RMIT University. She is an experienced undergraduate and Higher Degrees by Research (HDR) Program Manager with a demonstrated history of senior leadership in higher engineering education (most recently Head of the Discipline of Electrical and Biomedical engineering) and engineering research. Elena's research expertise includes bioengineering, biomedical devices, biomaterials, microfluidic systems technology, bioelectromagnetics, and biosignal processing. Professor Pirogova has established successful research collaborations with colleagues at Aikenhead Centre for Medical Discovery (ACMD), Australia's premier biomedical engineering research translation centre located at St Vincent's Hospital, Melbourne; The Baker Heart & Diabetes Institute; the University of Wollongong, and the University of Melbourne. Her research is fundamental and applied, interdisciplinary and impactful. It is funded by Australian Government Category 1 grants, philanthropic organizations and directly by industry. Her research aims to advance medical technologies for improving healthcare in Australia.

Margaret Lech

Margaret Lech holds an MSc in Physics from the University of Maria Curie-Sklodowska (UMCS) in Poland and a PhD in Electrical Engineering from the University of Melbourne. She worked as a Research Fellow at Monash University and the Bionic Ear Institute. In 1998, she joined RMIT and progressed to her current position as a professor. She has co-authored over 160 research papers in the fields of artificial intelligence, machine learning, and signal processing. Her research team contributed groundbreaking techniques for automatically detecting emotion and clinical depression from speech signals. For her work in this area, she was awarded an international patent and won the Telstra Innovation Challenge 2010. Her pioneering work extends to modelling and analyzing emotional interactions in conversations, detecting interpersonal trust and modelling cognitive load. Margaret has co-supervised over 30 PhD students and four Postdoctoral Fellows. She received the Vice-Chancellor's Research Supervision Excellence Award in 2013 and the RMIT Award for Excellence in Graduate Research in 2019. Her past research grants include VPAC, ARC Linkage, DSI, AOARD, and DSTG. She is currently a co-investigator on the Office of National Intelligence Discovery and ARC Discovery grants.

Preface

The continuous monitoring of human physiological signals has become a foundation of modern personalized healthcare. Physiological signals, such as brain waves (EEG), cardiac signals (ECG), and heart rate, provide critical insights into human wellness and are particularly vital for elderly individuals and those living with chronic conditions. With the advent of wearable technologies, it is now possible to measure these parameters in real-time, continuously, and non-intrusively. Coupled with the rapid growth of digital health platforms and Artificial Intelligence (AI), these innovations are transforming healthcare delivery, enabling timely interventions, improving the quality of care, and facilitating valuable data-driven decision-making for patients, practitioners, hospitals, and governments alike.

This Special Issue, "Sensors for Physiological Monitoring and Digital Health", brings together diverse scientific perspectives to explore these exciting developments. It highlights contributions at the intersection of biomedical signal processing, wearable technologies, machine learning, health informatics, mobility research, bioinformatics, and sports science. Our goal is to foster interdisciplinary dialogue and provide a platform for highly innovative researchers to share their findings in this rapidly evolving field.

The motivation behind this reprint is the recognition of both the urgent healthcare needs of today and the vast opportunities afforded by advances in microfabrication, flexible electronics, nanomaterials, and wireless communication technologies. The global market for wearable medical devices reflects this momentum, having grown significantly in recent years, and the demand for innovative solutions is stronger than ever. By curating the latest research, we aim to showcase the transformative potential of sensors and digital health in redefining healthcare practices.

This Special Issue is intended for a broad audience, including academic researchers, healthcare professionals, industry innovators, and policy makers interested in the future of healthcare. We are deeply grateful to the authors for their valuable contributions and to the reviewers for their thoughtful evaluations, which ensured the high quality of this collection. We also extend our sincere appreciation to the editorial team of Sensors for their support in bringing this reprint to fruition.

As Guest Editors, we are honoured to present this Special Issue and hope it serves as both an inspiration and a resource for continued innovation in the field of physiological monitoring and digital health.

Ganesh R. Naik, Elena Pirogova, and Margaret Lech
Guest Editors

sensors

MDPI

Article

SenseHunger: Machine Learning Approach to Hunger Detection Using Wearable Sensors

Muhammad Tausif Irshad [1,2,*], Muhammad Adeel Nisar [1,2], Xinyu Huang [1], Jana Hartz [1], Olaf Flak [3], Frédéric Li [1], Philip Gouverneur [1], Artur Piet [1], Kerstin M. Oltmanns [4] and Marcin Grzegorzek [1,5]

1 Institute of Medical Informatics, University of Lübeck, Ratzeburger Allee 160, 23562 Lübeck, Germany
2 Department of IT, University of the Punjab, Katchery Road, Lahore 54000, Pakistan
3 Department of Management, Faculty of Law and Social Sciences, Jan Kochanowski University of Kielce, ul. Żeromskiego 5, 25-369 Kielce, Poland
4 Section of Psychoneurobiology, Center of Brain, Behavior and Metabolism, University of Lübeck, Ratzeburger Allee 160, 23562 Lübeck, Germany
5 Department of Knowledge Engineering, University of Economics in Katowice, Bogucicka 3, 40-287 Katowice, Poland
* Correspondence: m.irshad@uni-luebeck.de Tel.: +49-451-3101-5612

Abstract: The perception of hunger and satiety is of great importance to maintaining a healthy body weight and avoiding chronic diseases such as obesity, underweight, or deficiency syndromes due to malnutrition. There are a number of disease patterns, characterized by a chronic loss of this perception. To our best knowledge, hunger and satiety cannot be classified using non-invasive measurements. Aiming to develop an objective classification system, this paper presents a multimodal sensory system using associated signal processing and pattern recognition methods for hunger and satiety detection based on non-invasive monitoring. We used an Empatica E4 smartwatch, a RespiBan wearable device, and JINS MEME smart glasses to capture physiological signals from five healthy normal weight subjects inactively sitting on a chair in a state of hunger and satiety. After pre-processing the signals, we compared different feature extraction approaches, either based on manual feature engineering or deep feature learning. Comparative experiments were carried out to determine the most appropriate sensor channel, device, and classifier to reliably discriminate between hunger and satiety states. Our experiments showed that the most discriminative features come from three specific sensor modalities: Electrodermal Activity (EDA), infrared Thermopile (Tmp), and Blood Volume Pulse (BVP).

Keywords: hunger; satiety; physiological signals; non-invasive sensing; multimodal sensing; machine learning; artificial neural network

1. Introduction

Hunger and satiety perception occurs within the hypothalamic areas of the brain, processing a number of endocrine signals coming from peripheral organs such as the stomach, liver, pancreas, intestine, or fat tissue [1]. Differentiating between hunger and satiety is crucial to maintaining stable body weight and preventing malnutrition. Specifically, overweight and obesity are known to be associated with a gradually advanced loss of this perception, leading to overeating, underlying the disease [2]. According to the World Health Organization (WHO), 39% of adults aged 18 years and older were overweight, and 13% were obese in 2016 [3]. So far, common methods to determine hunger and satiety are invasive, i.e., via hormonal analyses from blood samples, or based on self-assessment, such as Visual Analog Scales (VAS) [4,5]. The latter records subjective sensations such as the desire to eat, hunger, satiety, and nausea [6,7] and by nature, underlies several external factors influencing the test results (e.g., stress level, environmental temperature, etc.). In contrast, invasive methods—mostly used in experimental settings—measuring blood concentrations of relevant hormones are not practicable in everyday life. In order to develop a therapeutic device that may assist people to train hunger and satiety perception, objective and non-invasive measurements are necessary.

The detection of hunger and satiety with multimodal physiological sensor signals using supervised machine learning (ML) is a worthy investigation. This is because ML has already shown promising results on physiological sensor signals in a various applications in other fields such as biology, medicine, and psychology [8–11]. An important step in a ML process is *feature extraction*, which consists of computing some values from the data—referred to as *features*—that are meaningful for the problem to solve. Feature extraction approaches map the data from a high-dimensional space to a low-dimensional one to lower the complexity of the ML problem. There are two main families of feature extraction, namely feature engineering and feature learning. Feature engineering refers to the manual crafting of features, either based on expert knowledge or on simple transformation functions (e.g., arithmetic operators and/or aggregation operators) applied to the sensor signals.

Feature learning, on the other hand, designates the automated learning of features from the data. One of the most popular feature learning approaches nowadays is deep learning that is based on Artificial Neural Networks (ANNs). They work in an end to end fashion and have already shown promising results in a large number of health-related applications [12–16]. ANNs are modeled after their biological counterparts and can be implemented on computers as software applications. The basic elements of ANNs are artificial neurons, which are interconnected in form of layers. Sensor signals are provided to the input layer, and then they move to the output layer via interconnected neurons. An ANN, which consists of more than three layers, i.e., an input layer, an output layer, and several hidden layers, is called a Deep Neural Network (DNN). DNNs can be trained with appropriate data to create a useful model that converts inputs into outputs [17,18].

Developing an objective system to predict hunger and satiety using multimodal sensory signals is a complex task. However, such a problem has not been explored extensively in the past literature. More specifically, all past studies either used invasive sensor modalities or investigated a related but different problem than the recognition of hunger and satiety. In this work, we therefore hypothesize that modern non-invasive wearable sensors can allow us to distinguish hunger and satiety states. We perform an ML study involving the comparison of several state-of-the-art feature extraction and classification approaches. We also investigate various sensor modalities recording physiological data to determine which one(s) contribute the most to this problem.

To summarize, we make the following contributions:

1. We investigate the use of non-invasive multimodal sensors in the context of hunger and satiety detection and develop a state-of-the-art machine learning model, which learns hunger and satiety patterns from multimodal sensors data and classifies them into hunger and satiety classes.
2. We analyze and compare wearable devices and sensor channels to select the most relevant physiological signals for an accurate classification of hunger and satiety data.
3. We perform a comparative analysis of feature extraction approaches and machine learning algorithms to identify the best features in achieving optimal classification results.
4. We also provide a brief review of related approaches.

The rest of the article is structured as follows. Section 2 presents the current state-of-the-art in hunger and satiety detection. Section 3 describes the materials and methods used to analyze multimodal signals for assessing hunger and satiety. Section 4 presents the experimental results. Section 5 provides a discussion, and finally, Section 6 concludes this work.

2. Related Work

In recent years, some hunger detection methods have been applied for clinical and behavioral assessments [4,19–25]. Table 1 lists the sensors and systems used in the reviewed studies.

Table 1. Sensors and systems for the assessment of hunger in the literature.

Study	Sensors/System	Dataset Information	Features	Detection
Barajas-Montiel and Reyes-Garcia [25]	Microphone	1627—samples of hunger and pain cries (acoustic data of infants)	Acoustic features by means of frequencies	Hunger cry, no-hunger cry, pain cry and no-pain cry
Krishnan et al. [4]	VAS	13—subjects plasma concentrations of satiety hormones from blood samples	Feature learning (ANN)	VAS responses from satiety hormone values
Bellmann et al. [19]	In vitro gastrointestinal model	Gastric viscosity and intestinal digestion from tiny-TIMagc	-	Fullness vs. Hunger
Rahman et al. [20]	Microsoft Band, Affectiva Q sensor, Microphone	8—subjects (3 female, 5 male) from 26 to 54 years	Statistical features	Time until the next eating event, and about-to-eat
Al-Zubaidi et al. [21]	fMRI	24—male subjects from 20 to 30 years (fMRI data)	3—features (DC, ReHo and fALFF)	Neuronal resting state alterations changes during hunger and satiety
Lakshmi et al. [22]	EEG	EEG signals	-	Hunger, thirst, and rest-room sensations
Maria and Jeyaseelan [23]	Microphone	Synthetically collected audio signals through mobile phones	SF, CDF and GCC	Growling vs. Burp sound
Gogate and Bakal [24]	EDA	35—patients (20 of them used as control group)	-	Hunger vs. Stress

VAS: Visual analog scales; ANN: Artificial neural network; fMRI: Functional magnetic resonance imaging; DC: Degree of centrality; ReHo: Regional homogeneity; fALFF: Fractional amplitude of low-frequency fluctuations; EEG: Electroencephalography; SF: Spectral features; CDF: Cepstral domain features; GCC: Gammatone cepstral coefficients; EDA: Electrodermal activity; tiny-TIMagc: In vitro gastrointestinal model.

To the best of our knowledge, physiological signals acquired from multimodal sensors have not yet been used for the prediction of hunger and satiety responses using machine learning. For example, Barajas-Montiel and Reyes-Garcia [25] applied traditional signal processing and pattern classification methods to detect hunger cries, no-hunger cries, pain cries, and no-pain cries from infant acoustic data. Here, the detection of hunger cries and no hunger cries is based on acoustic features in the form of frequencies. The model proposed in this paper [25] is specific to infants and could not be generalized to the young and elderly population to detect hunger and satiety. They did not describe feature learning or the use of wearable physiological sensors for hunger and satiety detection.

Interestingly, Maria and Jeyaseelan [23] used audio signals generated by the stomach to identify growls that can describe hunger well. The synthetic audio signals were recorded using mobile phones and pre-processed using smoothing methods and median filtering. Spectral features were calculated to classify the signals into growls and burps.

Krishnan et al. [4] used ANN to model the feelings of hunger and satiety after food intake. They trained their model with a dataset relating concentration–time courses of plasma satiety hormones to VAS assessments. The proposed model successfully predicted VAS responses from the dataset of satiety hormones obtained in experiments with different food compositions. They also revealed that the predicted VAS responses for the test data separated the satiety effects of highly satiating foods from less satiating foods, for both oral and ileal infusion. However, their approach is time-consuming and invasive because they used plasma hormone levels, which are not easy to obtain compared to physiological signals detected by smart sensor devices.

Bellmann et al. [19] claimed that human clinical trials are time-consuming and costly. Therefore, they developed a gastrointestinal model in conjunction with ANN to predict feelings of hunger and satiety after the ingestion of different meals. They trained their model with a series of training datasets to create a prediction set and link the model measurements to VAS scores for hunger and satiety. Although gastrointestinal-based modeling is still in its infancy, it is evident that the development of machine learning approaches has the potential to transform such models into powerful predictive tools, which can predict physiological responses to food. However, the acquisition of physiological responses by miniaturized sensors is state-of-the-art.

Rahman et al. [20] proposed that predicting eating events can enable users to adopt better eating behaviors. As a consequence, they used a set of sensor devices to record physical activity, location, heart rate, electrodermal activity, skin temperature, and calories ingested while eight users were eating. They extracted 158 window-level features, followed by correlation-based feature selection (CFS), and trained a classifier to predict the about-to-eat event. Time until the next eating event was predicted using regression analysis. However, the use of motion sensors such as accelerometers and gyroscopes is questionable for the "time until the next eating" event. Additionally, they did not provide any comparison between sensor modalities to determine the best optimal device.

Al-Zubaidi et al. [21] investigated the influence of hunger and satiety on resting-state functional magnetic resonance imaging (rs-fMRI) using connectivity models, i.e., local connectivity, global connectivity, and the amplitude of rs-fMRI signals. They extracted the connectivity parameters of ninety brain regions for each model and used the sequential forward sliding selection strategy in conjunction with a linear support vector machine classifier to determine which connectivity model best discriminated between metabolic states (hunger vs. satiety). They claimed that the amplitude of the rs-fMRI signals, with a classification accuracy of 81%, is slightly more accurate than the local and global connectivity models in detecting changes in the resting state of the brain during hunger and satiety. However, they did not show results with the state-of-the-art supervised feature learning approach.

Gogate and Bakal [24] presented a hunger- and stress-monitoring system using galvanic skin response data from 35 patients using proprietary data processing and classification techniques. They claimed an overall accuracy of the system of 86.6%. However, they did neither specify a method for data processing and feature extraction, nor did they use classical or modern classification methods.

Lakshmi et al. [22], proposed a method to detect hunger specifically in physically disabled people. The main goal was to communicate using the brain's thoughts without muscle control, specifically for severely paralyzed people with a non-invasive approach to make the task less complex and more convenient. In this approach, a single-channel electrode was placed on a person's scalp to detect human sensations of hunger, thirst, and toilet using images placed in front of it. The final result was obtained by analyzing the person's attention level. The attention levels of each image were compared to the corresponding image in MATLAB, and the resulting attention level value was obtained.

In general, there are very few studies [4,19–25] on the subject that we investigate. However, each of them has some limitations; for example, the data collection method used by Krishnan et al. [4] was invasive, and the results of Bellmann et al. [19] were based on gastrointestinal models. Rahman et al. [20], used motion sensors for the "time until the next eating" event, which is questionable. Maria and Jeyaseelan [23], and Barajas-Montiel and Reyes-Garcia [25] used microphones to record the data, which can trigger a privacy risk. The authors in [21,22,24] used hand-crafted features, while feature learning can perform as well or better than state-of-the-art [26]. To-date, no automated system for detecting hunger and satiety using multimodal physiological signals has been evaluated, nor is there a public dataset.

3. Materials and Methods

In this section, we present the aspects of the sensor modalities accumulated for data acquisition, the process of data acquisition, and discuss the experimental settings. The entire process from data acquisition to analysis consists of a series of steps as shown in Figure 1, which has been extensively described in the past literature [9,27].

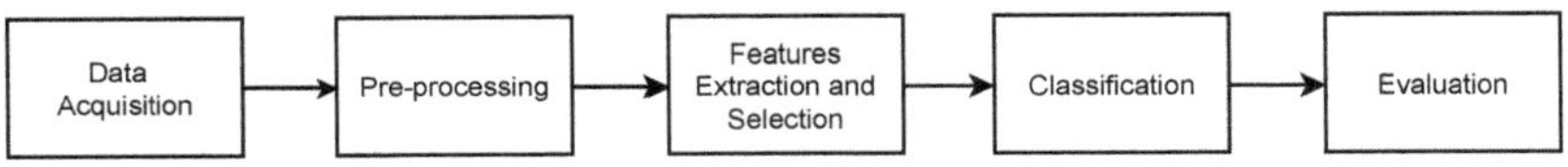

Figure 1. Standard approach to developing machine learning and pattern recognition systems. Each step should be optimized in parallel to achieve the best performance.

3.1. Dataset Acquisition

The hardware configuration of our proposed sense-hunger system is shown in Figure 2. We used the following wearable devices and sensor modalities to collect physiological hunger and satiety signals from five healthy individuals:

1. RespiBan (Plux Wireless Biosignals S. A., Lisboa, Portugal) [28]: Subjects wear the respiration belt on the chest, at the level of the thorax, with the electrode connectors facing forward. It contains the Respiration (Resp) sensor and also provides the possibility for connecting to other sensors such as Electrodermal activity (EDA), Electrocardiography (ECG), and Electromyography (EMG), as shown in Figure 2. The description of these sensors is as follows:
   - Resp: This sensor measures the respiration rate. It detects chest or abdominal expansion/contraction, and outputs a respiration signal. It is usually worn using a comfortable and flexible length-adjustable belt. It is sampled at 475 Hz.
   - EDA [29]: EDA of RespiBan (Eda_RB) consists of two electrodes placed on the front, in the middle of the index finger, and in the middle of the middle finger of subject's non-dominant hand. This sensor measures the galvanic skin response, i.e., the change in electrical conductivity of skin in response to sweat secretion. It is also sampled at 475 Hz.
   - ECG [30]: It consists of three electrodes placed on the subject's right upper pectoral, left upper pectoral, and at the left bottom thoracic cage. This sensor records the electrical impulses through the heart muscle, and it can also be used to provide information on the heart's response to physical exertion. It is also sampled at 475 Hz.
   - EMG [31]: This sensor is used to assess the electrical activity associated with muscle contractions and respective nerve cells, which control them. It is placed on the subject's abdomen above the belly button and is also sampled at 475 Hz.
2. Empatica E4 wristband (Emaptica Inc., Cambridge MA, USA) [32]: It contains photoplethysmogram (PPG), infrared thermopile (Tmp), and EDA sensors that allow

measurements of sympathetic nervous system activity and heart rate (HR) variability. The description of these sensors is as follows:

- PPG: This sensor measures blood volume pulse (BVP), which can be used to derive HR and inter-beat interval (IBI). It is sampled at 1 Hz.
- Tmp: This sensor records skin temperature. It is sampled at 5 Hz.
- EDA: EDA of Empatica E4 (Eda_E4) wristband measures the galvanic skin response, which is the change in the electrical conductivity of the skin in response to sweat secretion. It is sampled at 5 Hz.

3. JINS MEME smart glasses (Jins Inc., Tokyo, Japan) [33]: They can track not only where we look, but how often we blink and even whether we are about to relax or fall asleep. It uses electrooculography (EOG) electrodes placed in three locations on the frame. These electrodes can track blink duration and eye movements in different directions. It is sampled at 20 Hz.

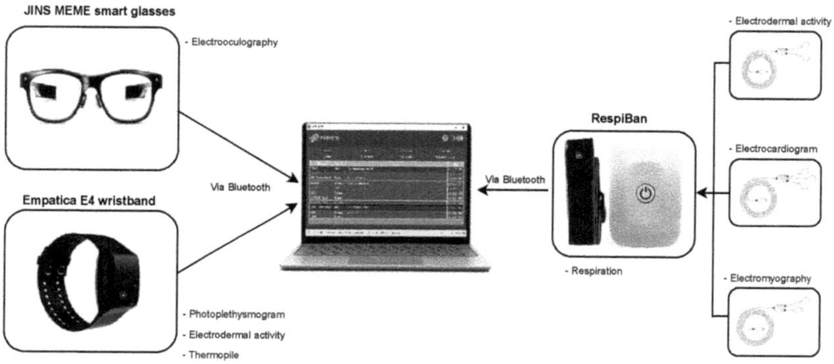

Figure 2. The SenseHunger system uses three sensory devices, namely, JINS MEME smart glasses, Empatica E4 wristband, and RespiBan. The Electrodermal activity (EDA), Electrocardiogram (ECG), and Electromyography (EMG) electrodes are plugged into the RespiBan device. Datasets from all devices are sent to the laptop for storage using a Bluetooth connection.

The data collection of hunger and satiety activities involved five healthy volunteers whose demographic information is provided in Appendix C. Subjects were asked not to eat anything for 16 h before data collection. However, drinking water was allowed. Data collection for each subject was divided into two phases, namely, the hunger and the satiety phase. In the hunger phase, data collection lasted for 5 min, using the sensory devices shown in Figure 2. After eating, the process was resumed for the satiety phase, which lasted for 30 min.

3.2. Pre-Processing

State-of-the-art machine learning (ML) algorithms can certainly derive knowledge from raw sensor data. However, their output generally depends on the quality of the datasets they are working with. If data are insufficient or contain extraneous and irrelevant information, ML algorithms may produce less accurate and less understandable results or discover nothing useful at all. Therefore, pre-processing of the data is an important step in the process of ML. The pre-processing step is necessary for solving various types of problems influencing data such as noise, redundancy, missing values, etc. [34]. In the first step, datasets from all sensor channels (as shown in Figure 2) are synchronized, resampled to a frequency of 100 Hz, and linearly interpolated to ensure that the channels shared a common repetition.

Based on our preliminary experiments, we segmented the data of each sensor channel using a Sliding Window Segmentation (SWS) in the following three settings with an overlapping window, to select the optimal setting: In the first setting, the length T and sliding stride (step size) ΔS of a time window are set to 10 and 5 s, respectively. The second setting is defined by length $T = 30$ s and sliding step $\Delta S = 15$ s, while in the third setting, the length T and the sliding step ΔS of a time window are set to 60 and 30 s, respectively. The experimental results with the mentioned window sizes and step sizes are presented in Section 4.

3.3. Feature Extraction and Selection

In a linear or nonlinear fashion, feature extraction approaches model the data from a high-dimensional space into a reduced dimensional space. In this study, we used two approaches to extract features, namely the hand-crafted features and automated feature learning.

Hand-crafted Features: We used 18 hand-crafted features [9,35] consisting of the statistical and frequency-related values of the input signals. These features are listed in Table 2. All features were computed independently for each axis of each sensor channel, following the suggestions of Cook and Krishnan [36]. They were subsequently concatenated to obtain a feature vector of size 18 × sensor (S). To remove the effects of discrepancies between the values of each feature, min-max normalization was performed for each feature to project its values into the interval $[0, 1]$. The normalization constants calculated on the training set were again used to calculate the features in the test set.

Table 2. Hand-crafted features calculated independently for each sensor channel.

Hand-Crafted Features	
Maximum	Minimum
Average	Standard deviation
Zero-crossing	Percentile 20
Percentile 50	Percentile 80
Interquartile	Skewness
Kurtosis	Auto-correlation
First-order mean	Second-order mean
Norm of the first-order mean	Norm of the second-order mean
Spectral energy	Spectral entropy

We applied feature selection on the features we manually computed to remove useless or redundant ones, and to decrease the complexity of our classification model. This can improve the performance of a model and determine the interdependence between features and class labels [36]. A common approach for feature selection is feature ranking, which quantifies the ability of the feature to predict the desired class. A Random Forest (RF) was used to select the most important hand-crafted features [37]. It is a tree-based learner that generally grows by applying the classification and regression tree method (CART) [38], where binary splits recursively partition the tree into homogeneous or nearly homogeneous terminal nodes. After a fair split, the data is moved from the root tree node to the child nodes, improving the homogeneity of the child nodes relative to the parent node [39]. Typically RF consists of a set of hundreds of trees, where each tree is grown using a sample of the dataset.

In RF, trees are generally grown non-deterministically using a two-step randomization procedure. Apart from the randomization applied by growing the tree using a sample of the primary data, a subsequent level of randomization is set at the node level as the tree grows. The objective of this two-step randomization is to decorrelate the trees, so that RF ensemble has low variance. Features ranked by RF are based on the quality of the purity improvement (which is the fraction of data items that belong to the class) of the node.

Given a node n and the estimated class probabilities $p(k|n)$ $k = 1, \ldots Q$. The Gini index can be defined by using the following equation [40].

$$G(n) = 1 - \sum_{k=1}^{Q} p(k|n)^2 \quad (1)$$

In Equation (1), Q is the total number of classes. In order to obtain the Gini index-based measure at each node, the Gini index decline is calculated for the variable used for partitioning. The Gini index-based measure of variable importance is then obtained by the average drop in the Gini index. For the comparison of manual feature selection approaches, see Appendix A.

Feature Learning: Feature learning involves learning features from labeled input data in an automated way without any human input. Feature learning has become increasingly popular over the past years with the popularization of ANNs and DNNs. During training, they are fed with raw input data to learn a mapping against each class in an end to end fashion. ANN and DNN models have been shown to perform well on various tasks (e.g., image classification [41], activity recognition [9,42], and sleep stage classification [8]). However, training such models can be challenging as it is computationally more expensive than training traditional models. Moreover, finding optimal architectures is a non-trivial process.

In the past, Multi-Layer Perceptrons (MLPs) [43] and Convolutional Neural Networks (CNNs) [44] have been used for various tasks. MLPs represent the most primitive type of ANN. In order to process 2D sensor data with its sensor axis (S) and time (T), the input data are first normalized using the batch-normalization layer [45], and then passed to fully connected layers that expect 1D input. A syntactic example of the MLP architecture can be seen in Figure 3.

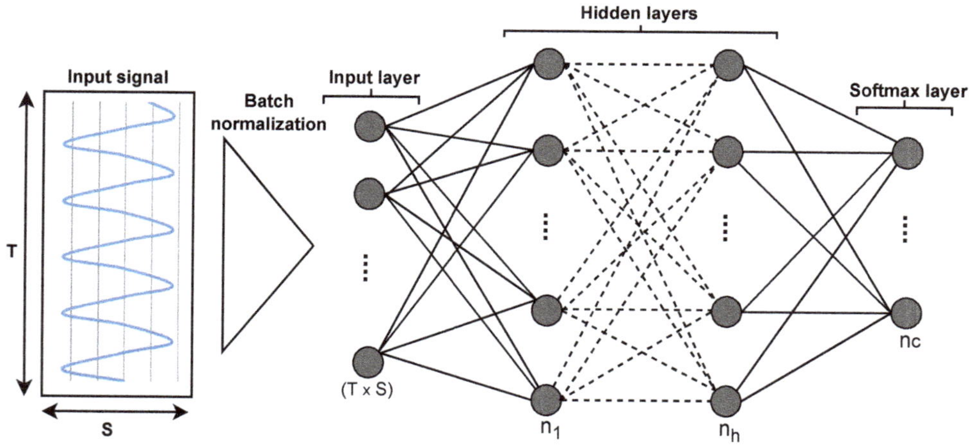

Figure 3. Illustration of a MLP where different sensor channels are converted into a (T×S) dimensional vector, which is passed to the different hidden layers (h) and output classes (c) as defined by the softmax layer.

In CNN architectures, the convolutional layers are the main building blocks normally used to perform convolutional operations between one or several convolutional filters (or kernels) learned during the training phase and the layer input. The convolution operation can be applied by sliding the convolution kernels over the input data. In this study, raw sensor data are given as 3D input (S× T× 1) to the CNN model for processing. After a series of convolutional and pooling layers, the output of the last convolutional layer is usually smoothed into a 1D vector and fed into the softmax layer. The Rectified Linear Unit (ReLU) is the most commonly used activation function for convolutional layers. It is also common to add multiple dense layers of a multilayer perceptron to the CNN architecture for classification problems. In that case, a softmax activation function is usually used to connect the aftermost dense layer to the output layer. An example of a CNN model can be seen in Figure 4.

In initial experiments (whose results are reported in Appendix B), various configurations for the window size (T), step size (ΔS), and learning rate (lr) parameters were examined. It was found that T = 60 s, ΔS= 5 s, and lr =10^{-4} yielded the best performances. Therefore, each sensor channel information was segmented into parts, resulting in data frames of the form ($N \times S \times 1$), where N is the number of segments, or more precisely, ($6000 \times 7 \times 1$) for each class.

The purpose of this study was to test the use of feature learning methods with a dual objective. The primary goal was to analyze the quality of MLP and CNN in automatically extracting features with different hyperparameters. The secondary objective was to examine and compare the results of human-generated features and automatic feature extraction. The results of classifying hunger and satiety using the above mentioned approaches are presented in the experimental results section.

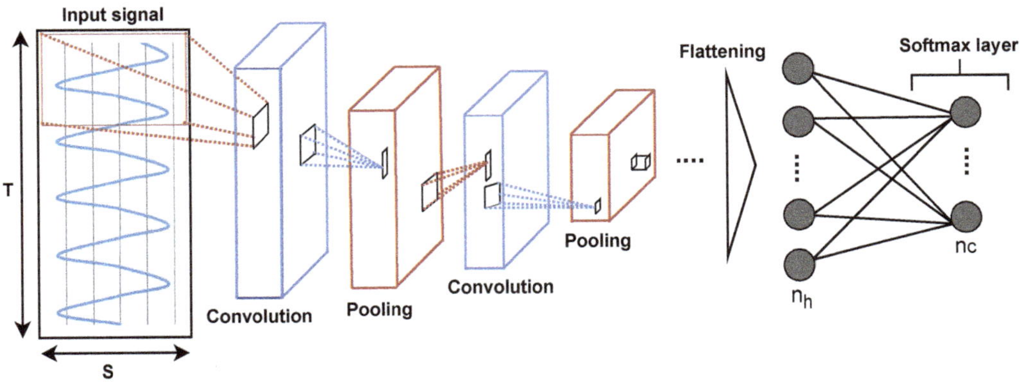

Figure 4. Illustration of a Convolutional Neural Network (CNN) model with convolutional layers, pooling layers, h dense layers, and c output classes represented by a softmax layer. Input data are processed by convolutional layers and pooling layers, and are passed to dense layers after extraction of profound features.

3.4. Classification

To provide a comparison between hand-crafted features and automatically learned features, we used two types of classification approaches. Traditional classifiers such as support vector machine (SVM), decision tree (DT), and RF were trained and tested on hand-crafted features, and ANN-based models such as MLP and CNN with softmax layers were applied to classify the automatically learned features into hunger vs. satiety classes. The description of these methods are as follows:

1. SVM: In pattern recognition, SVM is a supervised learning algorithm, which can be used for classification and regression tasks. Its robust performance on noisy and sparse data makes it a good choice for a variety of applications [42]. In a classification task, the SVM separates the labeled training data with a maximum margin hyperplane. Test data are then mapped to the same space to predict a class label. SVM can also efficiently map high-dimensional data to a high-dimensional dimension feature space to perform nonlinear classification [46].

2. DT: This is an approach to classification or regression analysis, in which a decision tree is constructed by recursively partitioning the feature space of the training set into smaller and smaller subsets. The final consequence is a tree with decision and leaf nodes. DT aims to find a set of decision rules that instinctively divide the feature space to build a instructive and robust classification model. A decision node has binary or multiple branches. A leaf node indicates a class or outcome. The top decision node in a tree points to the best predictor, which is called the root node [47].
3. RF: This is a popular ensemble learning method used for various types of classification problems such as activity recognition [35], where multiple DTs are created at training time [48–52]. In RF, each tree casts a unit vote by assigning each input to the most likely class label. RF is fast, robust to noise, and an effective ensemble, which can be used to identify nonlinear patterns in datasets. It can handle both numeric and categorical data. The biggest advantage of RF compared to DT is that it is significantly more resilient to overfitting [53].

3.5. Evaluation

The selection of the evaluation metric is very important and application-dependent, because an inadequately defined metric may lead to incorrect conclusions [54]. For this reason, the evaluation metrics were designed to be consistent with the state-of-the-art work in this field, and to facilitate comparison. It is worth mentioning that in all experiments of this work, cross-validation was used according to the Leave-One-Subject-Out (LOSO) protocol, in which each subject's data are used once as the test set, whereas the remaining data constitute the training set. In general, the overall performance is the average of the results gained for each tested subject. The LOSO cross-validation procedure guarantees that all models are tested on unknown subjects, which allows a realistic evaluation of the classification algorithms used in de-factor applications.

For the classification performance of the different models tested, we used accuracy assessed by the ratio of true predictions (i.e., true positive (t_p), true negative (t_n)) to all entries (i.e., true positive (t_p), true negative (t_n), false positive (f_p), false negative (f_n)) [55], as shown in Equation (2):

$$\text{Accuracy} = \frac{t_p + t_n}{t_p + t_n + f_p + f_n} \tag{2}$$

In addition to the accuracy, we used the averaged F1 (AF1) score (short for macro-averaged F1 score), which treats all classes equally and can be used to evaluate the class imbalance problem (as shown in Equation (6)). It can be defined by using Precision (Equation (3)), Recall (Equation (4)), and F1 score (Equation (5)) [55,56].

$$\text{Precision} = \frac{t_p}{t_p + f_p} \tag{3}$$

$$\text{Recall} = \frac{t_p}{t_p + f_n} \tag{4}$$

The F1 score combines the precision and recall into a single metric by taking its harmonic mean, as shown in Equation (5):

$$\text{F1 score} = \frac{2 \times \text{Precision} \times \text{Recall}}{\text{Precision} + \text{Recall}} \tag{5}$$

In our experiments, the AF1 score is given, which is the average of the F1 scores of all classes:

$$\text{AF1 score} = \frac{1}{c} \sum_{i=1}^{c} \text{F1 score}_i \tag{6}$$

In Equation (6), c represents the no. of classes and F1 $score_i$ represents the F1 score for the ith class.

4. Experimental Results

In our study, all algorithms and models were implemented using Python 3.9. For the algorithms SVM, DT, and RF, and the deep learning models MLP and CNN, the libraries sklearn and Keras with Tensorflow 2.2.0 backend were used. Adaptive Moment Estimation (ADAM) [57] was chosen as the optimizer for our deep learning model with an initial learning rate of 10^{-4}, and trained with 50 epochs at a batch size of 32. The categorical cross entropy was used as the loss function for the deep learning models. Since no automated method for the optimization of DNN hyper-parameters has been found so far, trial-and-error was used to obtain the best hyper-parameters for the DNNs we tested in our study. The configurations we tested are provided in Appendix B. The hyper-parameter values that were used in our experiments are provided in Tables 3 and 4 for MLP and CNN, respectively. It is worth mentioning that we decided not to report the result of a single LOSO cross-validation, but the average results obtained after performing it five times.

Table 3. MLP architecture with learning rate set to 10^{-4}.

Layer Name	Neurons/Dropout Rate	Activation
Dense	64	ReLU
Batch Norm	-	-
Dense	16	ReLU
Dropout	0.5	-
Flatten	-	-
Dense	8	ReLU
Dropout	0.5	-
Dense	2	Softmax

Table 4. CNN architecture with a fixed dropout rate of 0.5 and learning rate of 10^{-4}.

Layer Name	No. Kernels (Units)	Kernel (Pool) Size	Stride	Activation
Convolutional	64	(1,1)	(1,1)	ReLU
Batch Norm	-	-	-	-
Convolutional	32	(1,1)	(1,1)	ReLU
Convolutional	16	(1,1)	(1,1)	ReLU
Flatten	-	-	-	-
Dense	2	-	-	Softmax

Preliminary experiments with all hand-crafted features (i.e., without feature selection), and SVM, DT, and RF classifiers were carried out to determine the best segmentation parameters. The results of these experiments are shown in Table 5. It can be seen that the best performing configuration is obtain when using RF with T = 60 s and ΔS = 30 s, and largely outperforms the others that were tested. We therefore selected these segmentation parameters and classifier for the rest of our studies. However, the overall classification results remain mediocre, with a AF1 score of around 60%.

Table 5. Results of binary classification of hunger and satiety.

Classifier	Win Size (T)	Step Size (ΔS)	Acc. Hungry	Acc. Satiety	Acc	AF1 Score
SVM	10	05	20.90	70.37	56.89	45.63
DT	10	05	27.94	70.40	58.04	49.17
RF	10	05	30.97	71.75	59.90	51.36
SVM	30	15	21.61	68.86	55.43	45.24
DT	30	15	21.93	71.54	58.29	46.73
RF	30	15	**38.59**	73.23	62.71	55.91
SVM	60	30	13.19	69.50	55.00	41.34
DT	60	30	18.44	79.43	67.14	48.93
RF	**60**	**30**	36.36	**82.05**	**72.00**	**59.21**

DT: Decision tree classifier; RF: Random forest classifier; SVM: Support vector machine classifier; Acc: Accuracy; AF1 Score: Averaged macro F1 score.

To improve the initial classification results and verify the potential of each sensor channel, experiments were also conducted with each sensor channel separately. We monitored the classification accuracies of each sensor channel after the LOSO cross-validation to determine its relevance in detecting hunger and satiety. Figure 5 shows the boxplot, mean, and standard deviation (in dotted lines) of the obtained accuracies.

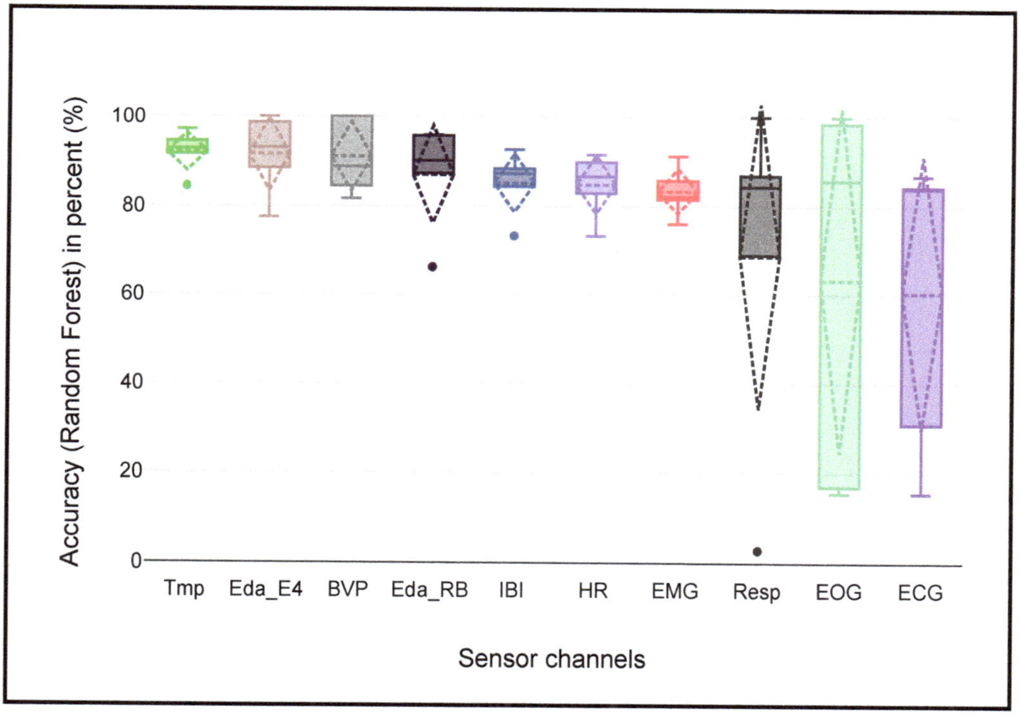

Figure 5. Importance of each sensor channel in recognizing hunger and satiety.

The standard deviations of Resp, ECG, and EOG are higher compared to the other sensors. The results in Table 6 show that these sensors are the least significant because their accuracy is less than 70%, and there is a very large variance among the different subjects. Therefore, we decided to exclude the Resp, ECG, and EOG sensors data for further experiments. Moreover, the literature also confirms the importance of Tmp, BVP, and EDA (Eda_E4 and Eda_RB) signals in the detection of hunger. For example, the research of Mandryk and Klarkowski [58] reveals that BVP increases in response to hunger and decreases in response to relaxation, He et al. [59] identifies changes in Tmp, EDA, and HR values following the ingestion of food. The authors in [24] had already used EDA for hunger detection. Furthermore, IBI and HR are directly related to BVP, since they are derived from it.

Table 6. Hunger and satiety classification results on each sensor channel using RF classifier.

Sensor	Acc. Hungry	Acc. Satiety	Acc	AF1 Score
Tmp	73.08	95.30	92.00	84.19
Eda_E4	70.59	94.98	91.43	82.79
BVP	67.35	94.68	90.86	81.02
Eda_RB	62.18	92.25	87.14	77.22
IBI	43.48	91.95	85.14	67.46
HR	40.45	91.33	84.86	65.89
EMG	30.95	90.58	83.43	60.77
Resp	29.30	79.56	68.29	54.43
EOG	39.25	73.25	62.86	56.25
ECG	21.59	73.66	60.57	47.63

RF: Random forest classifier; Acc: Accuracy; BVP: Blood volume pulse; Eda_E4: Electrodermal activity sensor of empatica E4 wristband; Tmp: Thermopile; IBI: Inter-beat interval; HR: Heart rate; Resp: Respiratory; Eda_RB: Electrodermal activity sensor of RespiBan; ECG: Electrocardiogram; EMG: Electromyography; EOG: Electrooculography. Note: For these experiments, we used a window size of 60 s and a step size of 30 s to compute the 18 hand-crafted features for each axis of the sensor channel.

Further experiments were performed with the best 18, 54, 72, 90, and 108 features of the selected sensor channels (i.e., excluding Resp, ECG, and EOG), ranked by their increasing Gini impurity scores. With the best 18 features, an Acc of 93.43% and an AF1 score of 87.86% were obtained, as shown in Table 7.

Table 7. Results of the classification of hunger and satiety using RF classifier based on the best features selected with feature importance ranking.

No. of Best Features	Acc. Hungry	Acc. Satiety	Acc	AF1 Score
18	**79.65**	**96.08**	**93.43**	**87.86**
54	66.02	94.14	90.00	80.08
72	68.18	95.42	92.00	81.80
90	68.00	94.67	90.86	81.33
108	67.33	94.49	90.57	80.91

Acc: Accuracy; AF1 Score: Averaged macro F1 score.

The results of our experiments shows that the best results could be obtained with just 18 hand-crafted features based on the FIR (as shown in Table 7). Moreover, there is not much difference in the classification results of the best 54, 72, 90, and 108 features. Furthermore, the results with 18 hand-crafted features are notably better than the results that were obtained using all sensors (see Table 5). It could be concluded that Resp, ECG, and EOG are the least informative sensors in this case, while BVP, Eda_E4, Tmp, HR, Eda_RB, and EMG are the most informative sensors and could be used to detect hunger and satiety.

To determine the relative relevance of each wearable device (i.e., Empatica E4 wristband, JINS MEME smart glasses, and RespiBan professional, with ECG, EMG, and EDA sensors) in detecting hunger and satiety, further experiments were also conducted with the RF classifier. Figure 6 shows the results of each device using the best 18 features in each case. Our experimental results show that Empatica appears to be the best wearable device, outperforms the other devices, and might be used as the only wearable device for monitoring hunger and satiety.

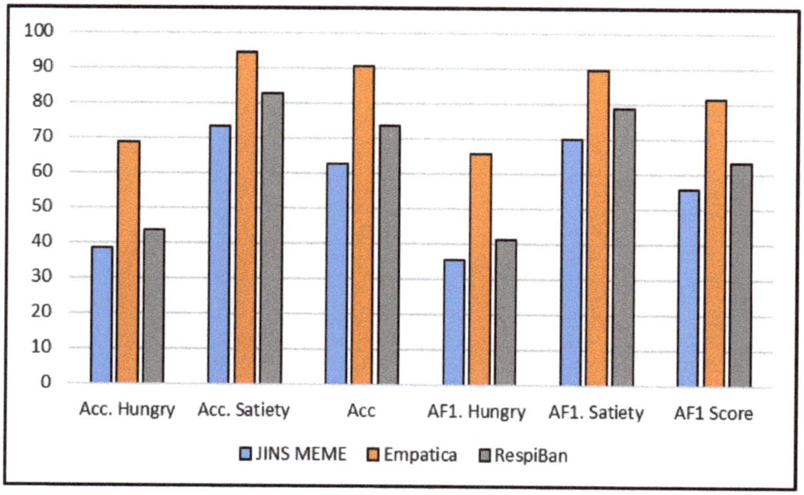

Figure 6. Comparison of sensor devices on the basis of accuracy (Acc) and averaged macro F1 score (AF1) for hungry and satiety classes. Empatica: Empatica E4 wristband; JIMS MEME: JINS MEME smart glasses; RespiBan: RespiBan professional device, including ECG, EMG, and EDA sensors.

To provide a comparison between feature engineering and feature learning approaches on our dataset, the experiments were also performed using CNN and MLP. With the CNN, an Acc of 82.90% and an AF1 score of 82.54% were obtained, as shown in Table 8. The segmentation technique mentioned above was not adequate for training a deep learning model. Therefore, we devised another segmentation technique using a window size of 60 seconds and a step size of 5 s for deep learning-based models.

Table 8. Results of the classification of hunger and satiety using feature learning approaches.

Classifier	Acc. Hungry	Acc. Satiety	Acc	AF1 Score
MLP	77.79	81.35	80.14	79.57
CNN	**81.37**	**83.70**	**82.90**	**82.54**

Acc: Accuracy; CNN: Convolutional Neural Network; MLP: Multi-Layer Perceptron.

5. Discussion

The following points provide a detailed discussion of the aforementioned results:

- One of the main objective of this paper was to develop a machine learning approach to classify hunger and satiety using wearable sensors. Therefore, we used wearable devices like the Empatica E4 wristband, JINS MEME smart glasses, and RespiBan professional with miniaturized sensors that provided sufficient quality data and that could capture physiological signals related to the perception of hunger and satiety in patients or people with occupational constraints, as opposed to invasive [4], gastrointestinal model [19], fMRI-based data [21], and gastric tone signals [23]. Our proposed non-invasive multimodal system with carefully selected sensor channels outperformed previous approaches with an accuracy of 93.43% and an average F1 score of 87.86%.
- Each classification algorithm is based on different mathematical models [60], and may produce different results for the same dataset. In order to obtain highly accurate results and to select the best classifier for further experiments, we not only conducted experiments with different classifiers, but also with different window sizes and step sizes. It was found that the RF classifier was best suited for hunger and satiety detection using hand-crafted features, and it outperformed the DT and SVM classifiers

in each scenario. It was also observed that the window size of 60 s and the step size of 30 were significant for each classifier.

- In the past, deep learning-based approaches have shown promising results in a variety of application domains such as biology, medicine, and psychology [8,12–15,42,61]. However, they are computationally expensive and also require a large number of training samples [62] to build successful models compared to traditional approaches using hand-crafted features. To compare the results of feature learning and feature engineering, we also computed 18 features independently for each axis of each sensor channel. They were subsequently concatenated to obtain a feature vector of the size of 18 × sensor (S) axis. It was found that well-engineered features can perform better than deep learning approaches in the case of a limited number of training samples.
- In this study, we used feature importance ranking (FIR), which measures the contribution of each input feature to the performance of the model. It turned out that the most accurate results can be obtained only with the best 18 hand-crafted features (as shown in Table 7) and the addition of other irrelevant and redundant features can introduce noise into the data, which can reduce the performance of a classifier. It can be pointed out that the top five features come exclusively from three different sensor channels (Eda_E4, BVP, and Tmp) and are either computing the mean or the 80th percentile of the data values. Percentile 80 provides an approximation of the maximum value in a data segment that is less sensitive to noise or outliers than the actual maximum computation. This would indicate that the average and upper data values in Eda_E4, BVP, and Tmp are of high importance to distinguish between hunger and satiety. This feature selection also validates our previous results to identify the importance of each sensor channel (Table 6), and seem to confirm findings from the literature that showed these sensor channels to be relevant in detecting hunger and satiety [24,58,59] (c.f. Figure 5). The overall selected best features can be seen in Figure 7.

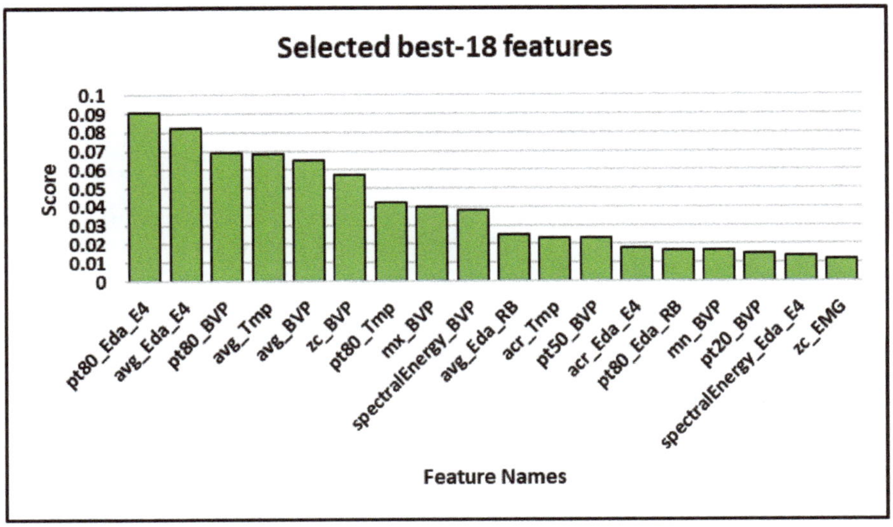

Figure 7. The overall 18 best features. Note: pt80: 80th percentile; avg: average; zc: zero crossings; mx: maximum; acr: auto-correlation; pt50: 50th percentile; mn: minimum; pt20: 20th percentile; BVP: Blood Volume Pulse; HR: Heart Rate; Tmp: Temperature; Eda: Electrodermal activity; RB: Respiration belt; E4: Empatica E4.

- Long-term monitoring with a large number of wearable sensors may be uncomfortable for users [63]. Therefore, eliminating irrelevant sensors can decrease the degree of discomfort and improve the robustness of the classification system by reducing the dimensionality and also save a lot of money [64]. In this work, we compared not only all sensors, but also wearable devices, to determine the most suitable sensors and wearable device for hunger and satiety detection. It was found that PPG (BVP, IBI, and HR), EDA (Empatica E4 and RespiBan), Tmp, and EMG were the appropriate sensor modalities for this study, and Resp, ECG, and EOG were the least appropriate. We also found that the Empatica E4 wristband was the most suitable device compared to the other devices.

6. Conclusions

In this paper, we introduced an objective and non-invasive machine learning model to detect hunger and satiety using physiological sensor data. Our proposed multimodal system enables the detection of hunger and satiety with an accuracy of 93.43%, and an average F1 score of 87.86% in LOSO configuration. The results of this study lead to the following conclusions: firstly, state-of-the-art wearable sensors provide good quality physiological data on hunger and satiety, and could be used to build a non-invasive and objective system. Furthermore, deep learning architectures do not necessarily perform well, especially when we have a limited number of training samples. In addition, feature selection could help to remove unnecessary and redundant features that lead to noise, which in turn leads to better results. Finally, the experiments of this study showed that the most discriminative features come from three specific sensor modalities: Electrodermal Activity (EDA), infrared Thermopile (Tmp), and Blood Volume Pulse (BVP). These sensors are part of the Empatica E4 wristband, which is the most influential device in this study and can be used as a standalone device. In order to learn more about the perception of hunger and satiety, further experiments with long-term hunger and satiety data are needed, which will not only help to train deep learning models well, but also further divide hunger and satiety into sub-classes to gain further insight, which is part of our future work.

Author Contributions: Conceptualization, M.G. and M.T.I.; methodology, M.T.I. and M.A.N.; software, M.T.I., M.A.N. and J.H.; validation, M.T.I., P.G. and J.H.; formal analysis, M.T.I. and X.H.; investigation, M.T.I., M.A.N., X.H. and O.F.; resources, O.F. and A.P.; data curation, A.P., F.L., P.G. and K.M.O.; writing—original draft preparation, M.T.I.; writing—review and editing, M.A.N., K.M.O. and F. L.; visualization, M.T.I. and X.H.; supervision, M.G. All authors have read and agreed to the published version of the manuscript.

Funding: Research activities leading to this publication have been financially supported by the DAMP foundation within the grant SENSE "Systemic Nutritional Medicine".

Informed Consent Statement: Informed consent was obtained from all subjects involved in the study.

Data Availability Statement: Data sharing is not applicable to this article.

Conflicts of Interest: The authors declare no conflict of interest.

Abbreviations

The following abbreviations are used in this manuscript:

VAS	Visual Analog Scales
ANN	Artificial Neural Networks
DNN	Deep Neural Networks
GSR	Galvanic Skin Response
EDA	Electrodermal Activity
EEG	Electroencephalography

fMRI	Functional Magnetic Resonance Imaging
DC	Degree of Centrality
ReHo	Regional Homogeneity
fALFF	Fractional Amplitude of Low Frequency Fluctuations
SF	Spectral Features
CDF	Cepstral Domain Features
GCC	Gammatone Cepstral Coefficients
CFS	Correlation-based Feature Selection
ECG	Electrocardiogram
EMG	Electromyography
PPG	Photoplethysmogram
TMP	Thermopile
EOG	Electrooculography
ML	Machine Learning
BVP	Blood Volume Pulse
MLP	Multi-layer Perceptrons
LSTM	Long Short-term Memory
CNN	Convolutional Neural Network
ReLU	Rectified Linear Unit
SVM	Support Vector Machine
DT	Decision Tree
RF	Random Forest
LOSO	Leave-one-subject-out
ADAM	Adaptive Moment Estimation
SWS	Sliding Window Segmentation
Acc	Accuracy
AF1	Averaged macro F1 score

Appendix A. Comparison of Manual Feature Selection Approaches

Feature selection (FS) is a process usually applied in machine learning studies that involve the computation of a large number of features. In particular, it is required to eliminate features that would not be the most discriminative for the classification problem to solve, and on the other hand, identify the most useful ones. We used in our study three commonly used FS methods: Boruta, eXtreme Gradient Boosting (XGB), and RF [65–67].

RF is an ensemble learner that works well with nonlinear data, handles large datasets efficiently, and is useful for feature selection. Most of the time, it provides better accuracy compared to other algorithms. However, RF can be slow in training when used with a large number of trees, and is sometimes not suitable for many sparse features [48–50,53,65].

Similar to RF, XGB is an ensemble machine learning algorithm that incorporates loss minimization using gradient descent to the RF framework. It is less prone to overfitting, can handle missing values, has minimal effects of outliers, and can also be used as a feature selector. However, it is more difficult to tune because there are many hyperparameters and overfitting is possible if the parameters are not set correctly [66,68].

Boruta is a wrapper feature selection approach based on RF that selects or eliminates features after computing an feature importance scores, so that the quality of its feature selection depends on the quality of the RF model. The sensitivity of Boruta can be improved by using a RF with a larger number of decision trees. However, increasing the number of trees in RF may increase the computation time of the Boruta algorithm, which limits the use of the algorithm for analyzing very large datasets [67].

In order to make a fair comparison between the manual FS approaches in this study, we selected the best 18, 54, 72, 90, and 108 features with Boruta, XGB, and RF, and classified them with XGB and RF classifiers. The best results of each classifier in each setting are shown in Table A1. The best configuration was obtained by using RF both for feature selection and classification.

Table A1. Results of the classification of hunger and satiety using RF and XGB classifier based on the best features selected with Boruta, XGB, and RF.

Classifier	FS Algorithm	No. of Best Features	Acc. Hungry	Acc. Satiety	Acc	AF1 Score
RF	**RF**	**18**	**79.65**	**96.08**	**93.43**	**87.86**
RF	Boruta	108	72.53	95.89	92.86	84.21
RF	XGB	54	73.12	95.88	92.86	84.50
XGB	RF	18	69.23	94.63	90.86	81.93
XGB	Boruta	54	53.33	93.11	88.00	73.22
XGB	XGB	18	63.92	94.20	90.00	79.06

RF: Random Forest; XGB: eXtreme Gradient Boosting; Acc: Accuracy; AF1 Score: Averaged macro F1 score.

Appendix B. Hyper-Parameter Selection for Feature Learning Approaches

Machine learning algorithms work with two types of parameters, namely learnable parameters and hyper-parameters. The learnable parameters are those that the algorithms learn themselves during training on a given dataset, while hyper-parameters are specified by engineers or scientists prior to the training in order to regulate how algorithms learn, and to change the performance of the model. In our study, the most impactful hyper-parameters on the final classification performances were the learning rate *(lr)*, window size *(T)*, and step size (ΔS).

The lr determines the rate at which the ANN training algorithm (backpropagation algorithm) updates the weights of the network during each training iteration. More specifically, each neural weight w_n at iteration $n \in \mathbf{N}^*$ is updated following the formula:

$$w_n = w_{n-1} - lr \times \frac{\partial L}{\partial w}(w_{n-1})$$

where L designates the loss function comparing the network outputs to the expected outputs.

The window size T and step size ΔS are both segmentation parameters that respectively determine how long in time the input of the network is, and how much time needs to pass between two consecutive windows of data. Both parameters control the rate at which the learning algorithm picks up new information.

Figure A1 shows the ANN performances obtained for the various combinations of hyper-parameters that were tested for the feature learning approaches (MLP and CNN) in this study. Since no automated method for optimizing the hyper-parameters of deep neural networks has proven its effectiveness in practice so far, the best values for these parameters in this study were determined through trial-and-error. The hyper-parameter T = 60 s, ΔS= 5 s, and lr =10^{-4} worked best for the MLP and CNN models of this study.

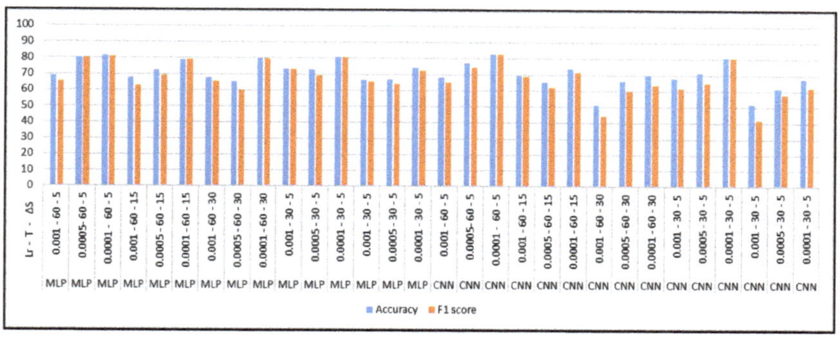

Figure A1. Selection of hyper-parameters for the feature learning approaches. lr: learning rate; T: window size; ΔS: step size.

Appendix C. Demographic Information about the Subjects

The following Table A2 shows the demographic data (such as sex, age, and weight) of the subjects used for data acquisition in this study.

Table A2. Demographic data of subjects used for data acquisition in this study.

Subject Name	Sex/Gender	Age (in years)	Weight (in kg)
S1	Female	23	65
S2	Male	29	71
S3	Male	37	72
S4	Male	26	81
S5	Male	27	75

kg: Kilograms; S1: Subject 1; S2: Subject 2; S3: Subject 3; S4: Subject 4; S5: Subject 5.

References

1. Jauch-Chara, K.; Oltmanns, K.M. Obesity–A neuropsychological disease? Systematic review and neuropsychological model. *Prog. Neurobiol.* **2014**, *114*, 84–101. [CrossRef]
2. Macpherson-Sánchez, A.E. Integrating fundamental concepts of obesity and eating disorders: implications for the obesity epidemic. *Am. J. Public Health* **2015**, *105*, e71–e85. [CrossRef] [PubMed]
3. WHO. Obesity and Overweight. 2016. Available online: https://www.who.int/news-room/fact-sheets/detail/obesity-and-overweight (accessed on 27 June 2021).
4. Krishnan, S.; Hendriks, H.F.; Hartvigsen, M.L.; de Graaf, A.A. Feed-forward neural network model for hunger and satiety related VAS score prediction. *Theor. Biol. Med. Model.* **2016**, *13*, 1–12. [CrossRef]
5. Parker, B.A.; Sturm, K.; MacIntosh, C.; Feinle, C.; Horowitz, M.; Chapman, I. Relation between food intake and visual analogue scale ratings of appetite and other sensations in healthy older and young subjects. *Eur. J. Clin. Nutr.* **2004**, *58*, 212–218. [CrossRef] [PubMed]
6. Sepple, C.; Read, N. Gastrointestinal correlates of the development of hunger in man. *Appetite* **1989**, *13*, 183–191. [CrossRef]
7. Rogers, P.J.; Blundell, J.E. Effect of anorexic drugs on food intake and the micro-structure of eating in human subjects. *Psychopharmacology* **1979**, *66*, 159–165. [CrossRef]
8. Huang, X.; Shirahama, K.; Li, F.; Grzegorzek, M. Sleep stage classification for child patients using DeConvolutional Neural Network. *Artif. Intell. Med.* **2020**, *110*, 101981. [CrossRef]
9. Li, F.; Shirahama, K.; Nisar, M.A.; Köping, L.; Grzegorzek, M. Comparison of feature learning methods for human activity recognition using wearable sensors. *Sensors* **2018**, *18*, 679. [CrossRef]
10. Di Lascio, E.; Gashi, S.; Debus, M.E.; Santini, S. Automatic Recognition of Flow During Work Activities Using Context and Physiological Signals. In Proceedings of the 2021 9th International Conference on Affective Computing and Intelligent Interaction (ACII), Nara, Japan, 28 September–1 October 2021; IEEE: Piscataway, NJ, USA, 2021; pp. 1–8.
11. Liaqat, S.; Dashtipour, K.; Arshad, K.; Ramzan, N. Non invasive skin hydration level detection using machine learning. *Electronics* **2020**, *9*, 1086. [CrossRef]
12. Roy, S.D.; Das, S.; Kar, D.; Schwenker, F.; Sarkar, R. Computer Aided Breast Cancer Detection Using Ensembling of Texture and Statistical Image Features. *Sensors* **2021**, *21*, 3628. [CrossRef]
13. Malmgren, H.; Borga, M. *Artificial Neural Networks in Medicine and Biology: Proceedings of the ANNIMAB-1 Conference, Göteborg, Sweden, 13–16 May 2000*; Springer Science & Business Media: Berlin, Germany, 2000.
14. Bustin, S.A. Nucleic acid quantification and disease outcome prediction in colorectal cancer. *Pers. Med.* **2006**, *3*, 207–216. [CrossRef]
15. Patel, J.L.; Goyal, R.K. Applications of artificial neural networks in medical science. *Curr. Clin. Pharmacol.* **2007**, *2*, 217–226. [CrossRef]
16. Rahaman, M.M.; Li, C.; Yao, Y.; Kulwa, F.; Rahman, M.A.; Wang, Q.; Qi, S.; Kong, F.; Zhu, X.; Zhao, X. Identification of COVID-19 samples from chest X-Ray images using deep learning: A comparison of transfer learning approaches. *J. X-ray Sci. Technol.* **2020**, *28*, 821–839. [CrossRef]
17. Shahid, N.; Rappon, T.; Berta, W. Applications of artificial neural networks in health care organizational decision-making: A scoping review. *PLoS ONE* **2019**, *14*, e0212356. [CrossRef] [PubMed]
18. Baxt, W.G. Application of artificial neural networks to clinical medicine. *Lancet* **1995**, *346*, 1135–1138. [CrossRef]
19. Bellmann, S.; Krishnan, S.; de Graaf, A.; de Ligt, R.A.; Pasman, W.J.; Minekus, M.; Havenaar, R. Appetite ratings of foods are predictable with an in vitro advanced gastrointestinal model in combination with an in silico artificial neural network. *Food Res. Int.* **2019**, *122*, 77–86. [CrossRef] [PubMed]

20. Rahman, T.; Czerwinski, M.; Gilad-Bachrach, R.; Johns, P. Predicting "about-to-eat" moments for just-in-time eating intervention. In Proceedings of the 6th International Conference on Digital Health Conference, Montréal, QC, Canada, 11–13 April 2016; pp. 141–150.
21. Al-Zubaidi, A.; Mertins, A.; Heldmann, M.; Jauch-Chara, K.; Münte, T.F. Machine learning based classification of resting-state fMRI features exemplified by metabolic state (hunger/satiety). *Front. Hum. Neurosci.* **2019**, *13*, 164. [CrossRef]
22. Lakshmi, S.; Kavipriya, P.; Jebarani, M.E.; Vino, T. A Novel Approach of Human Hunger Detection especially for physically challenged people. In Proceedings of the 2021 International Conference on Artificial Intelligence and Smart Systems (ICAIS), Coimbatore, India, 25–27 March 2021; IEEE: Piscataway, NJ, USA, 2021; pp. 921–927.
23. Maria, A.; Jeyaseelan, A.S. Development of Optimal Feature Selection and Deep Learning Toward Hungry Stomach Detection Using Audio Signals. *J. Control. Autom. Electr. Syst.* **2021**, *32*, 853–874. [CrossRef]
24. Gogate, U.; Bakal, J. Hunger and stress monitoring system using galvanic skin. *Indones. J. Electr. Eng. Comput. Sci.* **2019**, *13*, 861–865. [CrossRef]
25. Barajas-Montiel, S.E.; Reyes-Garcia, C.A. Identifying pain and hunger in infant cry with classifiers ensembles. In Proceedings of the International Conference on Computational Intelligence for Modelling, Control and Automation and International Conference on Intelligent Agents, Web Technologies and Internet Commerce (CIMCA-IAWTIC'06), Vienna, Austria, 28–30 November 2005; IEEE: Piscataway, NJ, USA, 2005; Volume 2, pp. 770–775.
26. Yu, D.; Seltzer, M.L.; Li, J.; Huang, J.T.; Seide, F. Feature learning in deep neural networks-studies on speech recognition tasks. *arXiv* **2013**, arXiv:1301.3605.
27. Irshad, M.T.; Nisar, M.A.; Gouverneur, P.; Rapp, M.; Grzegorzek, M. Ai approaches towards Prechtl's assessment of general movements: A systematic literature review. *Sensors* **2020**, *20*, 5321. [CrossRef] [PubMed]
28. respiBAN. Available online: https://plux.info/biosignalsplux-wearables/313-respiban-professional-820202407.html (accessed on 8 August 2021).
29. Electrodermal Activity (EDA). Available online: https://plux.info/sensors/280-electrodermal-activity-eda-820201202.html (accessed on 18 August 2021).
30. Electrocardiogram (ECG). Available online: https://plux.info/sensors/277-electrocardiogram-ecg-820201203.html (accessed on 18 August 2021).
31. Electromyography (EMG). Available online: https://plux.info/sensors/283-electromyography-emg-820201201.html (accessed 18 August 2021).
32. Empatica Wristband. Available online: https://www.empatica.com/research/e4/ (accessed on 8 August 2021).
33. JINS MEME: Eyewear That Sees Your EVERYDAY. Available online: https://jins-meme.com/en/ (accessed on 8 August 2021).
34. Kotsiantis, S.B.; Kanellopoulos, D.; Pintelas, P.E. Data preprocessing for supervised leaning. *Int. J. Comput. Sci.* **2006**, *1*, 111–117.
35. Amjad, F.; Khan, M.H.; Nisar, M.A.; Farid, M.S.; Grzegorzek, M. A Comparative Study of Feature Selection Approaches for Human Activity Recognition Using Multimodal Sensory Data. *Sensors* **2021**, *21*, 2368. [CrossRef] [PubMed]
36. Cook, D.J.; Krishnan, N.C. *Activity learning: Discovering, recognizing, and predicting human behavior from sensor data*; John Wiley & Sons: Hoboken, NJ, USA, 2015.
37. Genuer, R.; Poggi, J.M.; Tuleau-Malot, C. Variable selection using random forests. *Pattern Recognit. Lett.* **2010**, *31*, 2225–2236. [CrossRef]
38. Wu, X.; Kumar, V. *The Top Ten Algorithms in Data Mining*; CRC Press: Boca Raton, FL, USA, 2009.
39. Nguyen, C.; Wang, Y.; Nguyen, H.N. Random forest classifier combined with feature selection for breast cancer diagnosis and prognostic. *J. Biomed. Sci. Eng.* **2013**, *06*, 551–560. [CrossRef]
40. Breiman, L.; Friedman, J.H.; Olshen, R.A.; Stone, C.J. *Classification and Regression Trees*; Routledge: London, UK, 2017.
41. Nahid, A.A.; Mehrabi, M.A.; Kong, Y. Histopathological breast cancer image classification by deep neural network techniques guided by local clustering. *Biomed Res. Int.* **2018**, *2018*,2362108. [CrossRef]
42. Nisar, M.A.; Shirahama, K.; Li, F.; Huang, X.; Grzegorzek, M. Rank pooling approach for wearable sensor-based ADLs recognition. *Sensors* **2020**, *20*, 3463. [CrossRef]
43. Orhan, U.; Hekim, M.; Ozer, M. EEG signals classification using the K-means clustering and a multilayer perceptron neural network model. *Expert Syst. Appl.* **2011**, *38*, 13475–13481. [CrossRef]
44. Chen, Z.; Ma, G.; Jiang, Y.; Wang, B.; Soleimani, M. Application of deep neural network to the reconstruction of two-phase material imaging by capacitively coupled electrical resistance tomography. *Electronics* **2021**, *10*, 1058. [CrossRef]
45. Ioffe, S.; Szegedy, C. Batch normalization: Accelerating deep network training by reducing internal covariate shift. In Proceedings of the International Conference on Machine Learning, Lille, France, 7–9 July 2015; pp. 448–456.
46. Furey, T.S.; Cristianini, N.; Duffy, N.; Bednarski, D.W.; Schummer, M.; Haussler, D. Support vector machine classification and validation of cancer tissue samples using microarray expression data. *Bioinformatics* **2000**, *16*, 906–914. [CrossRef] [PubMed]
47. Myles, A.J.; Feudale, R.N.; Liu, Y.; Woody, N.A.; Brown, S.D. An introduction to decision tree modeling. *J. Chemom. J. Chemom. Soc.* **2004**, *18*, 275–285. [CrossRef]
48. Cutler, D.R.; Edwards Jr, T.C.; Beard, K.H.; Cutler, A.; Hess, K.T.; Gibson, J.; Lawler, J.J. Random forests for classification in ecology. *Ecology* **2007**, *88*, 2783–2792. [CrossRef]

49. Ghimire, B.; Rogan, J.; Miller, J. Contextual land-cover classification: Incorporating spatial dependence in land-cover classification models using random forests and the Getis statistic. *Remote Sens. Lett.* **2010**, *1*, 45–54. [CrossRef]
50. Gislason, P.O.; Benediktsson, J.A.; Sveinsson, J.R. Random forests for land cover classification. *Pattern Recognit. Lett.* **2006**, *27*, 294–300. [CrossRef]
51. Guo, L.; Chehata, N.; Mallet, C.; Boukir, S. Relevance of airborne lidar and multispectral image data for urban scene classification using Random Forests. *ISPRS J. Photogramm. Remote Sens.* **2011**, *66*, 56–66. [CrossRef]
52. Titapiccolo, J.I.; Ferrario, M.; Cerutti, S.; Barbieri, C.; Mari, F.; Gatti, E.; Signorini, M.G. Artificial intelligence models to stratify cardiovascular risk in incident hemodialysis patients. *Expert Syst. Appl.* **2013**, *40*, 4679–4686. [CrossRef]
53. Chaudhary, A.; Kolhe, S.; Kamal, R. An improved random forest classifier for multi-class classification. *Inf. Process. Agric.* **2016**, *3*, 215–222. [CrossRef]
54. Fatourechi, M.; Ward, R.K.; Mason, S.G.; Huggins, J.; Schloegl, A.; Birch, G.E. Comparison of evaluation metrics in classification applications with imbalanced datasets. In Proceedings of the 2008 seventh international conference on machine learning and applications, San Diego, CA, USA, 11–13 December 2008; IEEE: Piscataway, NJ, USA, 2008; pp. 777–782.
55. Hossin, M.; Sulaiman, M.N. A review on evaluation metrics for data classification evaluations. *Int. J. Data Min. Knowl. Manag. Process* **2015**, *5*, 1.
56. Takahashi, K.; Yamamoto, K.; Kuchiba, A.; Koyama, T. Confidence interval for micro-averaged F1 and macro-averaged F1 scores. *Appl. Intell.* **2022**, *52*, 4961–4972. [CrossRef]
57. Kingma, D.P.; Ba, J. Adam: A method for stochastic optimization. *arXiv* **2014**, arXiv:1412.6980.
58. Mandryk, R.; Klarkowski, M. Physiological measures for game evaluation. In *Game Usability*; CRC Press: Boca Raton, FL, USA, 2008; pp. 161–187.
59. He, W.; Boesveldt, S.; Delplanque, S.; de Graaf, C.; De Wijk, R.A. Sensory-specific satiety: Added insights from autonomic nervous system responses and facial expressions. *Physiol. Behav.* **2017**, *170*, 12–18. [CrossRef]
60. Dutta, N.; Subramaniam, U.; Padmanaban, S. Mathematical models of classification algorithm of Machine learning. In International Meeting on Advanced Technologies in Energy and Electrical Engineering; Hamad bin Khalifa University Press (HBKU Press): Doha, Qatar, January 2020; Volume 2019, No. 1, p. 3.
61. Peifer, C.; Pollak, A.; Flak, O.; Pyszka, A.; Nisar, M.A.; Irshad, M.T.; Grzegorzek, M.; Kordyaka, B.; Kożusznik, B. The Symphony of Team Flow in Virtual Teams. Using Artificial Intelligence for Its Recognition and Promotion. *Front. Psychol.* **2021**, *12*, 697093 [CrossRef]
62. Parisi, G.I.; Kemker, R.; Part, J.L.; Kanan, C.; Wermter, S. Continual lifelong learning with neural networks: A review. *Neural Netw.* **2019**, *113*, 54–71. [CrossRef] [PubMed]
63. Sweeney, K.T.; Ward, T.E.; McLoone, S.F. Artifact removal in physiological signals—Practices and possibilities. *IEEE Trans. Inf. Technol. Biomed.* **2012**, *16*, 488–500. [CrossRef]
64. Lan, T.; Erdogmus, D.; Adami, A.; Pavel, M.; Mathan, S. Salient EEG channel selection in brain computer interfaces by mutual information maximization. In Proceedings of the 2005 IEEE Engineering in Medicine and Biology 27th Annual Conference, Shanghai, China, 17–18 January 2006; IEEE: Piscataway, NJ, USA, 2006; pp. 7064–7067.
65. Chen, R.C.; Dewi, C.; Huang, S.W.; Caraka, R.E. Selecting critical features for data classification based on machine learning methods. *J. Big Data* **2020**, *7*, 1–26. [CrossRef]
66. Sang, X.; Xiao, W.; Zheng, H.; Yang, Y.; Liu, T. HMMPred: Accurate prediction of DNA-binding proteins based on HMM profiles and XGBoost feature selection. *Comput. Math. Methods Med.* **2020**, *2020, 1–10* . [CrossRef]
67. Rudnicki, W.R.; Wrzesień, M.; Paja, W. All relevant feature selection methods and applications. In *Feature Selection for Data and Pattern Recognition*; Springer: Berlin/Heidelberg, Germany, 2015; pp. 11–28.
68. Chang, Y.C.; Chang, K.H.; Wu, G.J. Application of eXtreme gradient boosting trees in the construction of credit risk assessment models for financial institutions. *Appl. Soft Comput.* **2018**, *73*, 914–920. [CrossRef]

sensors

MDPI

Article

Simultaneous Sleep Stage and Sleep Disorder Detection from Multimodal Sensors Using Deep Learning

Yi-Hsuan Cheng †, Margaret Lech *,† and Richardt Howard Wilkinson †

School of Engineering, RMIT University, Melbourne, VIC 3000, Australia
* Correspondence: margaret.lech@rmit.edu.au
† These authors contributed equally to this work.

Abstract: Sleep scoring involves the inspection of multimodal recordings of sleep data to detect potential sleep disorders. Given that symptoms of sleep disorders may be correlated with specific sleep stages, the diagnosis is typically supported by the simultaneous identification of a sleep stage and a sleep disorder. This paper investigates the automatic recognition of sleep stages and disorders from multimodal sensory data (EEG, ECG, and EMG). We propose a new distributed multimodal and multilabel decision-making system (MML-DMS). It comprises several interconnected classifier modules, including deep convolutional neural networks (CNNs) and shallow perceptron neural networks (NNs). Each module works with a different data modality and data label. The flow of information between the MML-DMS modules provides the final identification of the sleep stage and sleep disorder. We show that the fused multilabel and multimodal method improves the diagnostic performance compared to single-label and single-modality approaches. We tested the proposed MML-DMS on the PhysioNet CAP Sleep Database, with VGG16 CNN structures, achieving an average classification accuracy of 94.34% and F_1 score of 0.92 for sleep stage detection (six stages) and an average classification accuracy of 99.09% and F_1 score of 0.99 for sleep disorder detection (eight disorders). A comparison with related studies indicates that the proposed approach significantly improves upon the existing state-of-the-art approaches.

Keywords: machine learning; distributed networks; multimodal classification; multilabel classification; sleep stage detection; sleep disorder detection; decision-making networks

1. Introduction

Sleep is an integral part of human life. Poor sleep quality can lead to various physiological and mental health problems. Sleep experts identify two major stages of wakefulness and sleep, with sleep further subdivided into light sleep, deep sleep, and rapid eye movement (REM) behavior [1]. Good sleep quality is characterized by the deep sleep stage occupying a relatively high proportion of the sleep duration [2]. Therefore, accurate detection and analysis of sleep stages carry a heavy weight in the general assessment of a patient's health. Traditional sleep assessment requires the patient to sleep in a testing room while wearing a set of sensors collecting physiological data of different modalities, such as electroencephalograms (EEG), electrocardiograms (ECG), and electromyographs (EMG). A typical recording time is eight hours. The physiological data are manually analyzed (scored) offline by at least two qualified assessors identifying sleep stage intervals and sleep anomalies indicating possible sleep disorders. The sleep scoring procedure follows the American Academy of Sleep Medicine [3] or the Rechtschaffen and Kales [4] standards. It is costly, time-consuming, and requires highly qualified human resources [5]. Therefore, despite their importance, sleep diagnosis centers have limited availability. A solution to this dilemma could be given by an automatic sleep scoring algorithm that can automatically analyze the multimodal recordings and identify sleep stages and sleep disorders [6].

Early sleep scoring studies have exhaustively analyzed feature-based approaches and classical classifiers such as the support vector machine (SVM), random forest (RF), or artificial neural networks (ANNs); for example, Ref. [7] reviewed sleep stage classification systems using ANNs. The performance varied depending on the recognized stages. A comparative study was presented in [8] that aimed to identify the most effective features and the most efficient algorithm to classify sleep stages. An accuracy of 98% was reported. In [9], a single EEG channel was used to identify optimal machine learning (ML) and feature extraction. Spectral linear features and an RF classifier led to the best classification performance, while ensuring real-time online processing. An extensive review of the current literature on automated sleep scoring can be found in [10,11].

Although systematic research progress towards automatic sleep classification has been observed for almost two decades, the recent advancement in machine learning technology offered a leap into new and exciting opportunities for designing highly effective sleep diagnosis algorithms. The majority of recent sleep scoring studies investigate single-label cases where the algorithm has a task to identify either the sleep stage or the sleep disorder modality. This task is predominantly conducted using single-modality data, most often EEG. There is also an emerging line of research where the scoring is derived from multiple modalities such as EEG and ECG. We refer to these methods as multimodal. Only a small number of papers challenged the simultaneous sleep stage and sleep disorder recognition task. We refer to these methods as multilabel. Limited studies have been published on the combination of multimodal- and multilabel sleep techniques.

An example of a single-modality sleep stage classification approach is given in Kim et al. [12]. The heart rate variability (HRV) signals were classified to identify three sleep stages (wake, light sleep, and deep sleep). After denoising, the fractal property feature of the HRV signals led to a 72% classification accuracy using pairwise correlation analysis. Another example is available in Fernández-Varela et al. [13], who used two EEG, one EOG, and two EMG channels to detect five sleep stages. An assembly of five CNNs, one for each modality, was used to classify the input time waveforms. Validation results based on the Sleep Heart Health Study (SHHS) [14,15] resulted in an F_1 score of 0.76. Phan et al. [16] used spectrogram features and a multitask CNN to detect the five classes of sleep stages. The Sleep EDF database [17,18] was used to detect five sleep stages. Accuracies of 82% to 83% were reported using the Sleep EDF database [17,18]. Rui et al. [19] used a multitask 2D-CNN to detect five sleep stages based on the time series features. A testing accuracy of 85% was achieved using the SHHS [14,15] and Sleep-EDF [17,18] data.

While there is a relatively large body of research on sleep stage detection, research into sleep disorder classification has resulted in a smaller number of publications. Zhuang and Ibrahim [20] developed a multi-channel Deep Learning (DL-AR) model where a set of CNNs was applied to six channels of raw signals of different modalities, including three channels of EEG (electroencephalogram) signals and one channel each of EMG (electromyogram), ECG (electrocardiogram), and EOG (electrooculogram) signals. The model was tested on the PhysioNet CAP Sleep database [18,21], yielding specificity and sensitivity scores of around 95% for eight sleep disorders. Sharma et al. [22] used wavelet-based features extracted from EOG and EMG signals to identify six sleep disorders from the PhysioNet CAP Sleep database [18,21]. The Hjorth transform parameters were classified using ensemble bagged trees, resulting in a testing accuracy of 94.3%.

1.1. Paper Contributions

Current multimodal sleep classification methods have a single-label character, i.e., the combined modalities are used to classify either a sleep stage or a sleep disorder. To our knowledge, our experiments are the first attempt to conduct a simultaneous multimodal- and multilabel classification of sleep data. There are no similar studies classifying sleep data on such a large scale, which includes six sleep stages, eight sleep disorders, and three data modalities (EEG, ECG, and EMG). This paper presents one of the first research studies in this area. To accomplish such a vast task, we introduce a new Multimodal and Multilabel Decision-Making System (MML-DMS) consisting of multiple interconnected classifiers identifying either the sleep stage or the sleep disorder from different sensor modalities. The information generated by these classifiers is then passed to two decision-making neural networks: one to identify the sleep stage and the other to identify the sleep disorder. The proposed method is tested by simultaneously identifying six sleep stages and eight sleep disorders from three different sensor modalities using the PhysioNet CAP Sleep database [18,21]. Despite the significant complexity of this task, the system offers a high performance that can be largely attributed to its distributed and modular character.

1.2. Paper Structure

Section 2 provides a detailed description of the proposed MML-DMS system for automatic sleep scoring. Section 3 describes the data and experiments used to validate the MML-DMS. The results are discussed in Section 4, and the paper is concluded in Section 5.

2. Materials and Methods

2.1. Proposed Multimodal and Multilabel Decision-Making System (MML-DMS)

The MML-DMS is a system of interconnected independent neural network classifiers or units. The connections are determined by the flow of information between the units. Each classifier conducts its own individual task and uses a different type or modality of input data. However, as a whole, the system performs the main task of simultaneous identification of a sleep stage and sleep disorder. The system modules are relatively simple in their architectures, can be independently trained in a time- and data-efficient manner, and can eventually be reused in other similar systems.

In this study, we describe three experiments designed to gradually increase the system complexity and validate the system components. All experiments have a similar first step: splitting time waveforms of different modalities into short intervals, transferring each block into a logarithmic spectrogram array, and converting it into a corresponding color RGB image. Figures 1–3 illustrate how the MML-DMS concept was developed by gradually increasing its complexity and changing the interconnections between component modules. In its final form, as shown in Figure 3, the MML-DMS version, denoted as MML-DMS2, is a two-level classification procedure. At the first-level, there is an ensemble of six parallel CNN classifiers, including three networks classifying the sleep stage (one for each modality—EEG, ECG, and EMG) and three networks classifying the sleep disorder (one for each modality—EEG, ECG, and EMG).

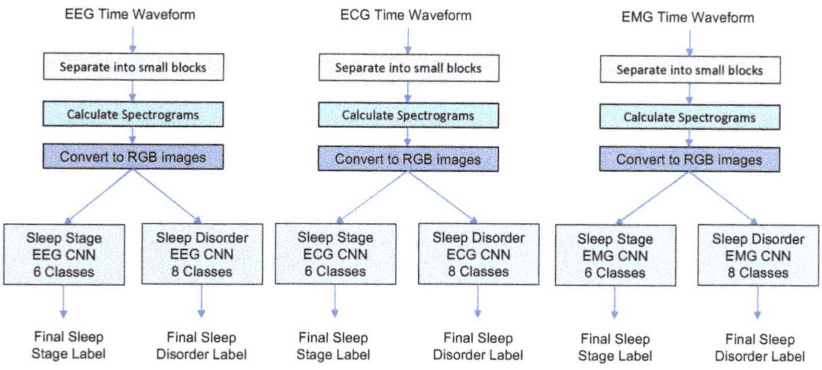

Figure 1. Experiment 1: Sleep stage and sleep disorder classification using a baseline approach.

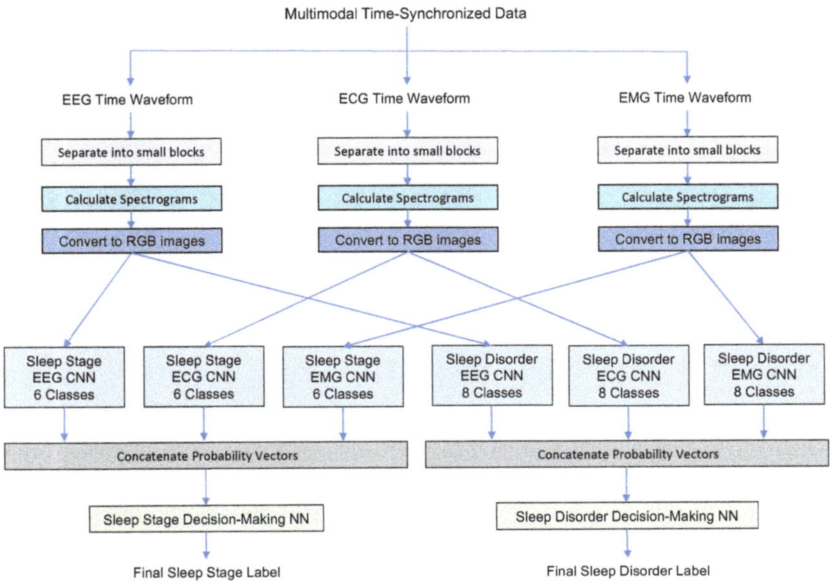

Figure 2. Experiment 2: Sleep stage and sleep disorder classification using MML-DMS1.

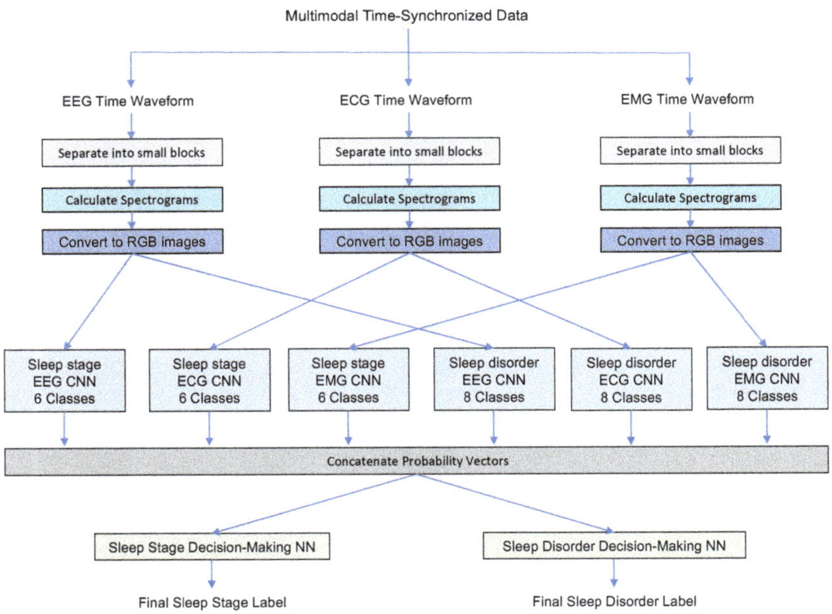

Figure 3. Experiment 3: Sleep stage and sleep disorder classification using MML-DMS2.

The CNNs act as independent evaluators, directly analyzing the physiological data coming from the sensors. The probability vectors given by all six CNNs are concatenated and passed to two second-stage decision-making classifiers designed as fully connected shallow neural networks (NNs). One of the networks is trained to provide the final identification of the sleep stage and the other to identify the sleep disorder. Both stages identify the sleep stage and the sleep disorder. The difference is that in the first stage, each CNN makes decisions based on single-modality physiological data with only one label representing either the sleep stage or the sleep disorder. In contrast, the second-stage

NNs use integrated sleep stage and sleep disorder information. Since the first-level CNN assessors use limited single-modality information, assessment results may vary between assessors, and their decisions may not always be correct. However, during the second stage of the classification process, the secondary NN evaluators compensate for the first-level limitations by using two-dimensional label information and arbitrating between the primary evaluators to arrive at the final sleep stage and sleep disorder labels.

2.2. Pre-Processing of Multimodal Data

The pre-processing steps followed were consistent across all three data modalities (EEG, ECG, and EMG). The pre-recorded time waveforms synchronized across modalities were first transformed to have the same bandwidth of 256 Hz and a sampling frequency of 512 Hz for all three modalities. The time waveforms were then divided into short-duration blocks to conduct block-by-block processing. Raw data signals sourced from the PhysioNet CAP Sleep database [18,21] represented at least eight hours of recordings labeled every 30 s with sleep stage- and sleep disorder information. However, when using 30-s non-overlapping intervals, the number of intervals was insufficient for training CNN models. Therefore, each 30-s sample was divided into overlapping 10-s intervals with a 1-s stride between subsequent blocks, resulting in a 90% overlap. The same approach was applied to all three modalities. Having such a short stride, we could generate a relatively large number of training data intervals. Since records are labeled sample-by-sample, a given interval was assumed to have the same label as the corresponding data sample. A two-dimensional spectrogram array was calculated for each interval.

2.3. Calculation of Amplitude Spectrograms and RGB Images

A two-dimensional amplitude spectrogram array was calculated for each 10 s interval using the Short-Time Fourier Transform (STFT). It was conducted the same way for all modalities to facilitate synchronized processing. By comparing the linear and the logarithmic frequency scales, it was experimentally determined that the logarithmic frequency scale led to better classification outcomes. Therefore, the spectrograms were generated using the logarithmic frequency scale, while the time scale was linear. Finally, the spectrogram arrays were converted into color RGB images using the "jet" colormap [23]. The color intensity values of the RGB images were normalized separately for each modality, with the minimum and maximum values corresponding to the average minima and maxima calculated for all images representing a given modality. Figure 4 shows examples of the original waveforms for different modalities and the corresponding RGB images representing different sleep stages and disorders. The RGB images were used to train the first-level classifiers of the proposed MML-DMS. Through visual inspection of these images, differences can be observed between the visual patterns for sleep stages and sleep disorders. These differences are difficult to comprehend by human observers. However, this study shows that CNNs can learn these differences to provide an automatic classification of sleep data.

It should be noted that the wavelet transform [24,25] is a very interesting alternative to the STFT. We used the STFT as it could be more efficiently implemented in real-time, and it is an industry-standard for real-time processing with widely available processing platforms and tools.

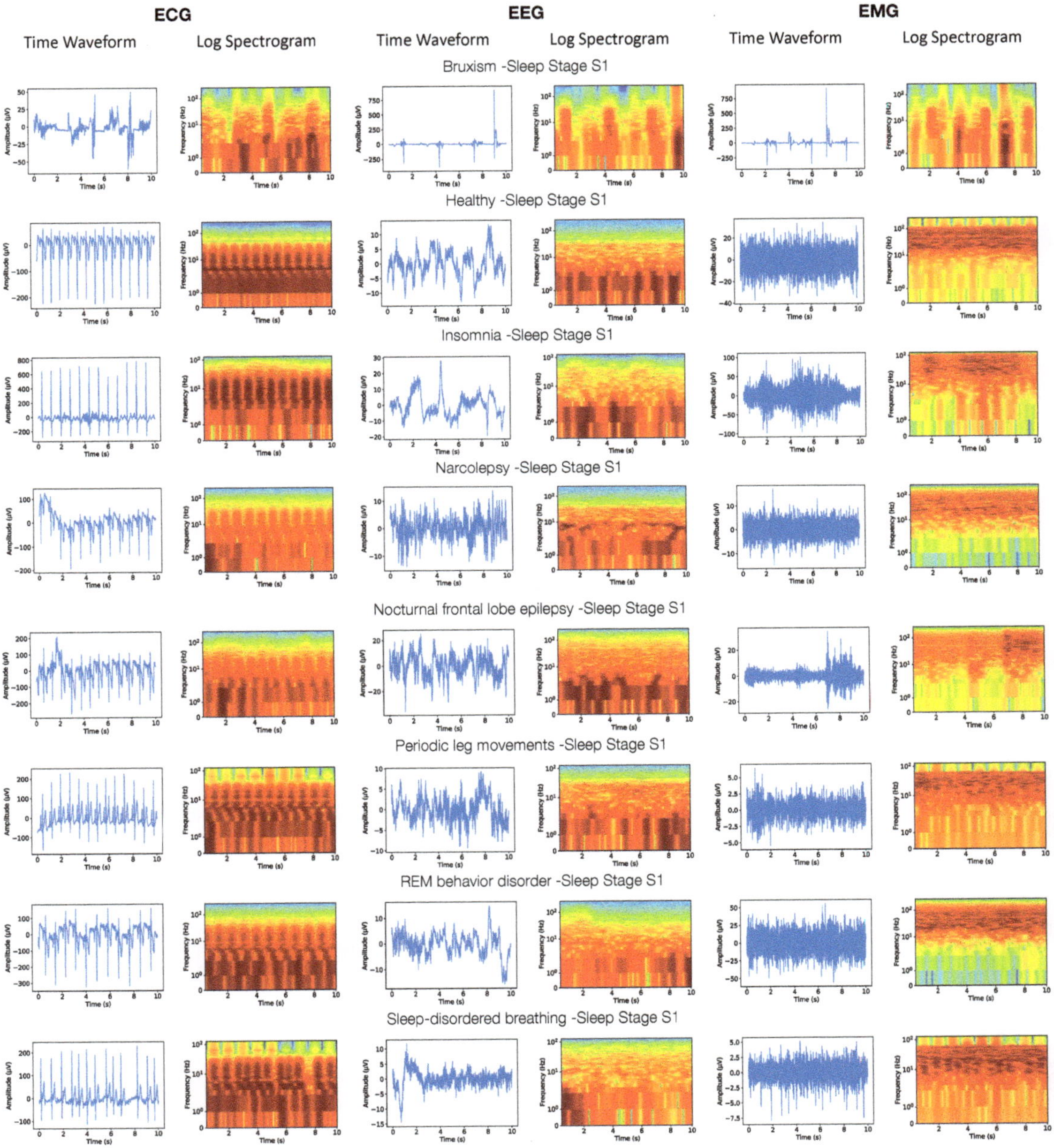

Figure 4. Examples of ECG-, EEG-, and EMG time waveforms and the corresponding logarithmic spectrograms for sleep stage S1 across different sleep disorders.

2.4. CNN Classifiers

The MML-DMS included six CNN classifiers. Each classifier was trained to recognize either a sleep stage or a sleep disorder from a single modality (EEG, ECG, or EMG). The sleep stage identification included six categories: wake (W), four sleep levels (from light sleep to deep sleep denoted S1, S2, S3, and S4, respectively), and rapid eye movement (R). At the same time, the sleep disorder identification included eight categories: normal sleep (N), Bruxism (B), insomnia (I), narcolepsy (Na), nocturnal frontal lobe epilepsy (Nf), periodic leg movements (P), REM behavior disorder (Rd) and sleep-disordered breathing (S).

The VGG16 architecture was chosen experimentally after evaluating different CNN classifiers, e.g., Inception-v3, ResNet50, and VGG16 structures, using a single classifier scenario. From the tested structures, VGG16 offered the highest classification accuracy at a reasonable computational time. In general terms, the MM-DMS is a modular classification system concept that can be implemented using different architectures for the component modules.

For all CNN models, the VGG16 CNN network structure [26,27] was used. It consisted of thirteen two-dimensional convolutional layers and three fully connected layers. The activations were rectified using a rectified linear unit (ReLu) activation function, and the learning rate was set to 0.001. All CNNs were trained from scratch; no transfer learning was applied. The VGG16 architecture was chosen experimentally after evaluating several alternative options. The VGG16 structure offered the highest accuracy at a reasonable computational time.

2.5. Concatenation of Probability Vectors

The final decision-making networks of the MML-DMS were trained on the soft probability vectors generated by the CNN classifiers. These vectors were concatenated and passed as inputs to the NNs. For example, given K data categories, M independent CNN classifiers, and N images, the probability vector generated by the jth CNN ($j = 1, \ldots, M$) for image i ($i = 1, \ldots, N$) was $P_{i,j} = [p_{i,j,1}, \ldots, p_{i,j,K}]$. Therefore, the concatenated probability vectors C_i were given as:

$$\begin{aligned} C_i = [&p_{i,1,1}, \ldots, p_{i,1,K}, \\ &p_{i,2,1}, \ldots, p_{i,2,K}, \\ &\ldots \\ &p_{i,M,1}, \ldots, p_{i,M,K}]. \end{aligned} \tag{1}$$

The concatenated probability vectors and the corresponding "ground truth" data labels were passed to the decision-making NN. It was trained to provide the final sleep stage categorization label. The probability merging process required having the same number of representative images for each modality. Since the available data contained different numbers of spectrogram images for different modalities (see Table 1), the number of training images was reduced in order to have the same number of images per modality. The NN training and testing runs were repeated three times, and the average values of the performance parameters were calculated.

Table 1. Number of spectrogram images calculated for six sleep stages (W: wake, S1–S4: sleep sub-stages, and R: rapid eye movement), and three modalities (ECG, EEG, and EMG).

Sleep Stage	ECG	EEG	EMG
R	38002	83345	38002
S1	10405	19326	10405
S2	79338	168825	79338
S3	25229	51083	25229
S4	28179	63765	28179
W	45552	97925	45552
Total	226705	484269	226705

2.6. Decision-Making Neural Network (NN)

Two shallow NNs have been trained to determine the final decision: one for the final sleep stage label; and the other for the final sleep disorder label. Both NNs consisted of an input layer containing 18 nodes, 2 hidden layers, each with 128 nodes, and an output layer with 6 nodes. The ReLu function was applied to the activations from the input and hidden layers, and the SoftMax function to the activations from the output layer. To enhance its performance, the sleep stage detection NN was trained using transfer learning from a VGG16 network pre-trained on the ECG data, as described in [23]. The sleep disorder NN on the other hand was trained from scratch, and no pre-training was applied.

2.7. Classical Decision-Making Methods

As shown in Figures 2 and 3, when arbitrating between the outcomes of different CNN classifiers, the MML-DMS used a shallow decision-making NN. To validate the NN performance, a comparison was made by replacing the NN with other classical decision-making approaches, i.e., maximum probability, average probability, and majority voting.

When using the maximum probability method, the final label was assigned to the label indicated by the largest probability across all CNN classifiers. The majority voting approach would evaluate the categories suggested by each CNN classifier and make a decision based on the category that achieved the highest vote. When all assessors disagreed, the maximum probability criterion was used. The average probability method would average the voting provided by all CNNs for all categories and choose the category that scored the highest.

2.8. Performance Measures

The assessment of the MML-DMS performance was based on the classification accuracy, precision, recall, and F_1 score. Given the true positive (TP), true negative (TN), false-positive (FP), and the false-negative (FN) classification outcomes, the classification accuracy was calculated using:

$$A_{\text{classification}} = \frac{TP + TN}{TP + TN + FP + FN}. \tag{2}$$

Since the training data were unbalanced across categories, the F_1 score was estimated to indicate how well the classification accuracy was distributed across categories. It was calculated using:

$$F_1 = \frac{2 \cdot Recall \cdot Precision}{Recall + Precision}, \tag{3}$$

where the recall and precision values were defined as:

$$Recall = \frac{TP}{TP + FN} \tag{4}$$

$$Precision = \frac{TP}{TP + FP} \tag{5}$$

3. Experiments and Results

3.1. Data Description

The MML-DMS and the baseline approaches were tested using publicly available sleep data collected by the Sleep Disorders Center of the Ospedale Maggiore of Parma, Italy, available through the PhysioNet CAP Sleep database [18,21]. It is one of the most frequently used research databases. This choice was also motivated by the fact that the data represented recordings from multimodal sensors labeled with sleep stage as well as sleep disorder. Therefore, it provided a suitable testing bed for simultaneous multimodal- and multilabel sleep scoring. In addition, the number of available recordings was sufficient to train deep learning models. The data included synchronized waveforms representing three sensor modalities (ECG, EEG, and EMG). The total number of participants was 108. For all participants, the recordings were labeled with six sleep stages: wake (W), sleep sub stages (S1 to S4), and rapid eye movement (R). The data also included labels of normal sleep (N) from sixteen participants, and seven common sleep disorders: Bruxism (B) from two people, insomnia (I) from nine people, narcolepsy (Na) from five people, nocturnal frontal lobe epilepsy (Nf) from forty people, periodic leg movements (P) from ten people, REM behavior disorder (Rd) from twenty-two people, and sleep-disordered breathing (S) from four people.

Tables 1 and 2 list the numbers of RGB images of spectrograms across three modalities (EEG, ECG, and EMG) for the sleep stages and sleep disorders, respectively. It can be observed that the image data were imbalanced across the sleep stage and sleep disorder categories. For the sleep stage categories, the S2 category was represented by the largest number of images, followed by the W, R, S4, S3, and S1 categories. For the sleep disorder categories, the N class was represented by the largest number of images, followed by the I, Nf, Rd, P, Na, S, and B categories.

Table 2. Number of spectrogram images calculated for eight sleep disorders (N: normal sleep, B: Bruxism, I: insomnia, Na: narcolepsy, Nf: nocturnal frontal lobe epilepsy, P: periodic leg movements, Rd: REM behavior disorder, S: sleep-disordered breathing) and three modalities (ECG, EEG, and EMG).

Sleep Disorder	ECG	EEG	EMG
B	1423	25536	1423
I	18132	125116	18132
N	25599	89244	25599
Na	16764	39350	16764
Nf	58705	74328	58705
P	27330	41544	27330
Rd	67826	67575	67826
S	10926	21576	10926
Total	226705	484269	226705

The EEG recordings included signals collected from sixteen electrodes (P1-P16) placed on the patient's head at different positions, as shown in [18,21]. The ECG signals were collected from two electrodes, ECG1 and ECG2, placed on the patient's chest, as shown in [18,21]. The EMG samples included EMG measurements of the submentalis muscle and bilateral anterior tibial EMG [18,21].

3.2. Training, Validation and Testing Procedures

The MM-DMS modules were trained in a person-independent way. However, all participants were represented in training and testing data to achieve a fair representation of person-related diversity. For each participant and for each sleep stage, the data were split into training/validation (90%) and testing (10%) subsets. These subsets were then grouped across all subjects into the total training/validation and testing sets for the sleep stage and sleep disorder classification. The training and testing of the final trained model procedure was repeated three times, each time using different training/validation and testing subsets based on the three-fold cross-validation technique. The classification results were calculated as an average of these three repeats. The experiments were conducted using the Python programming platform with 90% of the training/validation dataset used to train the model hyperparameters and 10% of the training/validation dataset to perform validation of the training process. The hyperparameters are summarized in Table 3.

The MML-DMS is a modular system of neural networks. At the first level of classification, we have convolutional neural networks (CNNs), and at the second level, we have shallow perceptron neural networks (NNs). Each network was trained independently using standard neural network training algorithms and the same set of ground truth labels (either sleep stage or sleep disorder depending on the classification task). There was no external optimization loop with an objective function for the whole system.

For the CNNs, the objective function was the standard cross entropy loss, CE, between the ground truth probabilities $p(x)$ and network output probabilities $q(x)$, where x represents the training data vectors.

$$CE = -\sum_{x} p(x) \log q(x) \tag{6}$$

The optimization method used was stochastic gradient descent (SGD). For the shallow NNs, the objective functions and the optimization methods were the same as for CNNs, and both levels of classification used the same ground truth labels given either by the sleep stage or sleep disorder categories of the PhysioNet CAP Sleep database. The difference was that the first-level classifiers (CNNs) were trained on physical data from sensors, whereas the second-level decision-making NNs were trained on the metadata given as probability vectors generated by the first-level CNNs.

After training each of the CNNs, the output probabilities can be saved and used to train the shallow decision-making NNs. Unlike the CNNs, which classify using only a single label—either sleep stage or sleep disorder—the NNs have the advantage of making the decision based on information provided by both sleep stage and sleep disorder labels.

Table 3. Hyperparameters for the VGG16 CNNs and the Shallow NNs.

Parameters	CNN	DM-Shallow NN
Optimization	SGD *	SGD *
Initial learning rate	0.001	0.001
Batch size	10	3
Maximum epochs	100	10
Early Stopping	Yes	Yes

* Stochastic Gradient Descent.

3.3. Experimental Framework

To highlight the advantages of the MML-DMS and how it compares to baseline methods, three sleep stage and sleep disorder classification experiments were conducted. We started with a basic Experiment 1, testing the baseline CNN classifiers working with a single modality. In Experiment 2, we moved to a simplified form of the MML-DMS (denoted MML-DMS1) where there was no fusion of the sleep stage and sleep disorder information. Finally, we progressed to Experiment 3, where the sleep stage and sleep disorder information was fused at the final decision-making stage of the fully developed version of the MML-DMS (denoted MML-DMS2).

3.4. Experiment 1

In this experiment, a simple baseline system shown in Figure 1 was created with six CNNs working in parallel to classify either sleep stage or sleep disorder based on single-modality data (EEG, ECG, or EMG). No fusion of information was applied. The resulting classification accuracy and F_1 scores are presented in Table 4, and the examples of confusion matrices are shown in Figure 5.

Table 4. Experiment 1: Classification results for the baseline single-modality CNN classifiers.

	Sleep Stage Classification		Sleep Disorder Classification	
Modality	Accuracy (%)	F_1-Score	Accuracy (%)	F_1-Score
ECG	57.85%	0.50	93.74%	0.95
EEG	54.89%	0.43	79.21%	0.79
EMG	51.40%	0.40	74.91%	0.74

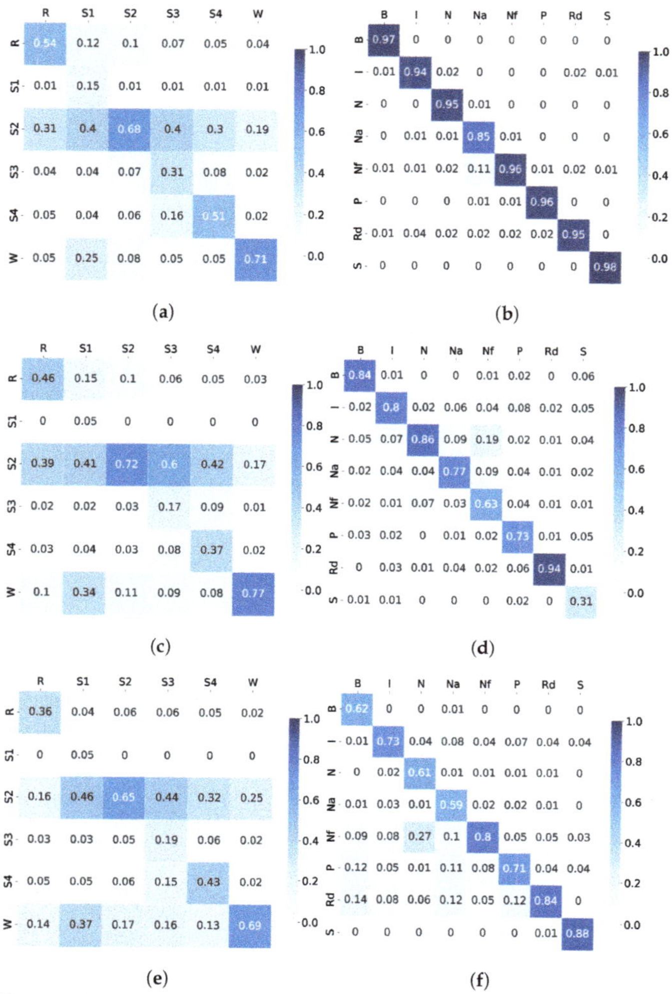

Figure 5. Experiment 1: Examples of confusion matrices for sleep stage and sleep disorder detection using baseline single-modality CNN classifiers: (a) ECG Sleep Stage detection confusion matrices; (b) ECG Sleep Disorder detection confusion matrices; (c) EEG Sleep Stage detection confusion matrices; (d) EEG Sleep Disorder detection confusion matrices; (e) EMG Sleep Stage detection confusion matrices; (f) EMG Sleep Disorder detection confusion matrices.

A comparison between sleep stage and sleep disorder detection shows that sleep disorder identification shows more than 20% higher accuracy and F_1 scores than sleep stage detection. While the sleep stage accuracy ranges between 51.4% and 57.85% and the F_1 scores from 0.4 to 0.5, for the sleep disorder, it is between 74.91% and 93.74% for the classification accuracy and between 0.74 and 0.95 for the F_1 scores. Similarly, the confusion matrices for sleep disorders show very clear diagonal patterns due to an even distribution of high accuracy across sleep disorder categories. Firstly, it could indicate that there are more distinct differences between spectral patterns of sleep disorders compared to that of sleep stages. Secondly, the data imbalances could play a less significant role in the training of disorder models than sleep stage models.

A comparison between different modalities shows that for both types of labels—sleep stage and sleep disorder—ECG signals show the highest performance, i.e., 57.85% accuracy for sleep stage and 93.74% for sleep disorder, followed by mid-performing EEG signals and finally by the lowest-performing EMG signals. It appears that ECG signals alone could be efficiently used to determine the sleep disorder. However, the sleep stage recognition scores were very low. Therefore, we needed to investigate ways of improvement to see if information fusion could be used to boost the sleep stage recognition accuracy.

3.5. *Experiment 2*

In this experiment, we test a simplified version of the MML-DMS denoted as MML-DMS1. As shown in Figure 2, it includes two levels of classification. At the first level, there are six CNN models. Three of these models are trained to identify sleep stages using only single-modality data (EEG, ECG, or EMG), and the other three to identify sleep disorders also using only single-modality data (EEG, ECG, or EMG). The probability vectors from the sleep stage classifiers are then concatenated and passed to the shallow NN (Sleep Stage Decision-making NN) trained to make the final sleep stage decision. At the same time, the probability vectors from the sleep disorder CNNs are concatenated and passed to another shallow NN (Sleep Disorder Decision-making NN) trained to decide the final sleep disorder label. The final decisions are made using a single-label approach since there is no fusion of sleep disorder information with sleep stage information.

The MML-DMS1 system allowed us to compare the multimodal information fusion with the single-modality approach used in Experiment 1. The MML-DMS1 accuracy and F_1 scores are presented in Table 5.

Table 5. Experiment 2: Classification results for MML-DMS1 with different final decision-making (DM) methods (MP: maximum probability; MV: majority voting; AP: average probability; PT-Shallow NN: pre-trained NN; Shallow NN: trained-from-scratch NN).

	Sleep Stage Classification		Sleep Disorder Classification	
DM-Methods	**Accuracy (%)**	**F_1-Score**	**Accuracy (%)**	**F_1-Score**
Shallow NN	73.42%	0.73	98.93%	0.99
PT-Shallow NN	91.06%	0.90	N/A	N/A
MP	65.09%	0.56	97.07%	0.97
MV	62.25%	0.52	94.27%	0.91
AP	42.21%	0.35	54.59%	0.53

At the same time, examples of confusion matrices are shown in Figure 6(a) and (b) for the sleep stage- and sleep disorder detection, respectively.

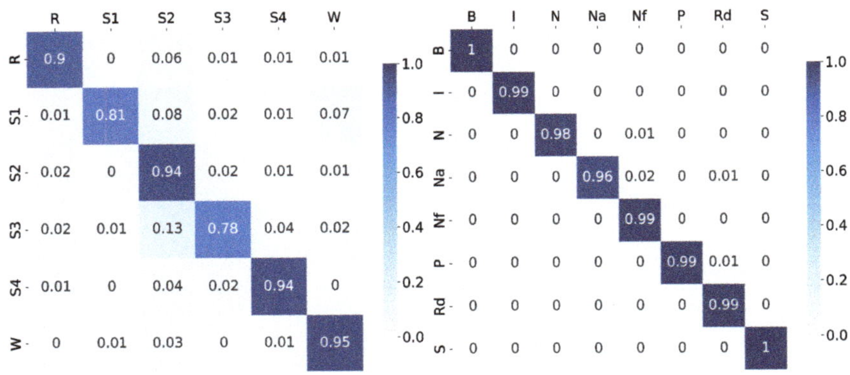

(a) (b)

Figure 6. Experiment 2: Examples of confusion matrices for (**a**) sleep stage using MML-DMS1 with pre-trained NN and (**b**) sleep disorder detection using MML-DMS1 with trained-from-scratch NN.

To determine the efficiency of NN-based decision making in comparison with other classical decision-making techniques, we have compared it with the maximum probability

(MP), majority voting (MV), and average probability (AP) methods. These methods were applied within the MML-DMS structure at the second level of classification by replacing the shallow NN. The first-level CNNs remained unchanged. The results are listed in Table 5. In the case of sleep stage classification, the shallow NN trained from scratch did not perform very well, showing only 73.42% accuracy (Table 5). Therefore, a pre-trained shallow NN (PT-Shallow NN) was applied to improve the performance. In the case of sleep disorder, no pre-training of the NN was used since the trained-from-scratch NN already provided high accuracy.

It can be observed from Table 5 that the MML-DMS1 clearly outperformed the single-modality classification tested in Experiment 1. However, the sleep stage detection improvement was more significant than for the sleep disorder. The sleep stage detection achieved 91.06% accuracy, improving upon the single modalities by about 30% to 40%, whereas the sleep disorder classification achieved 98.93% accuracy, improving upon the single modalities by about 6% to 20%. A clear improvement was also observed for the F_1 scores and the confusion matrices, indicating that the multimodal approach is more robust to the data imbalances across categories. Specifically, the examples of confusion matrices for the sleep stage, as shown in Figure 6, show a much stronger diagonal pattern of high classification accuracy for individual categories than the single-modality confusion matrices shown in Figure 5.

Based on the outcomes of Experiment 2, it can be concluded that the fusion of multimodal information led to the improvement of the classification results. The classification of sleep stages was somehow more challenging and led to slightly lower results than the classification of sleep disorders. The shallow NN outperformed other classical decision-making approaches.

3.6. Experiment 3

In this experiment, we tested a full version of the MML-DMS denoted as MML-DMS2. It represents a multimodal as well as a multilabel approach. As shown in Figure 3, it includes two classification levels. As for the MML-DMS1, at the first level, three CNN models are trained to identify sleep, each model using only single-modality data (EEG, ECG, or EMG). Similarly, three other CNN models are trained to identify the sleep disorder from single-modality data (EEG, ECG, or EMG).

The probability vectors from all sleep stage classifiers and all sleep disorder classifiers are then concatenated and passed to the shallow NN (Sleep Stage Decision-making NN) trained to make the final sleep stage decision as well as to another shallow NN (Sleep Disorder Decision-making NN) trained to decide the final sleep disorder label. Unlike in MML-DMS1, the final decisions in MML-DMS2 are made using both multimodal and multilabel approaches, which means that in addition to fusing the multi-sensor information (EEG, ECG, and EMG), the sleep disorder information is fused with the sleep stage information.

The implementation of MML-DMS2 allowed us to compare the combined multimodal and multilabel information fusion with the single-modality approach used in Experiment 1. In addition, we could investigate the effect of adding the multilabel fusion to the multimodal approach (MML-DMS1) used in Experiment 2.

The MML-DMS2 accuracy and F_1 scores are presented in Table 6. At the same time, the examples of the confusion matrices are shown in Figure 7(a) and (b) for the sleep stage- and sleep disorder detection, respectively. Like in Experiment 2, the shallow NN trained from scratch did not perform very well, giving only 84.89% accuracy (Table 6). Therefore, a pre-trained shallow NN (PT-Shallow NN) was applied to improve the system. No pre-training of the NN was applied for sleep disorder detection since the trained-from-scratch NN already led to high accuracy.

Table 6. Experiment 3: Classification results for MML-DMS2 using a shallow decision-making NN (PT-Shallow NN: pre-trained NN; Shallow NN: trained-from-scratch NN).

DM-Methods	Sleep Stage Classification Accuracy (%)	Sleep Stage Classification F_1-Score	Sleep Disorder Classification Accuracy (%)	Sleep Disorder Classification F_1-Score
Shallow NN	84.89%	0.77	99.09%	0.99
PT-Shallow NN	94.34%	0.92	N/A	N/A

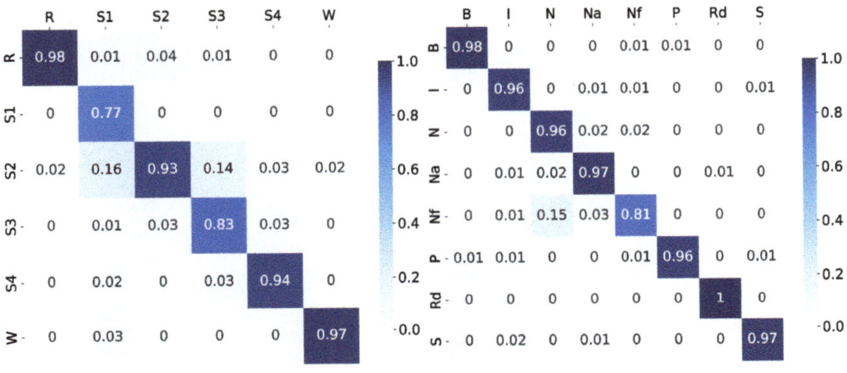

(**a**) (**b**)

Figure 7. Experiment 3: Examples of confusion matrices for (**a**) sleep stage using MML-DMS2 with pre-trained NN and (**b**) sleep disorder detection using MML-DMS2 with trained-from-scratch NN.

Table 6 shows that the MML-DMS2 achieved 94.34% accuracy for the sleep stage detection and 99.09% for the sleep disorder detection. It shows an improvement upon the MML-DMS1 of about 4% for the sleep stage and of 1% for the sleep disorder.

A clear improvement upon the MML-DMS1 was also observed for the F_1 scores and the confusion matrices, indicating that the combined multimodal and multilabel approach is even more robust to the data imbalances across categories. The examples of confusion matrices for the sleep stage, as shown in Figure 7, have very high classification accuracy for individual categories compared to the single-modality confusion matrices shown in Figure 5.

Based on the outcomes of Experiment 3, it can be concluded that the combined multimodal and multilabel information leads to an improvement in comparison with the multimodal approach and also in comparison with the single-modality baseline. The classification of sleep stages was more challenging and led to slightly lower results than the classification of sleep disorders.

4. Discussion

Figure 8 shows bar graphs summarizing the outcomes of this study. In Figure 8(a) and (c), the classification accuracy is presented for the sleep stage- and sleep disorder classification, respectively, while Figure 8(b) and (d) show the corresponding F_1 scores. Each bar corresponds to a different classification approach tested in our experiments.

In Figure 8(a) and (b), pertaining to the sleep stage recognition, ten approaches are listed, including three single-modality and single-label baseline classifiers (ECG CNN, EEG CNN, and EMG CNN), five versions of the MML-DMS1 system each with a different decision-making method (MML-DMS1 MP, MML-DMS1 MV, MML-DMS1 AP, MML-DMS1 NN, and MML-DMS1 PT-NN), and two versions of the MML-DMS2—one with the trained from scratch NN (MML-DMS2 NN) and the other with the pre-trained NN (MML-DMS2 PT-NN).

In contrast, in Figure 8(c) and (d), pertaining to the sleep disorder recognition, we only have eight approaches, including three single-modality and single-label baseline classifiers

(ECG CNN, EEG CNN, and EMG CNN), four versions of the MML-DMS1 system each with a different decision-making method (MML-DMS1 MP, MML-DMS1 MV, MML-DMS1 AP, and MML-DMS1 NN), and one version of the MML-DMS2 with the NN trained from scratch (MML-DMS2 NN).

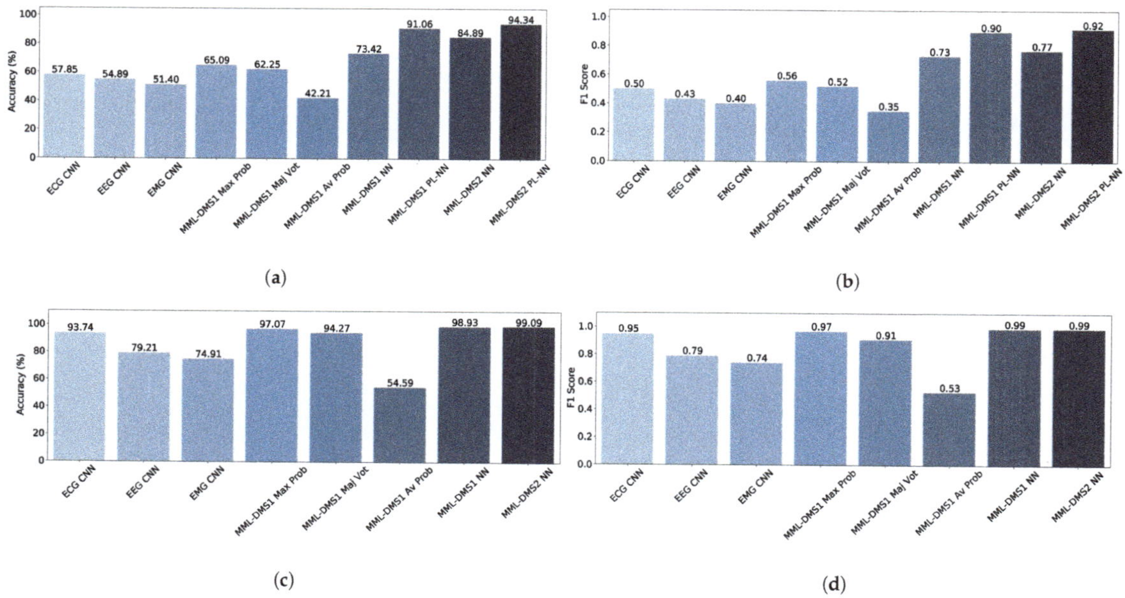

Figure 8. Comparison between all sleep stage and sleep disorder classification methods tested in this study: (**a**) Accuracy (%)—Sleep Stage Recognition; (**b**) F_1 Score (%)—Sleep Stage Recognition; (**c**) Accuracy (%)—Sleep Disorder Recognition; (**d**) F_1 Score (%)—Sleep Disorder Recognition.

The experiments demonstrated a clear advantage of combining not only the multimodal but also the multilabel information. It was confirmed by the highest performance resulting from the MML-DMS2 approach, which outperformed all other techniques and led to a 94.34% classification accuracy for the sleep stage recognition and 99.09% for the sleep disorder recognition. The F_1 scores and the confusion matrices were also consistently high, showing that the proposed modular system of networks has the capacity to compensate for the training data imbalance and give uniformly high recognition accuracy across all data categories. The second-best performance was achieved by the MML-DMS1 method offering a fusion of modalities but not the labels. It led to slightly lower classification accuracy values, i.e., 91.06% for sleep stage and 98.93% for sleep disorder classification. The highest difference was observed for the least-performing single-modality and single-label techniques. The CNN classifiers using EEG or EMG signals alone achieved around 51% to 55% accuracy for the sleep stage and about 75% to 79% for the sleep disorder recognition. Interestingly, ECG signals alone performed exceptionally well, yielding a 93.74% accuracy for the sleep disorder but only 57.85% for the sleep stage recognition. The F_1 scores and the confusion matrices corresponding to the single-modality methods were also consistently low, showing that a single CNN classifier cannot compensate for the training data imbalance.

One of the advantages of the MML-DMS is its distributed and modular character making it very versatile. The component modules are independent classifiers. Each of these classifiers uses a different combination of the input data and type of labels. The connections and data flow between modules determine the final output. It allows for either fusion or separation of specific data. Therefore, the system modules can be assembled in many different ways, and the trained units can be stored and reused depending on the task. It also means that the system can be trained with much less data, time, and lower hardware requirements compared to the large multi-branch stacked neural network structures frequently used in multimodal or multilabel problems.

One of the key factors leading to the overall high performance of the MML-DMS is the use of a shallow NN trained to arbitrate between the outcomes of an assembly of assessors (CNNs working with the single-modality data). As shown in our experiments, it outperforms other frequently used approaches, such as the maximum probability, majority voting, or average probability approaches. Each of these techniques makes certain arbitrary assumptions about how to judge the assessors. In contrast, this NN is free of such assumptions and learns directly from the data how to compensate for the potential mistakes made by the assembly of assessors.

Finally, we would like to compare the consistency of our results with other related studies. The majority of related multimodal classification methods have a single-label character, i.e., the combined modalities are used to classify either sleep stage or sleep disorder. Our experiments show one of the first attempts to conduct a simultaneous multimodal and multilabel classification of sleep data. Due to the lack of similar approaches, we present two separate tables. Table 7 shows a comparison with related sleep stage recognition studies, whereas Table 8 shows a comparison with sleep disorder classification works. We can see that for the sleep stage classification case, both of our methods outperform the best-performing study [19] by 6% (MML-DMS1) to 9% (MML-DMS2). Note that [19] classified five sleep stage categories, whereas our approach used six categories. Similarly, in sleep disorder classification, our approach outperformed the best results of [20] by 4% (MML-DMS1 and MML-DMS2).

Table 7. A comparison with related multimodal sleep stage classification studies.

Authors	Database	Modality	Classes	Features	Method	Accuracy (%)
Kim et al. (2017) [12]	CAP	ECG, HRV	2	DFA * alpha	k-fold cross validation (k = 13)	73.6%
Fernández-Varela et al. (2018) [13]	SHHS	EEG EOG EMG	5	Time series	1D-CNN	78%
Phan et al. (2019) [16]	Sleep EDF SHHS	EEG, EOG	5	Spectrogram	Multi-task CNN	82.3%
Rui et al. (2021) [19]	Sleep EDF	EEG, EOG, EMG, ECG	5	Time series	Multi-task 2D-CNN	85%
This study	CAP	EEG, ECG, EMG	6	Log Spectrogram	MML-DMS1 MML-DMS2	91.06% 94.34%

* Detrended Fluctuation Analysis.

Table 8. A comparison with related multimodal sleep disorder classification studies.

Authors	Database	Modality	Classes	Features	Method	Accuracy (%)
Zhuang et al. (2022) [20]	CAP	EEG, EMG, ECG, EOG	8	Spectrogram	DL-AR	95%
Sharma et al. (2022) [22]	CAP	EOG, EMG	6	Hjorth parameters	Ensemble Bagged Trees	94.3%
This study	CAP	EEG, ECG, EMG	8	Log Spectrogram	MML-DMS1 MML-DMS2	98.93% 99.09%

5. Conclusions

In this study, we investigated the simultaneous recognition of six sleep stages and eight sleep disorder conditions from three different sensor modalities: EEG, ECG, and EMG. We proposed a new multimodal and multilabel classification system (MML-DMS). The classification outcomes derived separately for each modality by a parallel set of CNNs identifying either sleep stages or sleep disorders were fused and passed to a shallow NN to make the final decision. The system was validated using the PhysioNet CAP Sleep database and achieved 94.34% classification accuracy for sleep stage recognition and 99.09% for sleep disorder recognition.

It has to be noted that the experimental testing setup presented in this study was limited to a closed-set scenario, where the training and testing sets of samples were mutually exclusive. However, both sets represented the same groups of patients. Future research will test if the system can be generalized to accurately categorize data from patients unseen in the training process.

We demonstrated that the fusion of multimodal and multilabel information significantly improves classification outcomes compared to single-classifier and single-modality methods. Most significantly, the MML-DMS improved not only the overall classification accuracy but also the confusion matrices, leading to a uniformly high classification accuracy across all data categories. It effectively canceled out the detrimental effect of class imbalance that crippled single-modality performance. A comparison with related studies shows a significant improvement upon existing state-of-the-art techniques.

The study provided a proof of concept for simultaneous multimodal and multilabel scoring using the MML-DMS method. Due to the high complexity of the multimodal and multilabel task, MML-DMS was validated on a single database using a single type of CNN and shallow NN structure. Future research will investigate different structures of the CNN and NN classifiers and validate the proposed approach on different databases. We will also investigate improvements to sleep stage classification as it was shown to be more challenging than sleep disorder recognition.

Author Contributions: Conceptualization, Y.-H.C., M.L., and R.H.W.; methodology, M.L. and Y.-H.C.; software, Y.-H.C.; validation, Y.-H.C.; formal analysis, Y.-H.C., M.L., and R.H.W.; investigation, Y.-H.C.; resources, Y.-H.C., M.L., and R.H.W.; data curation, Y.-H.C.; writing—original draft preparation, Y.-H.C.; writing—review and editing, M.L. and R.H.W.; visualization, Y.-H.C. and R.H.W.; supervision, M.L. and R.H.W.; project administration, Y.-H.C., M.L., and R.H.W. All authors have read and agreed to the published version of the manuscript.

Funding: This research was supported by an Australian Government Research Training Program Scholarship, Engineering Top-up Scholarship, and RMIT University Research Stipend.

Institutional Review Board Statement: Not applicable.

Informed Consent Statement: Not applicable.

Data Availability Statement: This study used the PhysioNet CAP Sleep database from the Sleep Disorders Center of the Ospedale Maggiore of Parma, Italy, as downloaded via physionet.org at https://physionet.org/content/capslpdb/1.0.0/ (accessed on 1 July 2020).

Acknowledgments: The PhysioNet CAP Sleep database from the Sleep Disorders Center of the Ospedale Maggiore of Parma, Italy was downloaded via physionet.org.

Conflicts of Interest: The authors declare no conflict of interest.

Abbreviations

The following abbreviations are used in this manuscript:

AP	Average Probability
B	Bruxism
CAP	Cyclic Alternating Pattern
CNN	Convolutional Neural Network
DM	Decision-making
ECG	Electrocardiogram
EEG	Electroencephalogram
EMG	Electromyogram
EOG	Electrooculogram
FN	False Negative
FP	False Positive
HRV	Heart Rate Variability
I	Insomnia
MML-DMS	Multimodal and Multilabel Decision-making System
MP	Maximum Probability
MV	Majority Voting
N	Normal - no sleep disorder
Na	Narcolepsy
Nf	Nocturnal frontal lobe epilepsy
NN	Neural Network
P	Periodic leg movements
PT	Pre-trained
Rd	REM behavior disorder
R	Rapid eye movement
RGB	Red, Green, and Blue
S	Sleep-disordered breathing
S1-S4	Sleep stages
SGD	Stochastic gradient descent
SHHS	Sleep Heart Health Study
TL	Transfer Learning
TN	True Negative
TP	True Positive
W	Wake

References

1. Walker, M. *Why We Sleep: The New Science of Sleep and Dreams;* Penguin Random House: London, UK, 2017.
2. Lee, S.; Kim, J.H.; Chung, J.H. The association between sleep quality and quality of life: A population-based study. *Sleep Med.* **2021**, *84*, 121–126. [CrossRef] [PubMed]
3. Berry, R.B.; Brooks, R.; Gamaldo, C.E.; Harding, S.M.; Marcus, C.; Vaughn, B.V. The AASM manual for the scoring of sleep and associated events. *Rules Terminol. Tech. Specif. Darien Illinois Am. Acad. Sleep Med.* **2012**, *176*, 2012.
4. Rechtschaffen, A.; Kales, A.; University of California Los Angeles Brain Information Service; NINDB Neurological Information Network (U.S.). *A Manual of Standardized Terminology, Techniques and Scoring System for Sleep Stages of Human Subjects;* Allan, R., Anthony, K., Eds.; NIH Publication, U.S. National Institute of Neurological Diseases and Blindness, Neurological Information Network: Bethesda, MD, USA, 1968.
5. Mansuri, L.E.; Patel, D. Artificial intelligence-based automatic visual inspection system for built heritage. *Smart Sustain. Built Environ.* **2021**, *11*, 622–646. [CrossRef]
6. Tsuneki, M. Deep learning models in medical image analysis. *J. Oral Biosci.* **2022**, *64*, 312–320. [CrossRef] [PubMed]
7. Ronzhina, M.; Janoušek, O.; Kolářová, J.; Nováková, M.; Honzík, P.; Provazník, I. Sleep scoring using artificial neural networks. *Sleep Med. Rev.* **2012**, *16*, 251–263. [CrossRef] [PubMed]
8. Şen, B.; Peker, M.; Çavuşoğlu, A.; Çelebi, F.V. A Comparative Study on Classification of Sleep Stage Based on EEG Signals Using Feature Selection and Classification Algorithms. *J. Med. Syst.* **2014**, *38*, 18. [CrossRef] [PubMed]
9. Radha, M.; Garcia-Molina, G.; Poel, M.; Tononi, G. Comparison of feature and classifier algorithms for online automatic sleep staging based on a single EEG signal. In Proceedings of the 2014 36th Annual International Conference of the IEEE Engineering in Medicine and Biology Society, Chicago, IL, USA, 26–30 August 2014; pp. 1876–1880. [CrossRef]

10. Alsolai, H.; Qureshi, S.; Iqbal, S.M.Z.; Vanichayobon, S.; Henesey, L.E.; Lindley, C.; Karrila, S. A Systematic Review of Literature on Automated Sleep Scoring. *IEEE Access* **2022**, *10*, 79419–79443. [CrossRef]
11. Fiorillo, L.; Puiatti, A.; Papandrea, M.; Ratti, P.L.; Favaro, P.; Roth, C.; Bargiotas, P.; Bassetti, C.L.; Faraci, F.D. Automated sleep scoring: A review of the latest approaches. *Sleep Med. Rev.* **2019**, *48*, 101204. [CrossRef] [PubMed]
12. Kim, J.; Lee, J.; Shin, M. Sleep stage classification based on noise-reduced fractal property of heart rate variability. *Procedia Comput. Sci.* **2017**, *116*, 435–440. [CrossRef]
13. Fernández-Varela, I.; Hernández-Pereira, E.; Moret-Bonillo, V. A convolutional network for the classification of sleep stages. *Proceedings* **2018**, *2*, 1174. [CrossRef]
14. Zhang, G.Q.; Cui, L.; Mueller, R.; Tao, S.; Kim, M.; Rueschman, M.; Mariani, S.; Mobley, D.; Redline, S. The National Sleep Research Resource: Towards a sleep data commons. *J. Am. Med. Inform. Assoc.* **2018**, *25*, 1351–1358. [CrossRef]
15. Quan, S.F.; Howard, B.V.; Iber, C.; Kiley, J.P.; Nieto, F.J.; O'Connor, G.T.; Rapoport, D.M.; Redline, S.; Robbins, J.; Samet, J.M.; et al. The sleep heart health study: Design, rationale, and methods. *Sleep* **1997**, *20*, 1077–1085. [PubMed]
16. Phan, H.; Andreotti, F.; Cooray, N.; Chén, O.Y.; De Vos, M. Joint Classification and Prediction CNN Framework for Automatic Sleep Stage Classification. *IEEE Trans. Biomed. Eng.* **2019**, *66*, 1285–1296. . [CrossRef]
17. Kemp, B.; Zwinderman, A.H.; Tuk, B.; Kamphuisen, H.A.; Oberyé, J.J. Analysis of a sleep-dependent neuronal feedback loop: The slow-wave microcontinuity of the EEG. *IEEE Trans. Biomed. Eng.* **2000**, *47*, 1185–1194. [CrossRef] [PubMed]
18. Goldberger, A.L.; Amaral, L.A.; Glass, L.; Hausdorff, J.M.; Ivanov, P.C.; Mark, R.G.; Mietus, J.E.; Moody, G.B.; Peng, C.K.; Stanley, H.E. PhysioBank, PhysioToolkit, and PhysioNet: Components of a new research resource for complex physiologic signals. *Circulation* **2000**, *101*, e215–e220. [CrossRef] [PubMed]
19. Yan, R.; Li, F.; Zhou, D.; Ristaniemi, T.; Cong, F. A Deep Learning Model for Automatic Sleep Scoring using Multimodality Time Series. In Proceedings of the 2020 28th European Signal Processing Conference (EUSIPCO), Amsterdam, The Netherlands, 18–21 January 2021; pp. 1090–1094. [CrossRef]
20. Zhuang, D.; Rao, I.; Ibrahim, A.K. A Machine Learning Approach to Automatic Classification of Eight Sleep Disorders. *arXiv* **2022**, arXiv:2204.06997. [CrossRef]
21. Terzano, M.G.; Parrino, L.; Sherieri, A.; Chervin, R.; Chokroverty, S.; Guilleminault, C.; Hirshkowitz, M.; Mahowald, M.; Moldofsky, H.; Rosa, A.; et al. Atlas, rules, and recording techniques for the scoring of cyclic alternating pattern (CAP) in human sleep. *Sleep Med.* **2001**, *2*, 537–553. [CrossRef]
22. Sharma, M.; Darji, J.; Thakrar, M.; Acharya, U.R. Automated identification of sleep disorders using wavelet-based features extracted from electrooculogram and electromyogram signals. *Comput. Biol. Med.* **2022**, *143*, 105224. [CrossRef]
23. Cheng, Y.H.; Lech, M.; Wilkinson, R. Sleep Stage Recognition from EEG Using a Distributed Multi-Channel Decision-Making System. In Proceedings of the 2021 15th International Conference on Signal Processing and Communication Systems (ICSPCS), Sydney, Australia, 13–15 December 2021; pp. 1–7. [CrossRef]
24. Vakharia, V.; Kiran, M.B.; Dave, N.J.; Kagathara, U. Feature extraction and classification of machined component texture images using wavelet and artificial intelligence techniques. In Proceedings of the 2017 8th International Conference on Mechanical and Aerospace Engineering (ICMAE), Prague, Czech Republic, 22–25 January 2017; pp. 140–144. [CrossRef]
25. Alturki, F.A.; AlSharabi, K.; Abdurraqeeb, A.M.; Aljalal, M. EEG signal analysis for diagnosing neurological disorders using discrete wavelet transform and intelligent techniques. *Sensors* **2020**, *20*, 2505. [CrossRef]
26. Qassim, H.; Verma, A.; Feinzimer, D. Compressed residual-VGG16 CNN model for big data places image recognition. In Proceedings of the 2018 IEEE 8th Annual Computing and Communication Workshop and Conference (CCWC), Las Vegas, NV, USA, 8–10 January 2018; pp. 169–175. [CrossRef]
27. Simonyan, K.; Zisserman, A. Very Deep Convolutional Networks for Large-Scale Image Recognition. *arXiv* **2015**, arXiv:1409.1556. [CrossRef]

sensors MDPI

Article

Sensor Selection for Tidal Volume Determination via Linear Regression—Impact of Lasso versus Ridge Regression

Bernhard Laufer [1,*], Paul D. Docherty [1,2], Rua Murray [3], Sabine Krueger-Ziolek [1], Nour Aldeen Jalal [1,4], Fabian Hoeflinger [5], Stefan J. Rupitsch [5], Leonhard Reindl [5] and Knut Moeller [1,2,5,*]

1 Institute of Technical Medicine (ITeM), Furtwangen University, 78054 Villingen-Schwenningen, Germany
2 Department of Mechanical Engineering, University of Canterbury, Christchurch 8041, New Zealand
3 School of Mathematics and Statistics, University of Canterbury, Christchurch 8041, New Zealand
4 Innovation Center Computer Assisted Surgery (ICCAS), University of Leipzig, 04109 Leipzig, Germany
5 Department of Microsystems Engineering, University of Freiburg, 79085 Freiburg, Germany
* Correspondence: b.laufer@hs-furtwangen.de (B.L.); moe@hs-furtwangen.de (K.M.); Tel.: +49-7720-307-4621 (B.L.)

Abstract: The measurement of respiratory volume based on upper body movements by means of a smart shirt is increasingly requested in medical applications. This research used upper body surface motions obtained by a motion capture system, and two regression methods to determine the optimal selection and placement of sensors on a smart shirt to recover respiratory parameters from benchmark spirometry values. The results of the two regression methods (Ridge regression and the least absolute shrinkage and selection operator (Lasso)) were compared. This work shows that the Lasso method offers advantages compared to the Ridge regression, as it provides sparse solutions and is more robust to outliers. However, both methods can be used in this application since they lead to a similar sensor subset with lower computational demand (from exponential effort for full exhaustive search down to the order of $O(n^2)$). A smart shirt for respiratory volume estimation could replace spirometry in some cases and would allow for a more convenient measurement of respiratory parameters in home care or hospital settings.

Keywords: wearables; smart clothing; sensor selection; linear regression; Lasso; Ridge regression; tidal volume

1. Introduction

Respiratory volumes and respiration-induced movements of the upper body are connected, and there is a desire to determine tidal volumes via surface motions of the human upper body. Respiration-induced motions were studied as early as 1848 by Sibson et al. [1]. Later, Wade et al. [2] used improved measurement methods and examined the respiratory-induced movements of the upper body, and recently, Laufer et al. [3] analyzed movement parameters of the upper body and their correlations with the respiratory volume in detail.

The pioneers who initiated the research field of determining tidal volumes from upper body movements were Konno and Mead [4]. They investigated the underlying relationships in more detail and published their first studies in the 1960s. The potential of such an approach was recognized, and many other studies followed. Unfortunately, only two measurement methods were able to establish themselves for clinical use and are still used sporadically today. One of these measurement methods is optoelectronic plethysmography [5,6]. The underlying principle of optoelectronic plethysmography is an optical motion tracking system (MoCap). The MoCap system detects respiration-induced movements on the upper body and determines respiration volumes. The disadvantages of an optoelectronic plethysmography are the acquisition costs and the complex procedure of use. It is nevertheless used in very sensitive areas of respiratory monitoring where breathing should not be influenced or impeded in any way by the measurement system—for example, in the respiratory monitoring of premature infants. The second established method is respiratory inductance plethysmography [7,8]. The respiratory inductance plethysmography measures respiratory-induced cross-sectional changes on the upper body inductively and thereby determines tidal volumes. The major disadvantage of respiratory inductance plethysmography is its reduced measurement accuracy [9].

Therefore, despite all efforts to date, tidal volumes are still determined by respiratory flow measurement using spirometers [10–12] or body plethysmographs [13–15]. For precise clinical respiratory flow measurements, patients under investigation must wear a face mask or breathe through a mouthpiece while the nose is blocked by a nose clip. This can be very inconvenient, especially for long-term measurements, and can falsify the measurement results themselves [16,17].

Hence, there remains a need for alternative methods for measuring respiratory volumes using upper body surface motion. A previous study [3] has shown that upper body movements are in some cases highly correlated with changes in respiratory volumes. This fact can be utilized for the determination of respiratory volumes via upper body movements, and some current approaches used inertial measurement units [18–20], others used strain gauges [21,22] or optical encoder systems, as in belts measuring changes in circumferences [23–25]. However, a real breakthrough has not been achieved yet despite the potential of new, improved and miniaturized sensors or sensor technologies [26,27]. In particular, the miniaturization and increased precision of sensors improves their integration into garments. In particular, smart shirts are increasingly used in medical diagnostics and therapy monitoring applications, where high accuracy is required [28–30]. To date, this has been mostly in the field of cardiovascular monitoring, e.g., heart rate monitoring or respiratory rate monitoring [19,31–36]. The Hexoskin Shirt (Montreal, QC, Canada) [37] is a newly launched smart shirt for monitoring vital signs and attempts to determine respiratory minute volumes in addition to common vital signs. However, various studies [38–40] have shown that the accuracy of measuring respiratory volumes are still outside the clinically relevant range.

In the development of new smart shirts, it is crucial to determine the optimal number, location and type of sensors to employ in the garment. Data from a MoCap system that tracks respiratory-induced movements at multiple points on the upper body were analyzed with different methods to select the optimal sensor sets for respiratory volume estimation. The MoCap system allows for the determination of various movement parameters of the upper body, such as accelerations, displacements and tilt angles at various surface points. Furthermore, upper body circumferences and local distance changes between the points can be determined [3]. These movement parameters can be measured via corresponding sensors.

In this work, two different regression methods were applied to map different subsets of displacement parameters, generated from the motion capture system data, to tidal volume. A preliminary analysis with five subjects indicated already the capabilities of the regression methods and provided accurate estimates of tidal volume [41]. The regression methods were exemplarily evaluated in this study on the displacement parameters; however, they are fully applicable to the other respiration induced motion parameters of the upper body. Such an analysis is essential to provide confidence in the subset selection for clinical use. Any approach that selects a small number of optimal sensors from a large set of sensors can be supported by the Lasso or Ridge regression, which results in a significant reduction of time and computing power at the cost of some loss in accuracy compared to an exhaustive search.

2. Materials and Methods

2.1. Measurement Setup

The study was based on the data recorded in Laufer et al. [3], where a motion capture system (MoCap) (Bonita, VICON, Denver, CO, USA) with nine infrared cameras (VICON

Bonita B10, firmware version 404) was used to measure the respiratory-induced movements of the human upper body via 102 highly reflective motion capture markers, attached at precise locations on a compression shirt. A schematic of the measurement system is shown in Figure 1. The markers were arranged in 8 different levels, where 48 were located ventrally, 18 laterally and 36 dorsally on the shirt (Figure 2). The highest MoCap marker (collar of the shirt) was located close to the C6 cervical vertebra and serves as a reference point (level 1). Since the cervical spine is barely exposed to respiratory movements, the reference marker can be used together with two other markers along the spine for a movement correction; non-respiratory movements can be eliminated via these 3 reference markers.

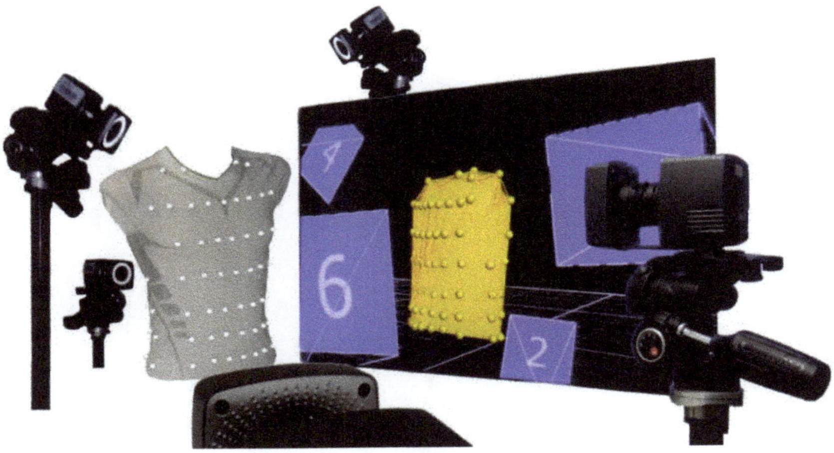

Figure 1. Schematic of the MoCap system. Five of the nine infrared cameras, the compression shirt with MoCap markers and the representation of the MoCap markers by the Vicon Systems on a screen. Figure published in [3].

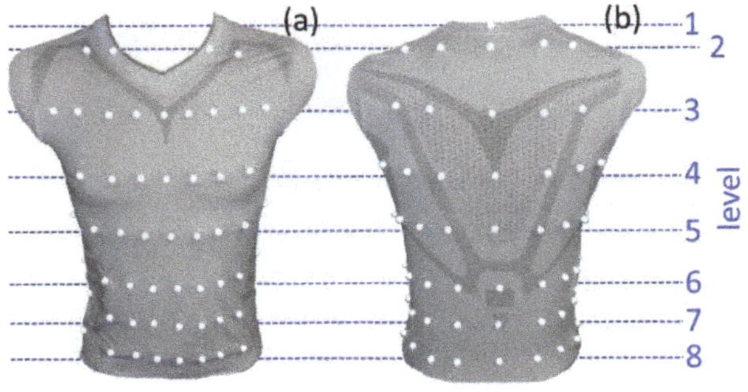

Figure 2. Compression shirt with 102 reflective MoCap markers–ventral view (**a**) and dorsal view (**b**). The markers are arranged in 8 distinct levels. Reference point in dorsal view ((**b**)—level 1) is the highest MoCap marker at the neck of the shirt.

As shown in Figure 2, level 2 was approximately located at the level of the thoracic vertebra T1 and at the level of the clavicula, respectively. Level 3 was at the height of T4, while level 4 was at the height of T7, caudally underneath the scapula. Level 5 was at the level of the thoracic vertebra T11, and level 6 was at the height of the lumbar vertebra L1, just at the caudal end of the arcus costalis. Level 7 was at the level of L3, and level 8 was at the height of L5. However, these levels are only approximations and were found to vary depending on the shape of the participants.

Subjects wearing the compression shirt and surrounded by the MoCap cameras performed different breathing patterns while breathing simultaneously through a spirometer

(SpiroScout and LFX Software 1.8, Ganshorn Medizin Electronic GmbH, Niederlauer, Germany). The spirometer served as a reference for tidal volume measurement. Flow and volume data were measured with the spirometer at a sampling frequency of 200 Hz. To reduce the dataset slightly, the sampling frequency was set to 40 Hz for the MoCap system. The MoCap system provided the spatial positions of all markers at each time point of the measurement, which were transferred via VICON Nexus software (version 1.8.5.6 1009h, Vicon Motion Systems Ltd., Denver, CO, USA) to MATLAB (R2022a, The MathWorks, Natick, MA, USA) for subsequent calculations.

During measurements, subjects sat as shown in Figure 3. To reduce non-respiratory movements of the upper body, the spirometer was attached to a rigid holder at the level of the subject's mouth. In this way, movements of the head and upper body were minimal, and the movement data obtained were almost entirely respiratory movements. Additionally, the subjects could rest their arms on that holder. This posture improved the optical detection of lateral markers in MoCap system and was more comfortable as reported by the subjects. To enhance marker detection, the subjects were asked to tie up long hair during the measurement.

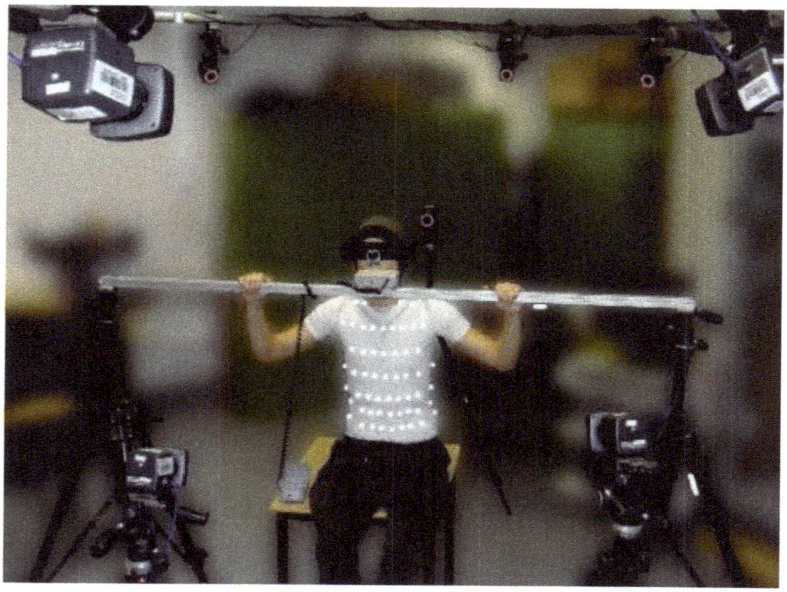

Figure 3. Measurement setup: A subject wearing the compression shirt with MoCap markers, breathing through the spirometer, which was fixed on the rigid mount and surrounded by the MoCap cameras. Figure published in [3].

2.2. Participants and Respiratory Manoeuvres

Ethical approval for this study was obtained from the University of Canterbury Ethics Committee HEC 2019/01/LR-PS and the Furtwangen University Ethics Committee. It was ensured that all measurements were performed in accordance with the principles of the Helsinki Declaration and that subjects were fully informed about the study prior to measurement. In addition, the subjects were informed about any risks, even if the risks associated with these measurements were minor and very unlikely. Signed informed consent was collected from each subject prior to experimentation. The subjects could stop the measurement at any time if they felt the slightest discomfort.

Participants were recruited via an email to the students of the Furtwangen University. Inclusion criteria included lung healthy students. Exclusion criteria included known lung disease, pregnant women and subjects aged under 18.

Three women and thirteen men participated in the measurements. The average height of the subjects was 1.76 ± 0.02 m, the average age was 25.7 ± 2.2 years and the average weight was 69.4 ± 2.0 kg. Further details are listed in Table 1.

Table 1. Details of the Participants. Table published in [3].

Subject	Height/[m]	Weight/[kg]	BMI/[kg/m^2]	Age/[years]	Gender
1	1.84	75	22.15	18	male
2	1.72	65	21.97	19	female
3	1.70	56	19.38	26	male
4	1.67	57	20.44	18	female
5	1.83	78	23.29	30	male
6	1.75	70	22.86	32	male
7	1.79	75	23.41	53	male
8	1.74	63	20.81	20	male
9	1.70	68	23.53	24	male
10	1.82	73	22.04	30	male
11	1.74	81	26.75	31	male
12	1.73	67	22.39	19	male
13	1.71	60	20.52	23	male
14	1.68	66	23.38	21	female
15	1.88	75	21.22	20	male
16	1.83	82	24.49	28	male

The subjects took different tidal volumes in order to capture as much of the respiratory spectrum as possible. For this purpose, the subjects reduced their breathing activity to a minimum and breathed shallow breaths. Afterwards, the subjects increased the tidal volume beyond the volume of normal spontaneous breathing (but not to the maximum), thus taking medium breaths, and finally, they breathed in and out as far as possible (maximal breaths). As shown in Table 2 and Figure 4, each of these breathing patterns was performed for approximately one minute.

Table 2. Performed respiratory patterns. Table published in [3].

Pattern Number	Duration [s]	Breathing Pattern
1	30	spontaneous breathing (normal)
2	60	shallow breathing
3	30	spontaneous breathing (normal)
4	60	medium breaths
5	30	spontaneous breathing (normal)
6	60	maximal breaths
7	30	spontaneous breathing (normal)

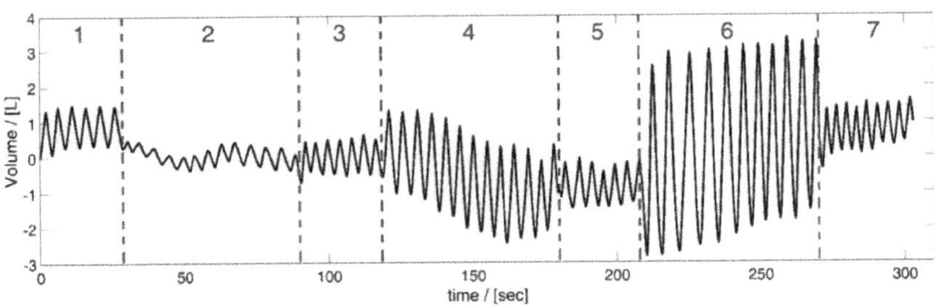

Figure 4. Respiratory patterns shown based on spirometer volume data from subject 5. Breathing of different tidal volumes—shallow (2), medium (4) and maximal breaths (6) between short ranges of normal spontaneous breathing ((1), (3), (5) and (7)). Figure published in [3].

Before and after each breathing pattern, subjects performed 30 s of normal spontaneous breathing to relax and to avoid risk of hyper/hypoventilation. The total measurement time was approximately 5 min, but the exact timing depended on the subject's breathing rhythm.

2.3. Data Processing

Motions of the MoCap markers were dimensionally reduced to their major axis using the methods of Laufer et al. [42], as they move predominantly on a specific line (Figure 5). By projecting the marker movements onto their major axis of movement, the dimension of the MoCap data was reduced by a factor of three.

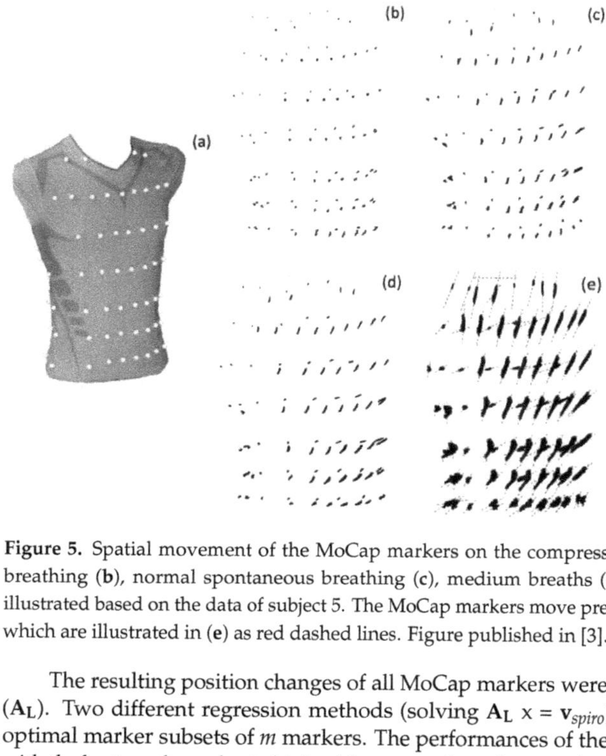

Figure 5. Spatial movement of the MoCap markers on the compression shirt (**a**) during shallow breathing (**b**), normal spontaneous breathing (**c**), medium breaths (**d**) and maximal breaths (**e**), illustrated based on the data of subject 5. The MoCap markers move predominantly on a specific line, which are illustrated in (**e**) as red dashed lines. Figure published in [3].

The resulting position changes of all MoCap markers were presented in matrix form ($\mathbf{A_L}$). Two different regression methods (solving $\mathbf{A_L}\ x = \mathbf{v}_{spiro}$) allowed for selection of optimal marker subsets of m markers. The performances of these subsets was compared with the best marker subset obtained from an exhaustive search of all possible combinations of m markers.

The analysis of all possible combinations is a computationally demanding and time-consuming process. However, unlike other methods that can only imply the optimal set based on probabilistic principles, the analysis of all possible combinations provides the best possible and thus optimal set of markers for the determination of the tidal volume. The number (N) of all combinations with k markers out of a set of n markers is given by:

$$N = \binom{n}{k} = \binom{102}{4} \approx 5 \times 10^6,$$
$$N = \binom{n}{k} = \binom{102}{5} \approx 8 \times 10^7 \qquad (1)$$
$$\text{or}$$
$$N = \binom{n}{k} = \binom{102}{6} \approx 1.4 \times 10^9$$

Apart from the analysis of all combinations, regression techniques allowed for faster selection of optimal markers/sensor locations. The first regression technique used was Ridge regression [43], which used a Tikhonov regularization term. Ridge regression finds the argument that minimizes both model error and parameter-squared magnitude (Equation (2)):

$$\mathbf{x}_{opt,R} = [x_1, \ldots x_m]^T_{opt,R} = \underset{\mathbf{x}}{\text{argmin}}\left(\|\mathbf{A_L x} - \mathbf{v}_{spiro}\|_2 + \alpha\|\mathbf{x}\|_2 \right) \quad (2)$$

where m is the number of chosen parameters and α is the regularization factor of the Tikhonov regularization term $\alpha\|x\|_2$.

For each parameter/MoCap marker of $\mathbf{A_L}$, an argument of $\mathbf{x}$ was determined. The value of the respective $\mathbf{x}$ corresponds to the significance of the parameter/the information content of the parameter with respect to the overall system. To reduce the marker set from n = 102 to m markers, the markers that were assigned the m highest absolute values of $\mathbf{x}$ were selected, because they carried the highest respiratory information of $\mathbf{v}_{spiro}$.

The second regression method used was the least absolute shrinkage and selection operator (Lasso) [44], which provided a sparse solution for $\mathbf{x}$, and solved:

$$\mathbf{x}_{opt,L} = [x_1, \ldots x_m]^T_{opt,L} = \underset{\mathbf{x}}{\text{argmin}}\left(\|\mathbf{A_L x} - \mathbf{v}_{spiro}\|_2 + \lambda\|\mathbf{x}\|_1 \right) \quad (3)$$

where m is the number of chosen parameters, and λ is the regularization factor of the penalty term of the regularization $\lambda\|\mathbf{x}\|_1$.

By a suitable selection of λ, the number of resulting MoCap markers was reduced to m. For comparison, the value of the (Lasso) regularization factor λ was also assigned to the regularization factor α (Ridge).

To increase the significance of this comparison, a bootstrapping resampling procedure was used. Using 16 data sets might be sufficient, but the additional bootstrapping resampling procedure provides more robust evaluation and reduces the relevance of outliers in the data. Hence, for m = 4 and m = 5, 250 random data segments (of random length) were selected from each of the 16 datasets, on which the analysis was performed separately. To obtain the corresponding data segments, two integer values from a discrete uniform distribution (*randi* function of MATLAB) were used as boundaries of the data segment. For m = 6, the number of bootstrapping steps/resampling was reduced to 50 due to time constraints. The analysis was done on a personal computer with a 12th Gen Intel (R) Core (TM) i7-12700K processor with 3.61 GHz (Intel Corporation, Santa Clara, CA, USA) and 64.0 GB RAM (Corsair Gaming Inc., Fremont, CA, USA).

Three MoCap markers along the spine (including the reference marker in the neck) were added to the marker set of m markers, chosen by the different approaches. These three MoCap markers/sensors can be used to compensate for non-respiration related movements, such as bending or twisting the upper body.

The final set of m + 3 MoCap markers provided by each method allowed for the calculation of the inspiratory volume:

$$\mathbf{v}_{m+3} = \mathbf{A_L} \cdot \mathbf{x}_{\text{opt}} \quad (4)$$

In each bootstrapping step, the target number of markers was selected for each of the three different approaches, which yielded a minimal volume error of $\mathbf{v}_{m+3}$ with respect to $\mathbf{v}_{spiro}$. The number of selected markers was according to the size of the targeted subsets of m = 4, m = 5 or m = 6 markers. Each time a MoCap marker was selected (amongst all subjects) the marker was noted. The number of times each marker occurs in all 16 subjects in the selected sensor is analyzed. Finally, the m markers with the highest notation amongst all bootstrapping steps and subjects were selected as most valuable MoCap markers.

3. Results

For all subjects, each of the 250 (respectively, 50 in a case of subsets of 6 sensors) random segments of measured data during bootstrapping was used to calculate the disparity between the volume estimations from the optimal models from the 3 methods and the gold standard $\mathbf{v}_{spiro}$ measurement. The resulting errors are illustrated in the box plot shown in Figure 6. The mean values of λ respectively α are given in Table 3. Based on a random data segment of 60 s, a computation time comparison of the three methods was performed, showing the time savings of the Lasso and Ridge regression regarding the calculation of all possible combinations. This time comparison is listed in Table 4. The sensor positions determined by the different optimization methods for m = 4, 5 and 6 are shown in Figures 7–9, respectively. In each figure, the added three datum markers along the spine are represented as red points while the m optimal locations are indicated in green dashed ellipses.

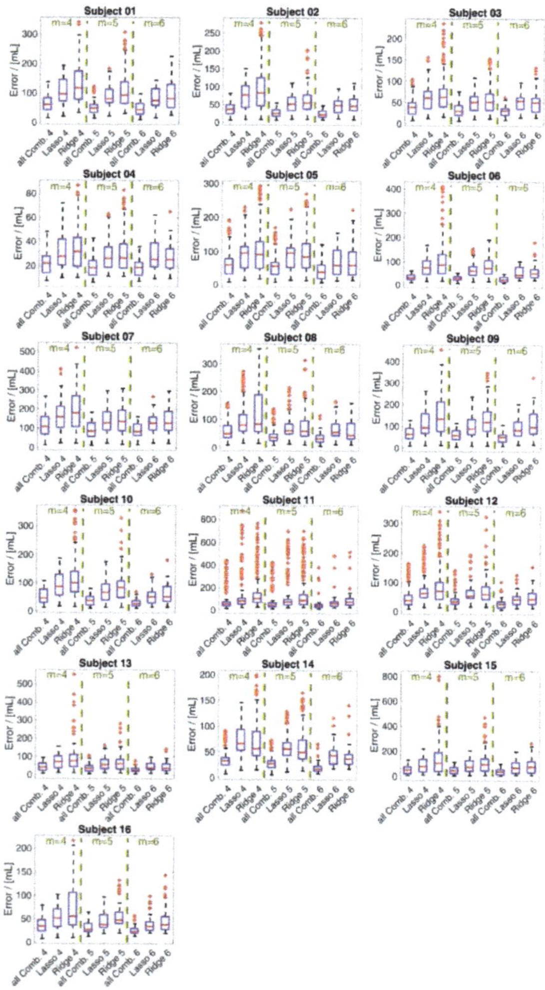

Figure 6. Box plot of the volume errors of $\mathbf{v}_{m+3}$ for the different approaches related to the spirometer volume $\mathbf{v}_{spiro}$ during bootstrapping. The errors are shown for subsets of 4, 5 and 6 markers for all 16 subjects. The box and whisker plot illustrate the minimum value, 25th percentile, median, 75th percentile and the maximum value, and the red + signs denote outliers.

Table 3. Mean values of the regularization factors λ (Lasso). The regularization factor α (Ridge) was set to the value of λ.

m	Mean (λ)
4	0.096
5	0.059
6	0.036

Table 4. Average calculation time required by Ridge regression and Lasso compared to the average time needed to analyse all combinations based on random data segments of 60 s.

	Average Required Time [s]		
m	**Ridge Regression**	**Lasso**	**All Combinations**
4	0.037	0.066	81
5	0.046	0.073	1573
6	0.047	0.112	46,886

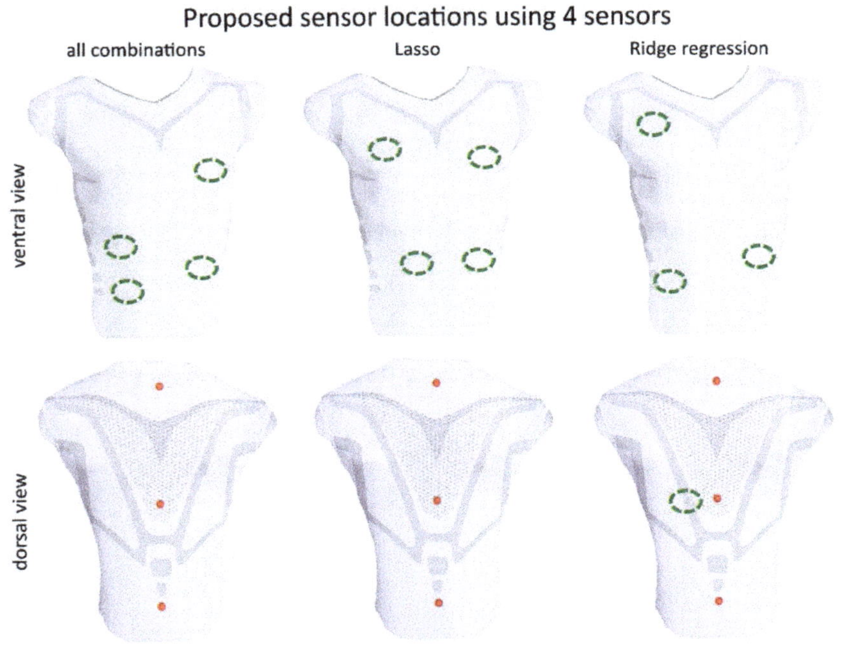

Figure 7. Visualization of the best sensor subset of 4 sensors (green dashed ellipses) by the analysis of all combinations (global optimal subset), Lasso and the Ridge regression–ventral view (**top**) and dorsal view (**bottom**). Red points represent the three datum markers.

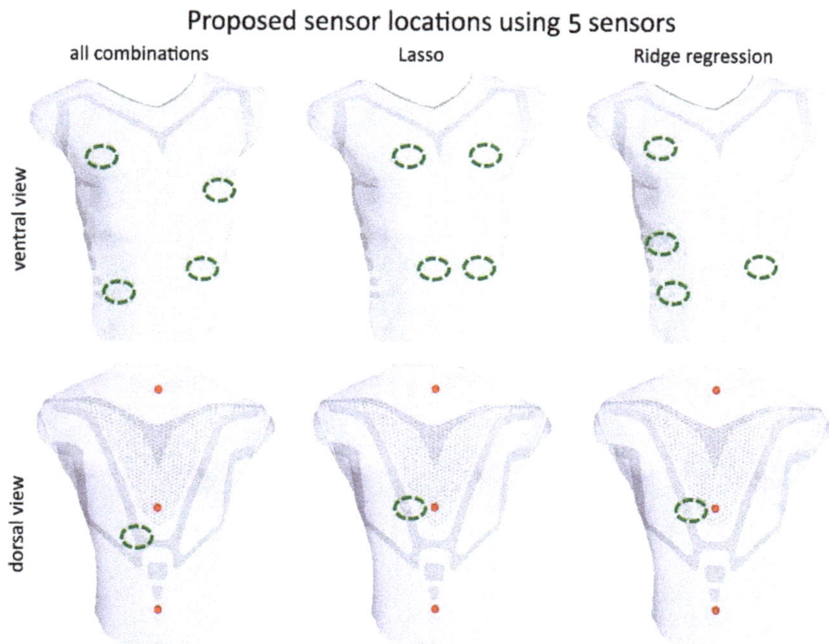

Figure 8. Visualization of the best sensor subset of 5 sensors (green dashed ellipses) by the analysis of all combinations (global optimal subset), Lasso and the Ridge regression–ventral view (**top**) and dorsal view (**bottom**). Red points represent the three datum markers.

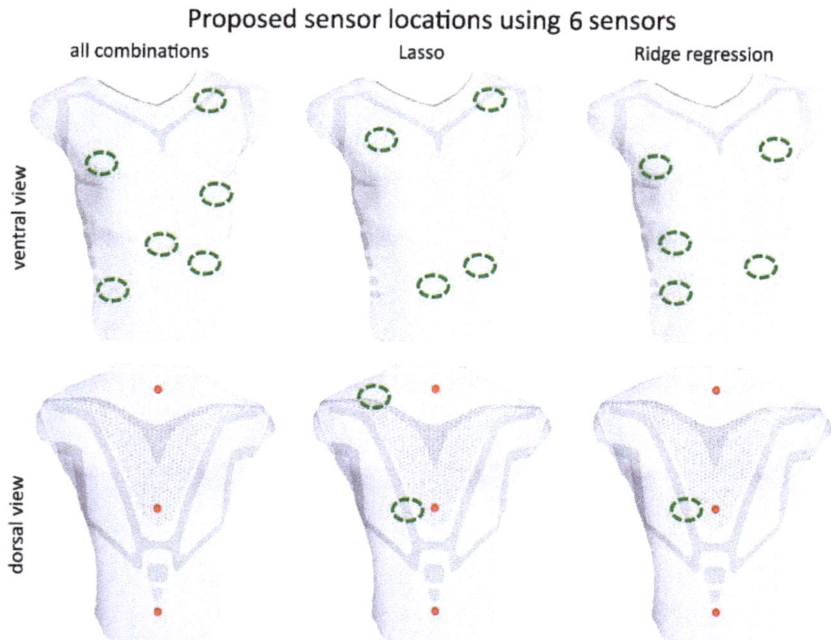

Figure 9. Visualization of the best sensor subset of 6 sensors (green dashed ellipses) by the analysis of all combinations (global optimal subset), Lasso and the Ridge regression–ventral view (**top**) and dorsal view (**bottom**). Red points represent the three datum markers.

4. Discussion

The use of optoelectronic plethysmography in clinical practice indicates that there is a need for alternatives to respiratory flow measurement via spirometers or body plethysmographs. A smart shirt to measure respiratory volume could be that alternative, would provide convenient measurement and could be used in many clinical scenarios—from sleep apnea monitoring to home care, from respiratory monitoring of comatose patients to exercise monitoring of competitive athletes.

In this study, we investigated the ability of different regression methods to determine the optimal, minimal sensor set that yields accurate inspiratory volume estimation. An optimal method could provide far-reaching support for sensor positioning in smart shirt development [42]. The performed breathing maneuvers (Table 2 and Figure 4) covered a broad range of clinically-relevant tidal volumes. Figure 6 shows the error in estimated tidal volumes of every method. The exhaustive search evaluated all possible combinations and suggested, consequently, the sensor subset that gave the lowest error. Thus, the considerable computational cost was able to yield the global optimal subset (assuming the original marker placement). The errors that occur even for the global optimal subset show that the tidal volumes of the spirometer $\mathbf{v}_{spiro}$ cannot be reproduced exactly with the chosen number of sensors and limited surface motion information.

In a previous study [45], deviations of tidal volumes measured by an optoelectronic plethysmography device from $\mathbf{v}_{spiro}$ were observed mainly for larger breaths. These deviations might be caused by pressure-induced compressions of the air in the thorax, whereas these compressions do not influence the flow measurement via the spirometer. These deviations are exemplarily shown based on the data of subject 15 in Figure 10. Apart from the maximum deviations, this seems to be mainly an underestimation of volumes, which could be caused by filtering effects (transfer function).

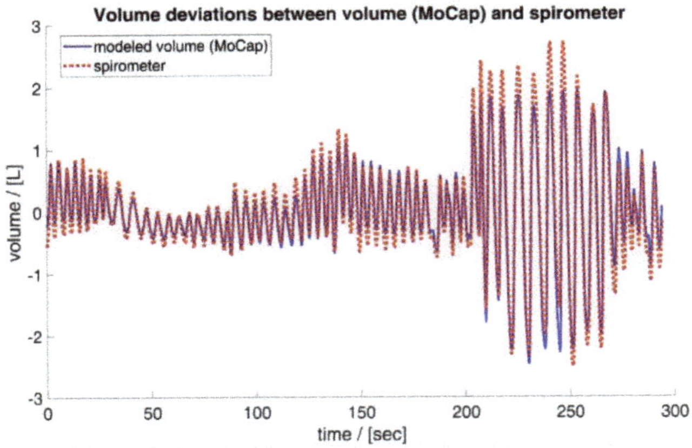

Figure 10. Deviations between the volume obtained by the MoCap system (blue) and the spirometer (red). Maximal deviations occur at maximal breaths—exemplarily illustrated based on the data of subject 15.

Expectedly, involving higher number of sensors enhances measurement of tidal volume and reduces the error (Figure 6), since any added information would improve a regressive estimation. Due to the bootstrapping process used to artificially expand the data set, the actual performance may differ slightly from the actual performance. In this respect, shorter data segments can lead to smaller errors because they typically have fewer divergent trends and features in respiratory curves and can be better fitted to $\mathbf{v}_{spiro}$. Figure 11 shows exemplarily two data segments of random length that were used for analysis during bootstrapping. It can be seen that shorter data segments have fewer divergent trends and features. In addition, it can be seen that the volumes determined via the movements of four

MoCap markers/sensors are highly correlated with $\mathbf{v}_{spiro}$, independent of the method used for selection of the MoCap markers/sensors.

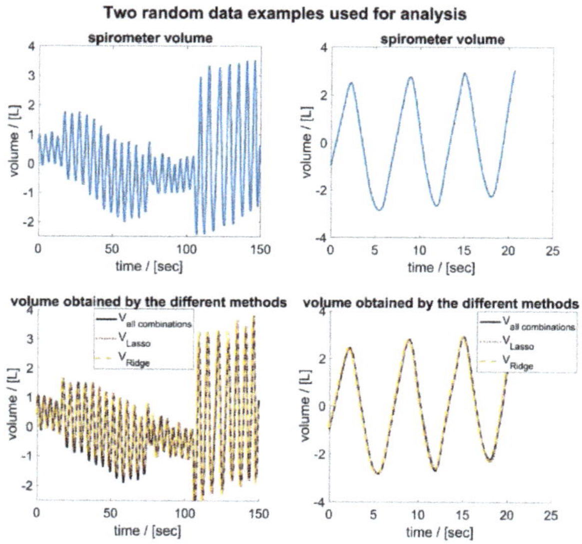

Figure 11. Two randomly selected areas of the data used for analysis during bootstrapping, illustrated based on the data of subject 5 and for $m = 4$. The upper part shows the volume curve of the spirometer, while the lower part shows the corresponding volume obtained by the three different methods.

Overall, the mean errors (Figure 6) of the two regression methods are of similar magnitude. The Lasso's mean errors in the case of $m = 4$ were slightly lower for 14 of the 16 subjects and in case of $m = 5$ for 13/16 subjects compared to the mean errors of the Ridge regression. For $m = 6$, the Lasso's mean errors were lower in 7/16 subjects and nearly equal in 5/16 subjects.

While in the Lasso, the value of λ was determined by the number of desired markers/sensors, the mean error of the Ridge regression can be influenced by the choice of α. A small α leads to smaller errors of the regression term $\|\mathbf{A}_L\mathbf{x} - \mathbf{v}_{spiro}\|_2$ while a larger α leads to faster convergence of the calculation. Thus, the choice of α affects the mean error of the calculation. Since α was assigned the value of λ in this study, a comparison is possible, but it is only indicative and should not be the decisive criterion for the choice between the Ridge and Lasso, as a change in the regularization factors may influence the determined errors.

Interestingly, the Lasso's mean errors as well as the Ridge's mean errors were consistently higher than the mean errors of the global optimal set in all cases. Compared to the Lasso and the global optimal subset, the Ridge regression has higher peak errors and higher deviations for nearly all subjects. Figure 6 indicates that the Ridge regression is much more susceptible to yielding outlier high errors than the Lasso regression. The results of this study are in agreement with the outcomes of Ng et al. [46] since in our case the Lasso method (L_1 norm) also showed clear advantages in terms of errors, robustness and outliers compared to the Ridge regression (L_2 norm). The Lasso approach is known to produce a sparse solution, prevent overfitting and remain robust to outliers. All these features of the Lasso method are advantageous when selecting sensors from a sensor set. In particular, the sparse solution supports the selection of the smallest possible subset, which reduces complexity, error-proneness and cost. In particular, the Lasso shows tremendous advantages in the investigation of respiration-induced upper body movements. Upper body movements during respiration show a high correlation with the respiratory volume itself.

The deeper a subject inhales the more the upper body expands. The high correlations of the movement parameters with the respiratory volume also imply high correlations of the respiratory parameters with each other. When the Lasso method is applied to data that are highly correlated with each other especially, it works well and provides a sparse solution.

The Ridge regression does not necessarily provide sparse solutions; on the contrary the regression is reducing the difference in the measurement positions and thus complicates the selection. However, the savings in both time (Table 4) and computational costs compared to the exhaustive search is considerable. The computational demand is reduced from an exponential effort for a full exhaustive search down to the order of $O(n^2)$ for the regression methods. Thus, in general, the comparatively light computational burden of the Ridge regression implies it has its legitimate benefit in some situations.

For a smart shirt as a medical product, an exhaustive search, although computationally intensive, provided significantly lower volume errors while the regressive models provided more consistent sensor sets. In practice, the maker location from such an analysis would be fixed and constant across patients. The regressive models could then be used to produce precise estimations of inspiratory volume. However, if more precise respiratory measurements were possible, the regression could be adapted to develop an individualized model for precise and accurate estimations of the inspiratory volume.

While there is general agreement in the optimal positions of MoCap markers/sensors in a smart shirt across regression methods, the regression methods did not yield exactly the same positions. It appears that the Ridge regression agrees with the positions of the best combination slightly more consistently than the Lasso. The positions obtained from the Ridge regression and exhaustive search are more lateral in the ventral region than the positions obtained by the Lasso. This is also evident for $m = 5$ (Figure 8) and $m = 6$ (Figure 9), where the Lasso method selects an area for a sensor in the central abdominal region.

When increasing the number of sensors from $m = 4$ (Figure 7) to $m = 5$ (Figure 8) then $m = 6$ (Figure 9), the previous positioning remains to a large extent consistent, usually only one marker/sensor is added, and the previous selection $(m-1)$ is preserved. In particular, the Ridge regression consistently reproduces previously selected positions. The Lasso method shows small shifts of the previously selected areas. The analysis of all combinations shows in this respect the biggest differences. The areas selected for smaller m are only partially preserved for larger m. Some sensors are no longer selected at all. For example, the dorsal region at $m = 5$ (Figure 8) is no longer selected when m is increased. This marker/sensor might be irrelevant due to the three fixed included sensors/datum markers along the spine.

Since the sensor positions did not differ significantly amongst the evaluated methods, both regression methods can support the development of smart shirts for respiratory volume estimation. For larger sensor subsets, the complex and exhaustive search is no longer possible and methods, such as the Ridge/Lasso, must be used.

There were some limitations in this study. One limitation was that the size of the shirt led to some error. This was clearly observed between tall and short participants (Figure 12). In particular, the positions of the markers were in slightly different positions on the upper body due to the uniform compression shirt and were not exactly in the same place. However, this error would also occur in a smart shirt, as the shirt is not individually tailored to the particular subject. Different shirt sizes can limit this error within certain limits; however, a tight fit of the shirt is essential in this context. Despite this fact, the results remained within acceptable bounds for these subjects.

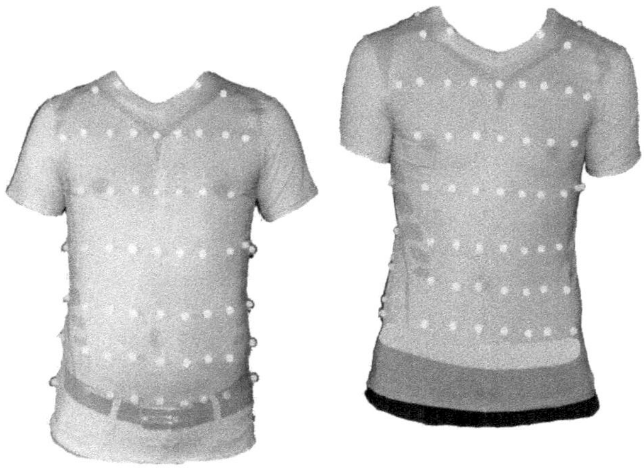

Figure 12. Illustration of variations in anatomical marker positions for subjects of different body shapes (visualized via subject 3 (**left**) and subject 1 (**right**)).

Another limitation was that the shirt could slip on the skin surface during respiration [47]. This error was only observed with very large breaths. Therefore, it represents a systematic error, which cannot be avoided without disturbing the subject. It would be possible to reduce the shirt-to-skin movement with a very tight fit of the smart shirt and/or an adhesive or clinging inner material in the shirt. However, such an approach may not improve results sufficiently to justify the irritation the subject may feel as a result of the adhesive. Multiple tissue interfaces exist between the alveoli and the skin surface, and these shift against each other during respiration. Adding another layer to the skin–shirt interface seems unlikely to be a confounding factor.

Further measurements with more subjects of different ages and body shapes should confirm the results of this study and provide better insights into the systematic nature of sensor selection. With more subjects, a subgroup analysis would also be possible (for example, to examine the effects of different breathing patterns, such as abdominal or chest breathing). Most participants in our study were male (13/16) and young adults (13/16 $\leq$ 30 years) in the healthy BMI range (15/16). This leads to bias that must be corrected prior to clinical application. A study with subjects with a lung disease, such as chronic obstructive pulmonary disease or cystic fibrosis, could provide further insight into optimal sensor selection. Additionally, extremely lung-sick patients who have only a small portion of their lung capacity available might be outside the range of tidal volumes covered by our subjects. In the case of subjects with lung disease, other aspects could play a decisive role that is not apparent in the case of lung-healthy subjects. In particular, the current study used subjects who did not have significant asymmetry in their pulmonary filling. In contrast, individuals with cystic fibrosis or other lung diseases may have significant asymmetries with respect to the left and right sides of the thorax and abdomen.

5. Conclusions

This study shows that the selection of sensors with linear regression depends on the regression method itself. The Lasso method is preferable to the Ridge regression because it provides both more robust and sparser solutions. However, both regression methods have their justification in this field of application, as they significantly reduce computation time and effort but with the disadvantage that their performance suffers compared to the performance of the optimal subset.

Both regression methods can support smart shirt development for respiratory volume estimation by guiding the type and optimal location of the required sensors. A smart shirt for respiratory volume estimation could replace spirometry and would allow for a more comfortable and long-term measurement of respiratory parameters in homecare or clinic.

Author Contributions: Conceptualization, B.L., P.D.D., F.H. and K.M.; methodology, B.L., P.D.D. and S.K.-Z.; software, B.L.; validation, B.L.; formal analysis, B.L.; investigation, B.L., N.A.J. and S.K.-Z.; resources, B.L.; data curation, B.L., and S.K.-Z.; writing—original draft preparation, B.L.; writing—review and editing, P.D.D., N.A.J., F.H., R.M., S.K.-Z., S.J.R., L.R. and K.M.; visualization, B.L.; supervision, P.D.D., R.M., S.J.R., L.R. and K.M.; project administration, K.M.; funding acquisition, K.M. All authors have read and agreed to the published version of the manuscript.

Funding: This research was partially supported by the German Federal Ministry for Economic Affairs and Climate Action (BMWi) (ZIM-Grant KK5151903BM1), the German Federal Ministry of Education and Research (MOVE, Grant 13FH628IX6) and by the European Commission H2020 MSCA Rise (#872488—DCPM).

Institutional Review Board Statement: The study was conducted in accordance with the Declaration of Helsinki and approved by the Human Ethics Committee of the University of Canterbury (HEC 2019/01/LR-PS) and of the Ethikkommission of the Furtwangen University.

Informed Consent Statement: A written informed consent was collected from each subject involved in the study.

Data Availability Statement: The data presented in this study are available on request from the corresponding author.

Acknowledgments: We would like to sincerely thank all the subjects who were willing to participate in our study despite the difficulties in the times of COVID-19.

Conflicts of Interest: The authors declare no conflict of interest.

Abbreviations

The following abbreviations are used in this manuscript:

Cx	Cervical vertebrae x ($1 \leq x \leq 7$)
Lasso	Least absolute shrinkage and selection operator
Lx	Lumbar vertebrae x ($1 \leq x \leq 5$)
MoCap	Motion capture system
Tx	Thoracic vertebrae x ($1 \leq x \leq 12$)
$\mathbf{v}_{m+3}$	Volume obtained via the selected MoCap marker subset of m MoCap markers and the additional 3 MoCap marker along the spine
$\mathbf{v}_{spiro}$	Volume obtained with spirometer

References

1. Sibson, F. On the Movements of Respiration in Disease, and on the Use of a Chest-Measurer. *Med. Chir. Trans.* **1848**, *31*, 353–498.3. [CrossRef]
2. Wade, O.L. Movements of the Thoracic Cage and Diaphragm in Respiration. *J. Physiol.* **1954**, *124*, 193–212. [CrossRef]
3. Laufer, B.; Hoeflinger, F.; Docherty, P.D.; Jalal, N.A.; Krueger-Ziolek, S.; Rupitsch, S.J.; Reindl, L.; Moeller, K. Characterisation and Quantification of Upper Body Surface Motions for Tidal Volume Determination in Lung-Healthy Individuals. *Sensors* **2023**, *23*, 1278. [CrossRef]
4. Konno, K.; Mead, J. Measurement of the Separate Volume Changes of Rib Cage and Abdomen during Breathing. *J. Appl. Physiol.* **1967**, *22*, 407–422. [CrossRef]
5. Parreira, V.F.; Vieira, D.S.; Myrrha, M.A.; Pessoa, I.M.; Lage, S.M.; Britto, R.R. Optoelectronic Plethysmography: A Review of the Literature. *Rev. Bras. Fisioter.* **2012**, *16*, 439–453. [CrossRef]
6. Massaroni, C.; Carraro, E.; Vianello, A.; Miccinilli, S.; Morrone, M.; Levai, I.K.; Schena, E.; Saccomandi, P.; Sterzi, S.; Dickinson, J.W.; et al. Optoelectronic Plethysmography in Clinical Practice and Research: A Review. *Respiration* **2017**, *93*, 339–354.
7. Heyde, C.; Mahler, H.; Roecker, K.; Gollhofer, A. A Wearable Respiratory Monitoring Device–the between-Days Variability of Calibration. *Int. J. Sports Med.* **2015**, *36*, 29–34. [CrossRef]
8. Kogan, D.; Jain, A.; Kimbro, S.; Gutierrez, G.; Jain, V. Respiratory Inductance Plethysmography Improved Diagnostic Sensitivity and Specificity of Obstructive Sleep Apnea. *Respir. Care* **2016**, *61*, 1033–1037. [CrossRef]

9. Heyde, C.; Leutheuser, H.; Eskofier, B.; Roecker, K.; Gollhofer, A. Respiratory Inductance Plethysmography-a Rationale for Validity during Exercise. *Med. Sci. Sports Exerc.* **2014**, *46*, 488–495.
10. Miller, M.R.; Hankinson, J.; Brusasco, V.; Burgos, F.; Casaburi, R.; Coates, A.; Crapo, R.; Enright, P.; van der Grinten, C.P.M.; Gustafsson, P.; et al. Standardisation of Spirometry. *Eur. Respir. J.* **2005**, *26*, 319–338. [CrossRef]
11. Hayes, D.J.; Kraman, S.S. The Physiologic Basis of Spirometry. *Respir. Care* **2009**, *54*, 1717–1726. [PubMed]
12. Criée, C.-P.; Baur, X.; Berdel, D.; Bösch, D.; Gappa, M.; Haidl, P.; Husemann, K.; Jörres, R.A.; Kabitz, H.-J.; Kardos, P.; et al. Leitlinie Zur Spirometrie. *Pneumologie* **2015**, *69*, 147–164. [CrossRef] [PubMed]
13. Coates, A.L.; Peslin, R.; Rodenstein, D.; Stocks, J. Measurement of Lung Volumes by Plethysmography. *Eur. Respir. J.* **1997**, *10*, 1415–1427. [CrossRef] [PubMed]
14. Criée, C.P.; Sorichter, S.; Smith, H.J.; Kardos, P.; Merget, R.; Heise, D.; Berdel, D.; Köhler, D.; Magnussen, H.; Marek, W.; et al. Body Plethysmography--Its Principles and Clinical Use. *Respir. Med.* **2011**, *105*, 959–971. [CrossRef]
15. Andersson, L.G.; Ringqvist, I.; Walker, A. Total Lung Capacity Measured by Body Plethysmography and by the Helium Dilution Method. A Comparative Study in Different Patient Groups. *Clin. Physiol.* **1988**, *8*, 113–119. [CrossRef]
16. Askanazi, J.; Silverberg, P.A.; Foster, R.J.; Hyman, A.I.; Milic-Emili, J.; Kinney, J.M. Effects of Respiratory Apparatus on Breathing Pattern. *J. Appl. Physiol. Respir. Env. Exerc. Physiol.* **1980**, *48*, 577–580. [CrossRef]
17. Gilbert, R.; Auchincloss, J.H.J.; Brodsky, J.; Boden, W. Changes in Tidal Volume, Frequency, and Ventilation Induced by Their Measurement. *J. Appl. Physiol.* **1972**, *33*, 252–254. [CrossRef]
18. Rahmani, M.H.; Berkvens, R.; Weyn, M. Chest-Worn Inertial Sensors: A Survey of Applications and Methods. *Sensors* **2021**, *21*, 2875. [CrossRef]
19. Karacocuk, G.; Höflinger, F.; Zhang, R.; Reindl, L.M.; Laufer, B.; Möller, K.; Röell, M.; Zdzieblik, D. Inertial Sensor-Based Respiration Analysis. *IEEE Trans. Instrum. Meas.* **2019**, *68*, 4268–4275. [CrossRef]
20. Monaco, V.; Giustinoni, C.; Ciapetti, T.; Maselli, A.; Stefanini, C. Assessing Respiratory Activity by Using IMUs: Modeling and Validation. *Sensor* **2022**, *22*, 2185. [CrossRef]
21. Chu, M.; Nguyen, T.; Pandey, V.; Zhou, Y.; Pham, H.N.; Bar-Yoseph, R.; Radom-Aizik, S.; Jain, R.; Cooper, D.M.; Khine, M. Respiration Rate and Volume Measurements Using Wearable Strain Sensors. *NPJ Digit. Med.* **2019**, *2*, 8. [CrossRef] [PubMed]
22. Rozevika, A.; Katashev, A.; Okss, A.; Mantyla, J.; Coffeng, R. *On the Monitoring of Breathing Volume, Using Textile Strain Gauges*; Lhotska, L., Sukupova, L., Lacković, I., Ibbott, G.S., Eds.; Springer: Singapore, 2019; pp. 921–925.
23. Laufer, B.; Krueger-Ziolek, S.; Docherty, P.D.; Hoeflinger, F.; Reindl, L.; Moeller, K. An Alternative Way to Measure Respiration Induced Changes of Circumferences: A Pilot Study. In Proceedings of the 2020 42nd Annual International Conference of the IEEE Engineering in Medicine & Biology Society (EMBC), Montreal, QC, Canada, 20–24 July 2020; pp. 4632–4635.
24. Laufer, B.; Krueger-Ziolek, S.; Docherty, P.D.; Hoeflinger, F.; Reindl, L.; Moeller, K. An Alternative Way to Measure Tidal Volumes. In *8th European Medical and Biological Engineering Conference*; Springer International Publishing: Cham, Switzerland, 2021; pp. 66–72.
25. Laufer, B.; Krueger-Ziolek, S.; Docherty, P.D.; Hoeflinger, F.; Reindl, L.; Möller, K. Tidal Volume via Circumferences of the Upper Body: A Pilot Study. In Proceedings of the 2019 41st Annual International Conference of the IEEE Engineering in Medicine and Biology Society (EMBC), Berlin, Germany, 23–27 July 2019; pp. 3559–3562.
26. Kaneko, H.; Horie, J. Breathing Movements of the Chest and Abdominal Wall in Healthy Subjects. *Respir. Care* **2012**, *57*, 1442. [CrossRef] [PubMed]
27. Khundaqji, H.; Hing, W.; Furness, J.; Climstein, M. Smart Shirts for Monitoring Physiological Parameters: Scoping Review. *JMIR mHealth uHealth* **2020**, *8*, e18092. [CrossRef] [PubMed]
28. Aliverti, A. Wearable Technology: Role in Respiratory Health and Disease. *Breathe* **2017**, *13*, e27–e36. [CrossRef]
29. Mannée, D.; de Jongh, F.; van Helvoort, H. The Accuracy of Tidal Volume Measured With a Smart Shirt During Tasks of Daily Living in Healthy Subjects: Cross-Sectional Study. *JMIR Form. Res.* **2021**, *5*, e30916. [CrossRef]
30. Liu, J.; Liu, M.; Bai, Y.; Zhang, J.; Liu, H.; Zhu, W. Recent Progress in Flexible Wearable Sensors for Vital Sign Monitoring. *Sensors* **2020**, *20*, 4009. [CrossRef]
31. Beck, S.; Laufer, B.; Krueger-Ziolek, S.; Moeller, K. Measurement of Respiratory Rate with Inertial Measurement Units. *Curr. Dir. Biomed. Eng.* **2020**, *6*, 237–240. [CrossRef]
32. Xu, D.; Yu, W.; Deng, C.; He, Z.S. Non-Contact Detection of Vital Signs Based on Improved Adaptive EEMD Algorithm (July 2022). *Sensors* **2022**, *22*, 6423. [CrossRef]
33. Jayarathna, T.; Gargiulo, G.D.; Lui, G.Y.; Breen, P.P. Electrodeless Heart and Respiratory Rate Estimation during Sleep Using a Single Fabric Band and Event-Based Edge Processing. *Sensors* **2022**, *22*, 6689. [CrossRef]
34. Vanegas, E.; Igual, R.; Plaza, I. Sensing Systems for Respiration Monitoring: A Technical Systematic Review. *Sensors* **2020**, *20*, 5446. [CrossRef]
35. Roudjane, M.; Bellemare-Rousseau, S.; Khalil, M.; Gorgutsa, S.; Miled, A.; Messaddeq, Y. A Portable Wireless Communication Platform Based on a Multi-Material Fiber Sensor for Real-Time Breath Detection. *Sensors* **2018**, *18*, 973. [CrossRef] [PubMed]
36. Cesareo, A.; Biffi, E.; Cuesta-Frau, D.; D'Angelo, M.G.; Aliverti, A. A Novel Acquisition Platform for Long-Term Breathing Frequency Monitoring Based on Inertial Measurement Units. *Med. Biol. Eng. Comput.* **2020**, *58*, 785–804. [CrossRef] [PubMed]
37. Hexoskin Hexoskin Smart Shirts-Cardiac, Respiratory, Sleep & Activity Metrics. Available online: https://www.hexoskin.com/ (accessed on 23 August 2022).

38. Feito, Y.; Moriarty, T.A.; Mangine, G.; Monahan, J. The Use of a Smart-Textile Garment during High-Intensity Functional Training: A Pilot Study. *J. Sports Med. Phys. Fit.* **2019**, *59*, 947–954. [CrossRef]
39. Elliot, C.A.; Hamlin, M.J.; Lizamore, C.A. Validity and Reliability of the Hexoskin Wearable Biometric Vest During Maximal Aerobic Power Testing in Elite Cyclists. *J. Strength Cond. Res.* **2019**, *33*, 1437–1444. [CrossRef] [PubMed]
40. Villar, R.; Beltrame, T.; Hughson, R.L. Validation of the Hexoskin Wearable Vest during Lying, Sitting, Standing, and Walking Activities. *Appl. Physiol. Nutr. Metab.* **2015**, *40*, 1019–1024. [CrossRef]
41. Laufer, B.; Jalal, N.A.; Docherty, P.D.; Krueger-Ziolek, S.; Hoeflinger, F.; Reindl, L.; Moeller, K. Sensor Selection for Tidal Volume Determination via Regression–Proof of Methodology. *Proc. Autom. Med. Eng.* **2023**, *2*, 734.
42. Laufer, B.; Murray, R.; Docherty, P.D.; Krueger-Ziolek, S.; Hoeflinger, F.; Reindl, L.; Moeller, K. A Minimal Set of Sensors in a Smart-Shirt to Obtain Respiratory Parameters. *IFAC-PapersOnLine* **2020**, *53*, 16293–16298. [CrossRef]
43. Hoerl, A.E.; Kennard, R.W. Ridge Regression: Biased Estimation for Nonorthogonal Problems. *Technometrics* **1970**, *12*, 55–67. [CrossRef]
44. Tibshirani, R. Regression Shrinkage and Selection Via the Lasso. *J. R. Stat. Soc. Ser. B (Methodol.)* **1996**, *58*, 267–288. [CrossRef]
45. Laufer, B.; Kretschmer, J.; Docherty, P.D.; Möller, K.; Höflinger, F.; Reindl, L. Sensor Placement in a Smart Compression Shirt to Measure Spontaneous Breathing. *Biomed. Tech.* **2017**, *62* (Suppl. S1), S127.
46. Ng, A.Y. Feature Selection, L1 vs. L2 Regularization, and Rotational Invariance. In Proceedings of the Twenty-First International Conference on Machine Learning, Banff, AB, Canada, 4–8 July 2004; Association for Computing Machinery: New York, NY, USA, 2004; p. 78.
47. Jayasinghe, U.; Hwang, F.; Harwin, W.S. Comparing Loose Clothing-Mounted Sensors with Body-Mounted Sensors in the Analysis of Walking. *Sensors* **2022**, *22*, 6605. [CrossRef] [PubMed]

sensors

MDPI

Article

Non-Invasive Blood Pressure Sensing via Machine Learning

Filippo Attivissimo, Vito Ivano D'Alessandro, Luisa De Palma, Anna Maria Lucia Lanzolla * and Attilio Di Nisio

Department of Electrical and Information Engineering, Polytechnic University of Bari, 70125 Bari, Italy; filippo.attivissimo@poliba.it (F.A.); v.dalessandro4@phd.poliba.it (V.I.D.); luisa.depalma@poliba.it (L.D.P.); attilio.dinisio@poliba.it (A.D.N.)

* Correspondence: anna.lanzolla@poliba.it

Abstract: In this paper, a machine learning (ML) approach to estimate blood pressure (BP) using photoplethysmography (PPG) is presented. The final aim of this paper was to develop ML methods for estimating blood pressure (BP) in a non-invasive way that is suitable in a telemedicine health-care monitoring context. The training of regression models useful for estimating systolic blood pressure (SBP) and diastolic blood pressure (DBP) was conducted using new extracted features from PPG signals processed using the Maximal Overlap Discrete Wavelet Transform (MODWT). As a matter of fact, the interest was on the use of the most significant features obtained by the Minimum Redundancy Maximum Relevance (MRMR) selection algorithm to train eXtreme Gradient Boost (XGBoost) and Neural Network (NN) models. This aim was satisfactorily achieved by also comparing it with works in the literature; in fact, it was found that XGBoost models are more accurate than NN models in both systolic and diastolic blood pressure measurements, obtaining a Root Mean Square Error (RMSE) for SBP and DBP, respectively, of 5.67 mmHg and 3.95 mmHg. For SBP measurement, this result is an improvement compared to that reported in the literature. Furthermore, the trained XGBoost regression model fulfills the requirements of the Association for the Advancement of Medical Instrumentation (AAMI) as well as grade A of the British Hypertension Society (BHS) standard.

Keywords: blood pressure (BP); digital health; machine learning (ML); physiological monitoring

1. Introduction

Hypertension is a health condition in which blood pressure (BP) at rest is higher than the physiological standards for a long time. It is one of the most common diseases; in fact, it affects about 20% of the adult population, representing one of the major clinical problems, and it is associated with chronic diseases and an increase in mortality and morbidity. BP is related to the force that blood exerts against the walls of blood vessels due to the pumping action carried out by the heart and its value depends on various factors. Moreover, BP is one of the so-called vital signs, also including respiratory rate, heart rate (HR), oxygen saturation (SpO_2), and body temperature, which require adequate monitoring on the general population.

For this reason, there is the spread of the development of practical and reliable telemedicine solutions [1–4] to guarantee monitoring at home and at hospital with the aim of ensuring early identification and prevention of cardiovascular diseases, hypertension, and other related diseases. As concerns BP measurement, traditional cuff-based devices have several disadvantages because they are not always accurate, they need appropriate calibration, and they do not allow continuous monitoring since performing a measurement requires about one minute or more. On the contrary, there is a strong tendency today to monitor health at home by using wearable, affordable, and small devices that are simple to use, non-invasive, and even wireless to obtain measurements continuously [5–7]. Hence, researchers are investigating ways to perform cuff-less and non-invasive BP measurements.

As a matter of fact, the monitoring of the health of individuals is also made possible by the spread of artificial intelligence in healthcare [8–10].

Nowadays, a measurement technique that is spreading for real-time monitoring of vital signs is photoplethysmography (PPG) [11–14]. Indeed, PPG is a simple, low-cost, and non-invasive optical measurement method that, in addition to the estimation of HR, SpO_2, and respiration rate, provides important health information regarding atherosclerosis and arterial stiffness. It is a type of plethysmography (PG) that exploits optical properties unlike other types of PG, such as those based on capacitive, inductive, and piezoelectric properties [15,16].

Recently, the use of PPG to also estimate BP values has become an active area of research. However, quite often, studies have focused on the simultaneous use of both electrocardiogram (ECG) and PPG signals or on the use of multi-site PPG acquisition [17,18] which introduces system complexity and the need for synchronization between those signals [19]. In fact, PPG for the estimation of BP presents criticalities and limitations, such as the development of multi-photodetectors, noise elimination, the event detection, the need of individual calibration, and calibration drift. A useful algorithm that can be used to overcome motion artifacts' problems is the adaptive neuro fuzzy inference system (ANFIS) that allows improvements in the signal to be obtained [20]. Moreover, this algorithm has proved to be versatile for other fields of application [21].

As a matter of fact, the single-site PPG signal approach has great potential even though it has some criticalities and limitations. Its deployment has also increased thanks to the encouraging results obtained by exploiting machine learning (ML) algorithms trained on purposely selected PPG signal features [22–28].

In a previous work carried out by the authors [29], PPG signals were analyzed to select the most significant features for BP estimation by using several selection algorithms, i.e., RReliefF [30,31], Correlation-based Feature Selection (CFS), and Minimum Redundancy Maximum Relevance (MRMR) [32,33]. That methodology has led to the justification of the application of the Maximal Overlap Discrete Wavelet Transform (MODWT) to enhance the single-site PPG signal and to the selection of new proposed features [29]. Following this line of research, in this paper, our focus is on the actual development of ML techniques to find the best algorithm to measure BP, showing the usefulness of the already analyzed features and, in particular, those selected by means of MRMR, including those obtained after the enhancement with MODWT. The novelty of the research is in the use of new extracted features from PPG signals, whose significance was evaluated by using several criteria, and in the use of ML algorithms.

For this purpose, eXtreme Gradient Boost (XGBoost) models with Bayesian optimization and Neural Network (NN) models were trained for regression using significant features selected with the MRMR algorithm. A comparison of results between XGBoost and NN models was presented and the improvements with respect to the literature, by using XGBoost models and the proposed features, are shown.

The paper is structured as follows: in Section 2, the description of the dataset used to train ML models is provided; in Section 3, the ML approach for both XGBoost and NN models is presented; in Section 4, the results obtained using the best model are reported and compared with the literature, focusing on standard medical protocols for performance assessment; and finally, there are the conclusions.

2. Dataset

In this work, the MIMIC-III Waveform Database [34–36] was used to obtain the dataset for training and validation following the same processing reported in detail in [29]. The MIMIC-III Waveform Database is a large and open access database where protected health information has been deidentified. It includes waveform records of digitized signals acquired at 125 Hz, such as arterial blood pressure (ABP) measured invasively, PPG, ECG, and respiration for neonatal and adult patients admitted to intensive care units and monitored with iMDsoft MetaVision ICU or Intellivue MP-70 monitors. Among these acquired data, ABP and PPG signals have proved useful for our work. Many processing steps, shown in Figure 1, were performed such as alignment between ABP and PPG signals, pre-processing of PPG signals with denoising, Z-score standardization, baseline correction, quality, similarity tests, and ABP and PPG pulses segmentation and labeling.

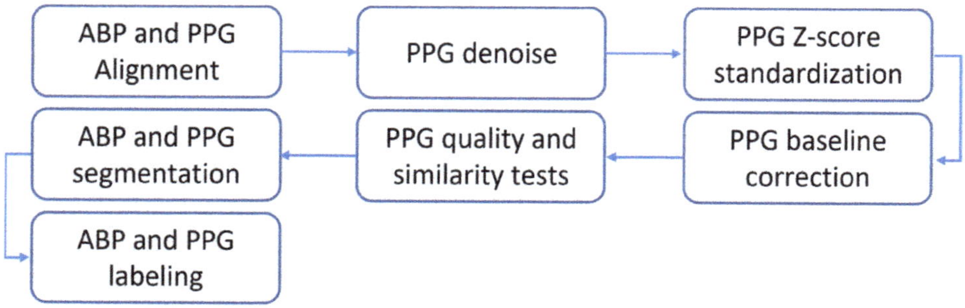

Figure 1. Workflow of the processing steps.

After the processing briefly described above, the features presented in [29] were calculated on the PPG signal. Many features were extracted in the time and frequency domain, others were related to the amplitude of the characteristic points (max slope point, systolic peak, dicrotic notch, inflection point, and diastolic peak), times and durations of characteristic points, areas, non-linear functions (logarithm of positions of dicrotic notch and inflection point), statistics (mean, STD, skewness, percentiles) and first and second derivatives. In this way, a dataset has been created containing, for each PPG pulse, 195 features and the target values of systolic blood pressure (SBP) and diastolic blood pressure (DBP) measured on the ABP signal. Then, the dataset was reduced to SBP in the range 80 mmHg to 180 mmHg and DBP in the range 60 mmHg to 110 mmHg to facilitate comparisons of the literature because similar distributions are used in other works [22,23,26,27,37–40]. Indeed, SBP under 80 mmHg and DBP under 60 mmHg correspond to a severe hypotension condition while SBP over 180 mmHg and DBP over 110 mmHg correspond to a severe hypertension condition and, in these cases, there were few observations in the initial dataset.

At the end of the processing, performed in MATLAB R2022a, the dataset contained 9.1×10^6 observations of PPG pulses from 1080 patients. The distribution of systolic and diastolic blood pressure values of the dataset processed in this work are shown in Figure 2. The described dataset was used to train and validate ML models developed in Python language, as discussed in the following sections. The dataset used to train and validate ML models included 9×10^6 observations; of these, the 90% constituted the training set and the 10% constituted the validation set. Instead, the test set included 100,000 observations.

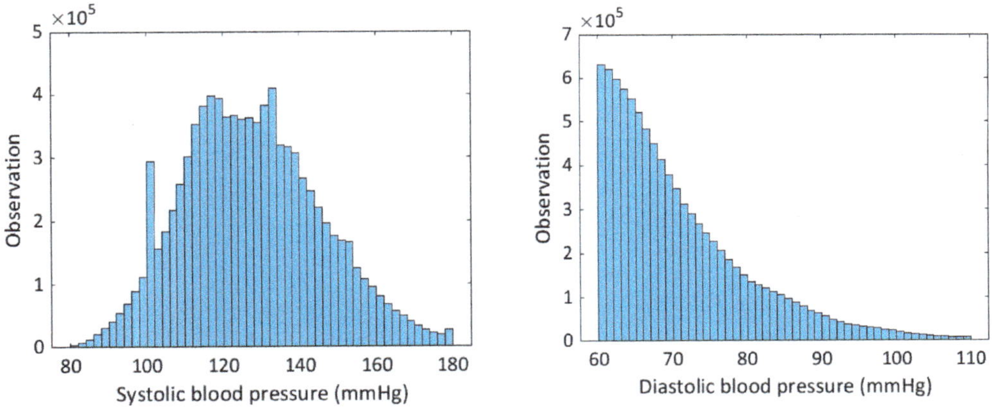

(a) (b)

Figure 2. (**a**) Systolic and (**b**) diastolic blood pressure occurrences in 2 mmHg bins. Only the observations with 80 mmHg ≤ SBP ≤ 180 mmHg and 60 mmHg ≤ DBP ≤ 110 mmHg were considered since outside these ranges there were few observations and, also, DBP less than 60 mmHg corresponds to a severe hypertension condition.

3. Machine Learning Models

ML offers powerful techniques to identify and evaluate cardiovascular risk and health conditions. In this paper, it has been exploited to train supervised regression models able to measure BP starting from features extracted from the PPG signal. For training purposes, each observation of the dataset is provided with systolic and diastolic labels obtained from the corresponding ABP signal, which serves as ground truth, as reported in [29].

In this paper, an XGBoost model was trained because of advantages such as execution speed and model performance, which have turned out to be suitable for our goal, while an NN model was trained to carry out a comparison of the results and it was chosen because it is an approach common to several researchers [27,28,37,41] and is characterized by higher training speed. Moreover, XGBoost models were used in the literature for a variety of purposes, such as wearable running monitoring [42], but recently also for PPG signal processing to estimate blood glucose levels [43], blood pressure (by using multisite PPG acquisition and Pulse Transit Time features) [44], and vascular aging [45].

XGBoost is an efficient open-source implementation of the gradient boosting algorithm and is also available in Python using the Scikit-learn library utilized in this work. Overall, gradient boosting refers to a class of ensemble ML algorithms that can be used both for classification and regression; ensembles, as a matter of fact, are based on decision tree models. In fact, trees are added to the ensemble to correct prediction errors made previously and these models are fitted using a differentiable loss function and a gradient descent optimization algorithm in order to minimize the loss gradient; moreover, this algorithm provides hyperparameters that can be tuned, such as the number of trees or estimators, the learning rate, the row and column sampling rate, the maximum tree depth, the minimum tree weight, and the regularization terms alpha and lambda. Indeed, XGBoost adds a regularization term in the objective function to make the model less vulnerable to overfitting.

Moreover, in this work, Bayesian hyper-parameter optimization [46] was used to tune the hyper-parameters of the XGBoost model in the chosen search space. Bayesian optimization allows the optimization of a proxy function rather than the true objective function and the search balances the exploration against exploitation, so at the beginning, it randomly explores to build the surrogate function with the objective of minimizing the cost function at a global level. In this work, the Bayesian Optimization implementation offered by the Python library Scikit-optimize was used. The Root Mean Square Error (RMSE) evaluation metric was defined using a Scikit-learn function to allow the conversion of optimization into a minimization problem as required by Scikit-optimize.

The Bayesian optimization was set providing the basic regressor, the search space, the evaluation metric, the cross-validation strategy (chosen to be 7-fold), the max number of trials, and the optimizer parameters for which the Gaussian Process (GP) was used. Then, the best hyper-parameters were obtained and used to instantiate the XGBoost model to be trained using the 10-fold cross-validation.

In the next paragraphs, there will be a focus on the XGBoost and NN models that were trained.

3.1. XGBoost Models

For both SBP and DBP, the entire dataset was used. The training and cross-validation were made using 9×10^6 observations (out of 9.1×10^6 observations). In total, 20 features for SBP and 25 features for DBP were used and selected in order of highest MRMR score among the 195 features listed in [29], which include those derived from the MODWT enhanced PPG signal. The number of features used to train the models has been chosen using the RReliefF algorithm for systolic and diastolic cases. In fact, using the RReliefF algorithm, the 20 features for SBP and the 25 features for DBP have an importance score greater than 0.001. We have considered lower scores as not significant because lower values are related to uncorrelated features to the output. That reduction in the number of features was operated to decrease the complexity of models and training; as a matter of fact, removing the noisy features helps with memory and computational cost but also helps avoid overfitting. Moreover, a normalization of columns into the range [0, 1] was carried out before the training.

Then, the first step consisted of finding of the best hyper-parameters in a specified search space for the Bayesian optimization using the selected features for both SBP and DBP measurements.

The search spaces and the best hyper-parameter values for SBP and DBP measurements are, respectively, shown in Tables 1 and 2.

Table 1. Search spaces and best values of hyper-parameters for SBP.

Hyper-Parameter	Range	Best
Learning rate	[0.01, 1.0]	0.226
Maximum tree depth	[2, 15]	15
Subsample	[0.1, 1.0]	0.894
Subsample ratio of columns by tree	[0.1, 1.0]	1.0
Lambda	$[1 \times 10^{-10}, 200]$	120.0
Alpha	$[1 \times 10^{-10}, 200]$	1×10^{-10}
Estimators	[50, 5100]	5000

Table 2. Search spaces and best values of hyper-parameters for DBP.

Hyper-Parameter	Range	Best
Learning rate	[0.01, 1.0]	0.136
Maximum tree depth	[2, 20]	15
Subsample	[0.1, 1.0]	0.894
Subsample ratio of columns by tree	[0.1, 1.0]	1.0
Lambda	$[1 \times 10^{-9}, 200]$	120.0
Alpha	$[1 \times 10^{-10}, 200]$	1×10^{-10}
Estimators	[50, 6000]	5200

An explanation of XGBoost hyper-parameters is reported below. The learning rate is the step size shrinkage used for the update to make the model more robust and to prevent overfitting by shrinking the feature weights; it is chosen in the range [0, 1] with typical values in [0.01, 0.2]. The maximum depth of a tree is used to control over-fitting as higher depth will make the model more complex and more likely to overfit; the value 0 is only accepted in a loss-guided growing policy while large values bring an aggressive consumption of memory. Any positive value is admissible, with typical values in [3, 10]; in this work, trial and error was used to modify the upper bound of the range to obtain better results. The subsample is, instead, the fraction of observations to be randomly sampled for each tree and is useful to prevent overfitting; in fact, lower values make the algorithm more conservative while too small values might lead to under-fitting. For this reason, the range is [0, 1] and typical values are in [0.5, 1]. The subsample ratio of columns by tree is the subsample ratio of columns when constructing each tree; this parameter has a range of [0, 1] and the default value of 1. Lambda is the L2 regularization term on weights and the increase in this value makes the model more conservative while Alpha is the L1 regularization term on weights and it is used in case of very high dimensionality so that the algorithm runs faster when implemented. Finally, estimators are the number of trees in an XGBoost model.

For the three last hyper-parameters, a trial and error method was used to define the range.

3.2. NN Models

In Python, TensorFlow 2.9.1 was used to define a sequential model with an input layer of size n, nine hidden layers, and an output layer. For all the layers, the activation function chosen was the Rectified Linear Unit (ReLU). The number of hidden layers and of neurons has been set making several trials. The NN model is shown in Figure 3. For SBP estimation, $n = 20$ while for DBP estimation, $n = 25$.

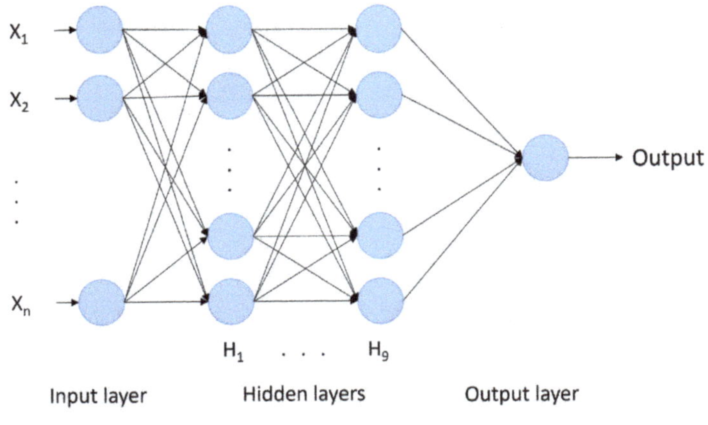

Figure 3. NN with nine hidden layers with 1024, 1024, 1024, 512, 512, 512, 128, 64, and 64 neurons.

Moreover, several optimizers were tested such as Adadelta, Adagrad, Adam, Adamax, Nadam, RMSprop, and SGD but the best result for both SBP and DBP estimations was obtained using the Nesterov-accelerated Adaptive Moment Estimation (Nadam) algorithm.

The fit was made using a batch size of 4096, 150 epochs, and a validation split of 0.2.

The NN architecture was chosen after trials and errors, by adding hidden layers since there was not an improvement in the results. The ReLU activation function was chosen because it is suitable for the normalized inputs and this function has allowed better results to be obtained. The batch size needs to fit the memory requirements of the GPU and the architecture of the CPU since too low values did not perform well while too high values were not allowed considering the memory requirements. Hence, the maximum possible batch size was set. The number of epochs was chosen in the range [50, 200] but beyond the 150 epochs there were not improvements.

4. Results and Discussion

In this section, the performance of ML algorithms will be shown. The two models, XGBoost and NN, were trained using the features selected by the MRMR algorithm and these features also include the new ones obtained on MODWT enhanced PPG pulses as reported in [29]. As pointed out in that previous work, it has been found that by using the MODWT, the PPG signal is enhanced, with an improvement in the identification of the characteristic points and making it more similar to the ABP signal.

The criteria used to evaluate the performance of ML models for estimating BP are the RMSE, Mean Absolute Error (MAE), correlation coefficient (R), and Mean Error (ME).

The results were then compared with other methods reported in the literature as well as with BP measurements standard guidelines focused on the classification of hypertension states. The predicted BP values from the regression model and the true values were used to verify the correct classification into the seven classes defined by the guideline considering the range of values of SBP and DBP. The classification results are evaluated by means of a confusion matrix.

4.1. Training and Test of XGBoost and NN Models

In this paragraph, the results obtained after training and validation are reported. In Table 3, XGBoost and NN results are reported considering the RMSE and MAE.

Table 3. Validation results for SBP and DBP estimations.

Model		RMSE (mmHg)	MAE (mmHg)
XGBoost	SBP	5.60	3.11
	DBP	3.92	2.09
NN	SBP	7.80	5.00
	DBP	5.56	3.53

After validation, a test was made for both models using a set of 100,000 new observations (out of the entire dataset of 9.1×10^6 observations) not included in the training set. The results were reported in Table 4 in which performance parameters are reported for SBP, DBP, and Mean Arterial BP (MAP).

Table 4. Test results using XGBoost and NN models.

Model		RMSE (mmHg)	MAE (mmHg)	R	ME (mmHg)
XGBoost	SBP	5.67	3.12	0.95	0.020
	DBP	3.95	2.11	0.91	−0.001
	MAP	3.24	2.01	0.93	0.006
NN	SBP	7.81	5.00	0.90	−0.420
	DBP	5.60	3.55	0.81	−0.250
	MAP	4.56	3.12	0.85	−0.310

In addition to SBP and DBP, MAP was considered because it is linked to the total peripheral resistance and to cardiac output and is associated with HR [47,48]. MAP is a popular BP parameter, and it is defined as the average pressure of the artery of a subject during one cardiac cycle (1). It is considered as a better indicator of perfusion to vital organs when compared with SBP [49].

$$\mathrm{MAP} = \frac{\mathrm{SBP} + 2\cdot\mathrm{DBP}}{3}, \quad (1)$$

The results reported in Tables 3 and 4 show that the use of XGBoost models rather than NN allows better results for both systolic and diastolic pressure measurement to be obtained.

Moreover, the results for XGBoost models obtained in the final test phase, shown in Table 4, are similar and confirm the ones obtained during the training and cross-validation phase, shown in Table 3.

Error probability densities of SBP, DBP, and MAP estimations are shown in Figure 4, where it is possible to notice that errors obtained using the XGBoost model have a narrower and more concentrated distribution around zero than the distribution obtained using the NN model. From regression plots reported in Figure 5, it is possible to notice that best predictions are obtained by using XGBoost models; in fact, R is in the three cases higher than those obtained using NN models.

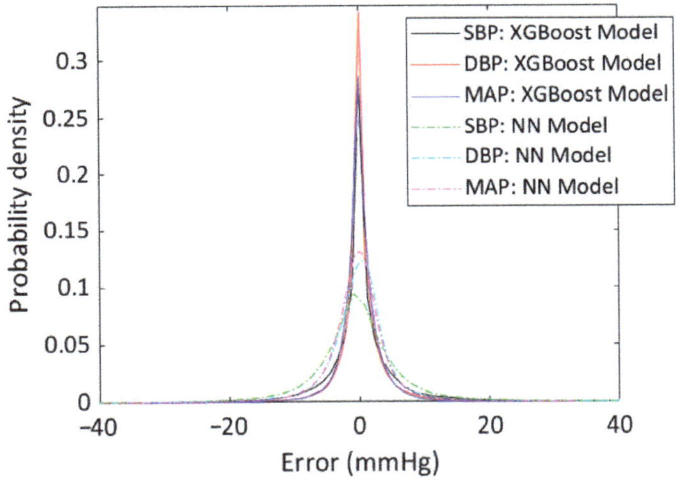

Figure 4. Error probability density of SBP, DBP, and MAP estimations. Errors were defined as the difference between the predicted pressures (using XGBoost model or NN model) and measured ones; then, their histograms were normalized to obtain the probability densities shown in the plot.

During the training phase, it was noticed that the training time for NN was smaller than the training time for the XGBoost models. The inference time was significantly reduced for XGBoost models so considering this aspect, it is possible to use the trained model for real time predictions useful for continuous monitoring.

Considering the computational complexity of current implementations for features extraction and ML models, onboard processing on a wearable device is not viable. So, a cloud-based solution would be required. The future aim is to streamline feature extraction by including only those selected in the present study and simplify models to permit onboard processing, reducing the computational complexity and assessing the minimal hardware requirements.

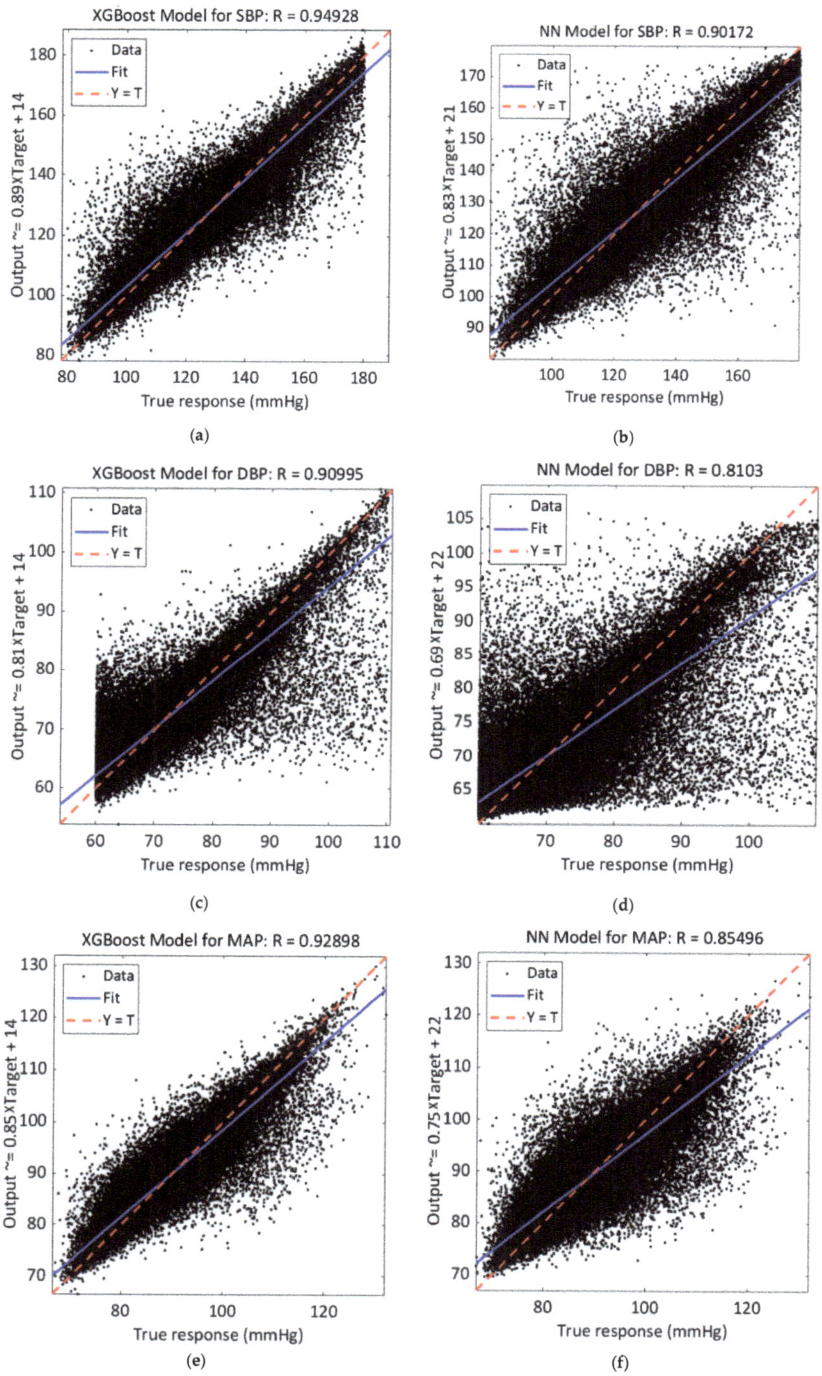

Figure 5. (**a**,**c**,**e**) Regression of the predicted output and true response for SBP, DBP, and MAP estimations using the XGBoost model; (**b**,**d**,**f**) Regression of the predicted output and true response for SBP, DBP, and MAP estimations using the NN model.

4.2. Comparison with Other Methods

A comparison of results with the literature is difficult due to the different evaluation criteria and the different datasets. In this paper, the type of the algorithms and the use of features have been used as the criteria to select and identify other works in the literature to make a comparison. In this context, the criterion is the training of ML algorithms with features extracted from the PPG signal, namely, the research's methodology.

In Table 5, the performance of other methods is shown.

Table 5. Comparison with other works.

Work	Method	Data Size	Performance Evaluation	SBP	DBP
Kachuee et al. [37]	Support vector machine (SVM)	MIMIC II (1000 subjects)	RMSE	/	/
			MAE	12.38	6.34
			R	/	/
			ME	/	/
Kim et al. [50]	ANN	180 recordings, 45 subjects	RMSE	/	/
			MAE	4.53	/
			R	/	/
			ME	/	/
Cattivelli et al. [51]	Proprietary algorithm	MIMIC database (34 recordings, 25 subjects)	RMSE	8.37	5.92
			MAE	/	/
			R	/	/
			ME	/	/
Zhang et al. [52]	SVM	7000 samples from 32 patients	RMSE	/	/
			MAE	11.64	7.62
			R	/	/
			ME	/	/
Zadi et al. [53]	Autoregressive moving average (ARMA) models	15 subjects	RMSE	6.49	4.33
			MAE	/	/
			R	/	/
			ME	/	/
Chowdhury et al. [24]	Gaussian process regression (GPR)	222 recordings, 126 subjects	RMSE	6.74	3.59
			MAE	3.02	1.74
			R	0.95	0.96
			ME	/	/
Hasanzadeh et al. [26]	AdaBoost	MIMIC II 942 subjects	RMSE	/	/
			MAE	8.22	4.17
			R	0.78	0.72
			ME	0.09	0.23
Kachuee et al. [38]	AdaBoost	1000 subjects	RMSE	/	/
			MAE	8.21	4.31
			R	/	/
			ME	/	/

Table 5. *Cont.*

Work	Method	Data Size	Performance Evaluation	SBP	DBP
Wang et al. [54]	ANN	58,795 PPG samples	RMSE	/	/
			MAE	4.02	2.27
			R	/	/
			ME	/	/
Kurylyak et al. [28]	ANN	15,000 PPG heartbeats	RMSE	/	/
			MAE	3.80	2.21
			R	/	/
			ME	/	/
Fleischhauer et al. [55]	XGBoost	MIMIC, Queensland, PPG BP (273 subjects and 259,986 single beats)	RMSE	/	/
			MAE	6.366	/
			R	0.874	/
			ME	/	/
Liu et al. [56]	SVR	MIMIC II 910 good PPG pules cycles	RMSE	/	/
			MAE	8.54	4.34
			R	/	/
			ME	/	/
Zhang et al. [57]	Gradient Boosting Regressor (GBR)	MIMIC II 2842 samples from 12,000 data points	RMSE	/	/
			MAE	4.33	2.54
			R	/	/
			ME	/	/
Proposed method	**XGBoost**	**MIMIC III 9.1×10^6 PPG pulses from 1080 subjects**	**RMSE**	**5.67**	**3.95**
			MAE	**3.12**	**2.11**
			R	**0.95**	**0.91**
			ME	**0.01**	**0.02**

The comparison with other works has shown that our models, based on the use of XGBoost, the MRMR selection algorithm, and features obtained on MODWT, enhanced PPG pulses, obtained small estimation errors for both systolic and diastolic blood pressure measurements [29]. In fact, XGBoost is derivative-free so it might have some advantage when the fitting problem has a lot of degrees of freedom. Moreover, the use of MODWT enhancement has allowed characteristic points of PPG pulses such as the diastolic point to be emphasized; these two aspects can be decisive in obtaining such results. As a matter of fact, for SBP measurement, the proposed method has allowed a smaller RMSE compared to the other works reported in the Table 5 to be obtained. Obviously, as mentioned at the beginning of this section, a comparison of results is difficult; in fact, as reported in Table 5, different datasets were used as well as different ML algorithms. For example, it should be noted that Chowdhury et al. [24] obtained a smaller RMSE for DBP, which may depend on the different dataset used and on the use of demographic features that are a powerful means to predict BP values because gender, age, and height are related to the shape of the PPG pulses and to the arterial stiffness. Considering Zhang et al. [57], they use a GBR algorithm obtaining slightly worse results than those reported in this paper as well as in Fleischhauer et al. [55] using XGBoost; as a matter of fact, in this paper, the best results are obtained implementing the Bayesian optimization for our XGBoost models and a different selection of features also obtained after the MODWT enhancement. This seems to be a better solution also compared with other ML algorithms as reported in Table 5.

4.3. Compliance to Standards and Classification Guidelines

The correct estimation of BP is critical for the detection of states of hypertension and health status and hence, accuracy requirements for BP measurement devices and methods have been standardized.

In this paper, the protocols proposed by the Association for the Advancement of Medical Instrumentation (AAMI) [58,59] and by the British Hypertension Society (BHS) [60] were considered to make a comparison with results reported in this paper as also made in [23–26,61–63].

Since the best results in this paper were obtained using the XGBoost models rather than using the NN models, the following comparisons regard only the XGBoost models.

As shown in Tables 6–9, the proposed method is compliant to AAMI and BHS grade A standards. The dataset included 1080 patients and a total of 9.1×10^6 observations of PPG pulses.

Table 6. Comparison of results for the validation set with AAMI standard.

		ME (mmHg)	STD (mmHg)
Results	SBP	0.009	5.60
	DBP	0.019	3.92
	MAP	0.0157	3.21
AAMI	SBP DBP	≤5	≤8

Table 7. Comparison of results for the test set with AAMI standard.

		ME (mmHg)	STD (mmHg)
Results	SBP	0.020	5.67
	DBP	−0.001	3.95
	MAP	0.006	3.24
AAMI	SBP DBP	≤5	≤8

Table 8. Comparison of results for the validation set with BHS standard.

		Cumulative Error Percentage		
		≤5 mmHg	**≤10 mmHg**	**≤15 mmHg**
Results	SBP	80.85%	93.00%	96.84%
	DBP	89.56%	96.86%	98.74%
	MAP	90.89%	98.18%	99.49%
BHS	Grade A	60%	85%	95%
	Grade B	50%	75%	90%
	Grade C	40%	65%	85%

Table 9. Comparison of results for the test set with BHS standard.

		Cumulative Error Percentage		
		≤5 mmHg	**≤10 mmHg**	**≤15 mmHg**
Results	SBP	80.96%	92.91%	96.73%
	DBP	89.48%	96.87%	98.68%
	MAP	90.84%	98.07%	99.44%
BHS	Grade A	60%	85%	95%
	Grade B	50%	75%	90%
	Grade C	40%	65%	85%

As is possible to notice in Tables 6 and 7, our results fulfill AAMI standard requirements; indeed, according to this protocol, the mean and the STD of the errors for both SBP and DBP estimations should not be more than 5 mmHg and 8 mmHg, respectively. Requirements of the BHS standard are also satisfied since the absolute error of more than 60% of the data is less than 5 mmHg, hence the method is considered as Grade A.

Moreover, as established in [26], another guideline was used to evaluate our regression models; for this purpose, the guideline [64] provided by the European Society of Hypertension (ESH) and the European Society of Cardiology (ESC) was considered. This guideline is focused on the state of hypertension and, in fact, categorizes it into seven classes:

- Optimal: if SBP < 120 mmHg and DBP < 80 mmHg;
- Normal: if 120 mmHg ≤ SBP ≤ 129 mmHg and/or 80 mmHg ≤ DBP ≤ 84 mmHg;
- High Normal: if 130 mmHg ≤ SBP ≤ 139 mmHg and/or 85 mmHg ≤ DBP ≤ 89 mmHg;
- Grade 1 Hypertension: if 140 mmHg < SBP ≤ 159 mmHg and/or 90 mmHg ≤ DBP ≤ 99 mmHg;
- Grade 2 Hypertension: if 160 mmHg ≤ SBP ≤ 179 mmHg and/or 100 mmHg ≤ DBP ≤ 109 mmHg;
- Grade 3 Hypertension: if SBP ≥ 180 mmHg and/or DBP ≥ 110 mmHg;
- Isolated Systolic Hypertension: if SBP ≥ 140 mmHg and DBP < 90 mmHg.

Since hypertension is a state of health of interest to be identified, we also used ESH/ESC guidelines to evaluate our regression models with a classification of the predicted values into seven classes. The BP ground truth and the BP predicted by the XGBoost model were labeled according to the previously described classification to evaluate the consistency between the classified predicted values and the classified true values in the different states of hypertension. The results are shown in Figure 6 and in Table 10. In the table, the accuracy, sensitivity, specificity, and F1-score are provided. There are two classes with a low sensitivity that are "Grade 3 Hypertension" and "Isolated Systolic Hypertension". The low sensitivity is due to the few training cases in the dataset. Indeed, "Grade 3 Hypertension" is a critical condition while "Isolated Systolic Hypertension" has low frequency in young and middle-aged subjects.

As is possible to see in Table 10, the average of accuracy, sensitivity, specificity, and F1-score are, respectively, 90.3%, 76.9%, 93.5%, and 77.0%.

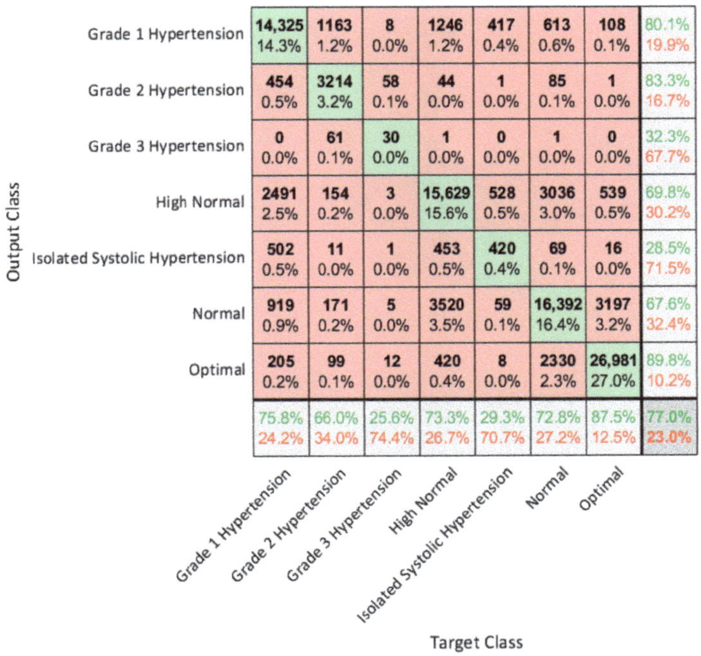

Figure 6. Confusion matrix for BP level classification according to ESH/ESC guidelines.

Table 10. Results of BP level classification according to ESH/ESC guidelines.

Class	Accuracy	Sensitivity	Specificity	F1-Score	Actual Class Members
Grade 1 Hypertension	91.9%	75.8%	95.6%	77.9%	18.9%
Grade 2 Hypertension	97.7%	66.0%	99.3%	73.6%	4.9%
Grade 3 Hypertension	99.8%	25.6%	99.9%	28.6%	0.1%
High Normal	87.5%	73.3%	91.4%	71.4%	21.3%
Isolated Systolic Hypertension	97.9%	29.3%	98.9%	28.9%	1.4%
Normal	86.0%	72.8%	89.8%	70.1%	22.5%
Optimal	93.1%	87.5%	95.6%	88.6%	30.8%
Average	90.3%	76.9%	93.5%	77.0%	

4.4. Bland–Altman Analysis

Finally, to test the validity of the prediction of the XGBoost models for SBP, DBP, and MAP, a Bland–Altman analysis was performed which was used to determine the limits of agreement (LOA) between two different measurements in clinical practice [65,66]. The mean and STD of the differences between two measurements are used for statistical limits. The mean bias (mean of the differences) and its LOA are provided by the Bland–Altman plot that is shown in Figure 7.

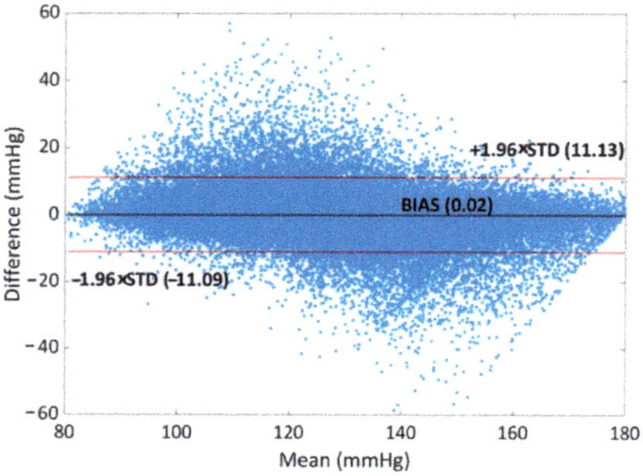

(**a**)

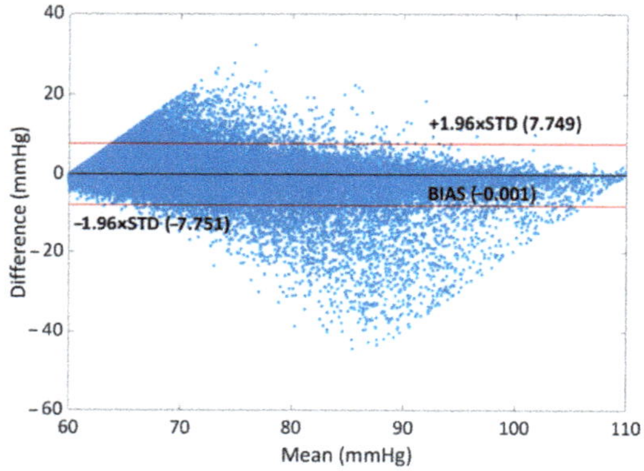

(**b**)

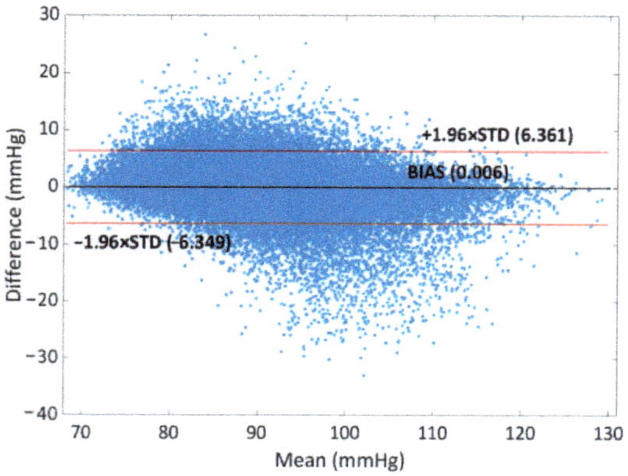

(**c**)

Figure 7. Bland–Altman plots for (**a**) SBP, (**b**) DBP, and (**c**) MAP.

The black line represents the mean of differences (BIAS) while the red lines represent the upper and lower limits (BIAS $\pm$ 1.96 $\times$ STD) of the LOA [67]. The LOA for errors of SBP is [-11.09, 11.13] mmHg and the percentage of points outside the LOA is 5.91%; the LOA for errors of DBP is [-7.75, 7.75] mmHg with a percentage of 5.08% points outside while for MAP the LOA for errors is [6.35, 6.36] mmHg with a percentage of 5.73% points outside. So, considering these results, it is possible to confirm the good accuracy of the proposed model.

5. Conclusions

The possibility of measuring BP by using PPG signals is advantageous for the monitoring of this vital sign since it avoids the use of cumbersome cuff-based devices, and it allows continuous monitoring. However, PPG for the estimation of BP has several criticalities and limitations, such as noise elimination, individual calibration, and calibration drift, that must be overcome.

In our previous work [29], the focus was on the extraction of new features from PPG signals, including those obtained after the enhancement with MODWT, whose significance was evaluated by using several criteria, such as MRMR. In this paper, the features selected by the MRMR algorithm were used to train ML models to estimate BP, giving improved results.

Among the ML models, the XGBoost model with Bayesian optimization proved to be suitable for estimating purposes, giving better results than an NN model trained on the same data; as a matter of fact, the XGBoost model combined with the use of novel features allowed an improvement for systolic blood pressure measurement with respect to the literature.

In addition, the SBP and DBP estimators proved to fulfill the requirements of the AAMI and BHS grade A standards, but also, good classification results were obtained according to the ESH/ESC guideline.

Considering these results, future work will focus on the realization of a portable measurement device to acquire PPG signals and implement the proposed BP estimator permitting onboard processing by reducing the computational complexity and assessing the minimal hardware requirements.

Author Contributions: Conceptualization, F.A., V.I.D., L.D.P., A.D.N. and A.M.L.L.; Software, L.D.P.; Writing—Original draft, F.A., V.I.D., L.D.P., A.D.N. and A.M.L.L.; Supervision, F.A. and A.D.N. All authors have read and agreed to the published version of the manuscript.

Funding: This research received no external funding.

Informed Consent Statement: Patient consent was waived because the project did not impact clinical care and all protected health information was deidentified.

Data Availability Statement: Publicly available datasets were analyzed in this study. This data can be found in [31]. The code developed and used in this work is available under request.

Conflicts of Interest: The authors declare no conflict of interest.

References

1. Fan, Y.; Xu, P.; Jin, H.; Ma, J.; Qin, L. Vital Sign Measurement in Telemedicine Rehabilitation Based on Intelligent Wearable Medical Devices. *IEEE Access* **2019**, *7*, 54819–54823. [CrossRef]
2. Pintavirooj, C.; Keatsamarn, T.; Treebupachatsakul, T. Multi-Parameter Vital Sign Telemedicine System Using Web Socket for COVID-19 Pandemics. *Healthcare* **2021**, *9*, 285. [CrossRef] [PubMed]
3. De Palma, L.; Attivissimo, F.; Di Nisio, A.; Lanzolla, A.M.L.; Ragolia, M.A.; Spadavecchia, M. Development of a web-based system for interfacing a portable Bluetooth vital sign monitor. In Proceedings of the 2022 IEEE International Symposium on Medical Measurements and Applications (MeMeA), Messina, Italy, 22–24 June 2022; pp. 1–6. [CrossRef]
4. Celler, B.G.; Sparks, R.S. Home Telemonitoring of Vital Signs-Technical Challenges and Future Directions. *IEEE J. Biomed. Health Inform.* **2015**, *19*, 82–91. [CrossRef] [PubMed]
5. Scarpetta, M.; Spadavecchia, M.; Andria, G.; Ragolia, M.A.; Giaquinto, N. Simultaneous Measurement of Heartbeat Intervals and Respiratory Signal using a Smartphone. In Proceedings of the 2021 IEEE International Symposium on Medical Measurements and Applications (MeMeA), Lausanne, Switzerland, 23–25 June 2021; pp. 1–5. [CrossRef]
6. Khoshmanesh, F.; Thurgood, P.; Pirogova, E.; Nahavandi, S.; Baratchi, S. Wearable sensors: At the frontier of personalised health monitoring, smart prosthetics and assistive technologies. *Biosens. Bioelectron.* **2021**, *176*, 112946. [CrossRef]
7. Arpaia, P.; Moccaldi, N.; Prevete, R.; Sannino, I.; Tedesco, A. A Wearable EEG Instrument for Real-Time Frontal Asymmetry Monitoring in Worker Stress Analysis. *IEEE Trans. Instrum. Meas.* **2020**, *69*, 8335–8343. [CrossRef]

8. D'Alessandro, V.I.; De Palma, L.; Attivissimo, F.; Di Nisio, A.; Lanzolla, A.M.L. U-Net convolutional neural network for multi-source heterogeneous iris segmentation. In Proceedings of the 2023 IEEE International Symposium on Medical Measurements and Applications (MeMeA), Jeju, Republic of Korea, 14–16 June 2023; pp. 1–5. [CrossRef]
9. Manickam, P.; Mariappan, S.A.; Murugesan, S.M.; Hansda, S.; Kaushik, A.; Shinde, R.; Thipperudraswamy, S.P. Artificial Intelligence (AI) and Internet of Medical Things (IoMT) Assisted Biomedical Systems for Intelligent Healthcare. *Biosensors* **2022**, *12*, 562. [CrossRef]
10. Cheng, Y.-H.; Lech, M.; Wilkinson, R.H. Simultaneous Sleep Stage and Sleep Disorder Detection from Multimodal Sensors Using Deep Learning. *Sensors* **2023**, *23*, 3468. [CrossRef]
11. Castaneda, D.; Esparza, A.; Ghamari, M.; Soltanpur, C.; Nazeran, H. A review on wearable photoplethysmography sensors and their potential future applications in health care. *Int. J. Biosens. Bioelectron.* **2018**, *4*, 195–202. [CrossRef]
12. Longmore, S.K.; Lui, G.Y.; Naik, G.; Breen, P.P.; Jalaludin, B.; Gargiulo, G.D. A Comparison of Reflective Photoplethysmography for Detection of Heart Rate, Blood Oxygen Saturation, and Respiration Rate at Various Anatomical Locations. *Sensors* **2019**, *19*, 1874. [CrossRef]
13. Tamura, T.; Maeda, Y.; Sekine, M.; Yoshida, M. Wearable Photoplethysmographic Sensors-Past and Present. *Electronics* **2014**, *3*, 282–302. [CrossRef]
14. López-Silva, S.M.; Giannetti, R.; Dotor, M.L.; Silveira, J.P.; Golmayo, D.; Miguel-Tobal, F.; Bilbao, A.; Galindo, M.; Martín-Escudero, P. Heuristic algorithm for photoplethysmographic heart rate tracking during maximal exercise test. *J. Med. Biol. Eng.* **2022**, *32*, 181–188. [CrossRef]
15. Qananwah, Q.; Dagamseh, A.; Alquran, H.; Ibrahim, K.S.; Alodat, M.D.; Hayden, O. A comparative study of photoplethysmogram and piezoelectric plethysmogram signals. *Phys. Eng. Sci. Med.* **2020**, *43*, 1207–1217. [CrossRef]
16. De Palma, L.; Scarpetta, M.; Spadavecchia, M. Characterization of Heart Rate Estimation Using Piezoelectric Plethysmography in Time- and Frequency-domain. In Proceedings of the 2020 IEEE International Symposium on Medical Measurements and Applications (MeMeA), Bari, Italy, 1 June–1 July 2020; pp. 1–6. [CrossRef]
17. Block, R.C.; Yavarimanesh, M.; Natarajan, K.; Carek, A.; Mousavi, A.; Chandrasekhar, A.; Kim, C.-S.; Zhu, J.; Schifitto, G.; Mestha, L.K.; et al. Conventional pulse transit times as markers of blood pressure changes in humans. *Sci. Rep.* **2020**, *10*, 16373. [CrossRef] [PubMed]
18. Geddes, L.; Voelz, M.; Babbs, C.; Bourl, J.; Tacker, W. Pulse transit time as an indicator of arterial blood pressure. *Psychophysiology* **1981**, *18*, 71–74. [CrossRef] [PubMed]
19. Elgendi, M.; Fletcher, R.; Liang, Y.; Howard, N.; Lovell, N.H.; Abbott, D.; Lim, K.; Ward, R. The use of photoplethysmography for assessing hypertension. *NPJ Digit. Med.* **2019**, *2*, 60. [CrossRef]
20. Tarvirdizadeh, B.; Golgouneh, A.; Tajdari, F.; Khodabakhshi, E. A novel online method for identifying motion artifact and photoplethysmography signal reconstruction using artificial neural networks and adaptive neuro-fuzzy inference system. *Neural Comput. Applic.* **2020**, *32*, 3549–3566. [CrossRef]
21. Arabameri, M.; Nazari, R.R.; Abdolshahi, A.; Abdollahzadeh, M.; Mirzamohammadi, S.; Shariatifar, N.; Barba, F.J.; Khaneghah, A.M. Oxidative stability of virgin olive oil: Evaluation and prediction with an adaptive neuro-fuzzy inference system (ANFIS). *J. Sci. Food Agric.* **2019**, *99*, 5358–5367. [CrossRef]
22. Slapničar, G.; Mlakar, N.; Luštrek, M. Blood Pressure Estimation from Photoplethysmogram Using a Spectro-Temporal Deep Neural Network. *Sensors* **2019**, *19*, 3420. [CrossRef]
23. Harfiya, L.N.; Chang, C.C.; Li, Y.H. Continuous Blood Pressure Estimation Using Exclusively Photopletysmography by LSTM-Based Signal-to-Signal Translation. *Sensors* **2021**, *21*, 2952. [CrossRef]
24. Chowdhury, M.H.; Shuzan, M.N.I.; Chowdhury, M.E.H.; Mahbub, Z.B.; Uddin, M.M.; Khandakar, A.; Reaz, M.B.I. Estimating Blood Pressure from the Photoplethysmogram Signal and Demographic Features Using Machine Learning Techniques. *Sensors* **2020**, *20*, 3127. [CrossRef]
25. Tjahjadi, H.; Ramli, K. Noninvasive Blood Pressure Classification Based on Photoplethysmography Using K-Nearest Neighbors Algorithm: A Feasibility Study. *Information* **2020**, *11*, 93. [CrossRef]
26. Hasanzadeh, N.; Ahmadi, M.M.; Mohammadzade, H. Blood Pressure Estimation Using Photoplethysmogram Signal and Its Morphological Features. *IEEE Sens. J.* **2020**, *20*, 4300–4310. [CrossRef]
27. Hsu, Y.C.; Li, Y.H.; Chang, C.C.; Harfiya, L.N. Generalized Deep Neural Network Model for Cuffless Blood Pressure Estimation with Photoplethysmogram Signal Only. *Sensors* **2020**, *20*, 5668. [CrossRef] [PubMed]
28. Kurylyak, Y.; Lamonaca, F.; Grimaldi, D. A Neural Network-based method for continuous blood pressure estimation from a PPG signal. In Proceedings of the 2013 IEEE International Instrumentation and Measurement Technology Conference (I2MTC), Minneapolis, MN, USA, 6–9 May 2013; pp. 280–283. [CrossRef]
29. Attivissimo, F.; De Palma, L.; Di Nisio, A.; Scarpetta, M.; Lanzolla, A.M.L. Photoplethysmography Signal Wavelet Enhancement and Novel Features Selection for Non-Invasive Cuff-Less Blood Pressure Monitoring. *Sensors* **2023**, *23*, 2321. [CrossRef] [PubMed]
30. Kira, K.; Rendell, L.A. The feature selection problem: Traditional methods and a new algorithm. *Assoc. Adv. Artif. Intell.* **1992**, *2*, 129–134.
31. Kononenko, I.; Robnik-Šikonja, M. Overcoming the myopia of inductive learning algorithms with RELIEFF. *Appl. Intell.* **1997**, *7*, 39–55. [CrossRef]

32. Roffo, G. Ranking to learn and learning to rank: On the role of ranking in pattern recognition applications. *arXiv* **2017**, arXiv:1706.05933.
33. Ding, C.; Peng, H. Minimum redundancy feature selection from microarray gene expression data. *J. Bioinform. Comput. Biol.* **2005**, *3*, 185–205. [CrossRef]
34. Moody, B.; Moody, G.; Villarroel, M.; Clifford, G.D.; Silva, I. MIMIC-III Waveform Database (version 1.0). *PhysioNet* **2020**. [CrossRef]
35. Johnson, A.E.W.; Pollard, T.J.; Shen, L.; Lehman, L.H.; Feng, M.; Ghassemi, M.; Moody, B.; Szolovits, P.; Celi, L.A.; Mark, R.G. MIMIC-III, a freely accessible critical care database. *Sci. Data* **2016**, *3*, 160035. [CrossRef]
36. Goldberger, A.L.; Amaral, L.A.; Glass, L.; Hausdorff, J.M.; Ivanov, P.C.; Mark, R.G.; Mietus, J.E.; Moody, G.B.; Peng, C.K.; Stanley, H.E. PhysioBank, PhysioToolkit, and PhysioNet: Components of a new research resource for complex physiologic signals. *Circulation* **2000**, *101*, E215–E220. [CrossRef] [PubMed]
37. Kachuee, M.; Kiani, M.M.; Mohammadzade, H.; Shabany, M. Cuff-less high-accuracy calibration-free blood pressure estimation using pulse transit time. In Proceedings of the 2015 IEEE International Symposium on Circuits and Systems (ISCAS), Lisbon, Portugal, 24–27 May 2015; pp. 1006–1009. [CrossRef]
38. Kachuee, M.; Kiani, M.M.; Mohammadzade, H.; Shabany, M. Cuffless blood pressure estimation algorithms for continuous health-care monitoring. *IEEE Trans. Biomed. Eng.* **2017**, *64*, 859–869. [CrossRef] [PubMed]
39. Chakraborty, A.; Goswami, D.; Mukhopadhyay, J.; Chakrabarti, S. Measurement of Arterial Blood Pressure Through Single-Site Acquisition of Photoplethysmograph Signal. *in IEEE Trans. Instrum. Meas.* **2021**, *70*, 4000310. [CrossRef]
40. Li, Z.; He, W. A Continuous Blood Pressure Estimation Method Using Photoplethysmography by GRNN-Based Model. *Sensors* **2021**, *21*, 7207. [CrossRef]
41. Pandey, R.K.; Lin, T.Y.; Chao, P.C.P. Design and implementation of a photoplethysmography acquisition system with an optimized artificial neural network for accurate blood pressure measurement. *Microsyst. Technol.* **2021**, *27*, 2345–2367. [CrossRef]
42. Guo, J.; Yang, L.; Bie, R.; Yu, J.; Gao, Y.; Shen, Y.; Kos, A. An XGBoost-based physical fitness evaluation model using advanced feature selection and Bayesian hyper-parameter optimization for wearable running monitoring. *Comput. Netw.* **2019**, *151*, 166–180. [CrossRef]
43. Prabha, A.; Yadav, J.; Rani, A.; Singh, V. Intelligent estimation of blood glucose level using wristband PPG signal and physiological parameters. *Biomed. Signal Process. Control* **2022**, *78*, 103876. [CrossRef]
44. Che, X.; Li, M.; Kang, W.; Lai, F.; Wang, J. Continuous Blood Pressure Estimation from Two-Channel PPG Parameters by XGBoost. In Proceedings of the 2019 IEEE International Conference on Robotics and Biomimetics (ROBIO), Dali, China, 6–8 December 2019; pp. 2707–2712. [CrossRef]
45. Shin, H. XGBoost Regression of the Most Significant Photoplethysmogram Features for Assessing Vascular Aging. *IEEE J. Biomed. Health Inform.* **2022**, *26*, 3354–3361. [CrossRef]
46. Gao, L.; Ding, Y. Disease prediction via Bayesian hyperparameter optimization and ensemble learning. *BMC Res. Notes* **2020**, *13*, 205. [CrossRef]
47. Gregg, M.E.; Matyas, T.A.; James, J.E. A new model of individual differences in hemodynamic profile and blood pressure reactivity. *Psychophysiology* **2002**, *39*, 64–72. [CrossRef]
48. Sherwood, A.; Dolan, C.A.; Light, K.C. Hemodynamics of blood pressure responses during active and passive coping. *Psychophysiology* **1990**, *27*, 656–668. [CrossRef]
49. DeMers, D.; Wachs, D. Physiology, mean arterial pressure. In *StatPearls*; StatPearls Publishing: Treasure Island, FL, USA, 2022.
50. Kim, J.Y.; Cho, B.H.; Im, S.M.; Jeon, M.J.; Kim, I.Y.; Kim, S.I. Comparative study on artificial neural network with multiple regressions for continuous estimation of blood pressure. In Proceedings of the 2005 IEEE Engineering in Medicine and Biology 27th Annual Conference, Shanghai, China, 17–18 January 2006; pp. 6942–6945.
51. Cattivelli, F.S.; Garudadri, H. Noninvasive cuffless estimation of blood pressure from pulse arrival time and heart rate with adaptive calibration. In Proceedings of the 2009 Sixth International Workshop on Wearable and Implantable Body Sensor Networks, Berkeley, CA, USA, 3–5 June 2009; pp. 114–119.
52. Zhang, Y.; Feng, Z. A SVM method for continuous blood pressure estimation from a PPG signal. In Proceedings of the 9th International Conference on Machine Learning and Computing, Singapore, 24–26 February 2017; pp. 128–132.
53. Zadi, A.S.; Alex, R.; Zhang, R.; Watenpaugh, D.E.; Behbehani, K. Arterial blood pressure feature estimation using photoplethysmography. *Comput. Biol. Med.* **2018**, *102*, 104–111. [CrossRef] [PubMed]
54. Wang, L.; Zhou, W.; Xing, Y.; Zhou, X. A Novel Neural Network Model for Blood Pressure Estimation Using Photoplethesmography without Electrocardiogram. *J. Healthc. Eng.* **2018**, *2018*, 7804243. [CrossRef] [PubMed]
55. Fleischhauer, V.; Feldheiser, A.; Zaunseder, S. Beat-to-Beat Blood Pressure Estimation by Photoplethysmography and Its Interpretation. *Sensors* **2022**, *22*, 7037. [CrossRef] [PubMed]
56. Liu, M.; Po, L.-M.; Fu, H. Cuffless blood pressure estimation based on photoplethysmography signal and its second derivative. *Int. J. Comput. Theory Eng.* **2017**, *9*, 202. [CrossRef]
57. Zhang, G.; Shin, S.; Jung, J.; Li, M.; Kim, Y.T. Machine learning Algorithm for Non-invasive Blood Pressure Estimation Using PPG Signals. In Proceedings of the 2022 IEEE Fifth International Conference on Artificial Intelligence and Knowledge Engineering (AIKE), Laguna Hills, CA, USA, 19–21 September 2022; pp. 94–97. [CrossRef]

58. Stergiou, G.S.; Alpert, B.; Mieke, S.; Asmar, R.; Atkins, N.; Eckert, S.; Frick, G.; Friedman, B. A universal standard for the validation of blood pressure measuring devices: Association for the Advancement of Medical Instrumentation/European Society of Hypertension/International Organization for Standardization (AAMI/ESH/ISO) Collaboration Statement. *Hypertension* **2018**, *71*, 368–374. [CrossRef]
59. *ANSI/AAMI SP10-2002/A1*; Association for the Advancement of Medical Instrumentation, American National Standard. Manual, Electronic or Automated Sphygmomanometers. Association for the Advancement of Medical Instrumentation: Arlington, VA, USA, 2003.
60. O'brien, E.; Waeber, B.; Parati, G.; Staessen, J.; Myers, M.G. Blood pressure measuring devices: Recommendations of the European Society of Hypertension. *BMJ* **2001**, *322*, 531–536. [CrossRef]
61. Rong, M.; Li, K. A multi-type features fusion neural network for blood pressure prediction based on photoplethysmography. *Biomed. Signal Process. Control* **2021**, *68*, 102772. [CrossRef]
62. Li, Y.H.; Harfiya, L.N.; Chang, C.C. Featureless Blood Pressure Estimation Based on Photoplethysmography Signal Using CNN and BiLSTM for IoT Devices. *Hindawi Wirel. Commun. Mob. Comput.* **2021**, *2021*, 9085100. [CrossRef]
63. Mousavi, S.S.; Firouzmand, M.; Charmi, M.; Hemmati, M.; Moghadam, M.; Ghorbani, Y. Blood pressure estimation from appropriate and inappropriate PPG signals using A whole-based method. *Biomed. Signal Process. Control* **2019**, *47*, 196–206. [CrossRef]
64. Mancia, G.; Fagard, R.; Narkiewicz, K.; Redon, J.; Zanchetti, A.; Böhm, M.; Christiaens, T.; Cifkova, R.; De Backer, G.; Dominiczak, A.; et al. 2013 ESH/ESC Guidelines for the management of arterial hypertension: The Task Force for the management of arterial hypertension of the European Society of Hypertension (ESH) and of the European Society of Cardiology (ESC). *Eur. Heart J.* **2013**, *34*, 2159–2219.
65. Altman, D.; Bland, J. Measurement in Medicine: The Analysis of Method Comparison Studies. *Statistician* **1983**, *32*, 307. [CrossRef]
66. Dogan, N. Bland-Altman analysis: A paradigm to understand correlation and agreement. *Turk. J. Emerg. Med.* **2018**, *18*, 139–141. [CrossRef] [PubMed]
67. Giavarina, D. Understanding Bland Altman analysis. *Biochem. Medica* **2015**, *25*, 141–151. [CrossRef] [PubMed]

sensors

MDPI

Article

Hybrid Integrated Wearable Patch for Brain EEG-fNIRS Monitoring

Boyu Li †, Mingjie Li †, Jie Xia, Hao Jin *, Shurong Dong * and Jikui Luo

Key Laboratory of Advanced Micro/Nano Electronic Devices & Smart Systems of Zhejiang, College of Information Science and Electronic Engineering, Zhejiang University, Hangzhou 310027, China; 12331032@zju.edu.cn (B.L.)

* Correspondence: hjin@zju.edu.cn (H.J.); dongshurong@zju.edu.cn (S.D.)

† These authors contributed equally to this work.

Abstract: Synchronous monitoring electroencephalogram (EEG) and functional near-infrared spectroscopy (fNIRS) have received significant attention in brain science research for their provision of more information on neuro-loop interactions. There is a need for an integrated hybrid EEG-fNIRS patch to synchronously monitor surface EEG and deep brain fNIRS signals. Here, we developed a hybrid EEG-fNIRS patch capable of acquiring high-quality, co-located EEG and fNIRS signals. This patch is wearable and provides easy cognition and emotion detection, while reducing the spatial interference and signal crosstalk by integration, which leads to high spatial–temporal correspondence and signal quality. The modular design of the EEG-fNIRS acquisition unit and optimized mechanical design enables the patch to obtain EEG and fNIRS signals at the same location and eliminates spatial interference. The EEG pre-amplifier on the electrode side effectively improves the acquisition of weak EEG signals and significantly reduces input noise to 0.9 μV_{rms}, amplitude distortion to less than 2%, and frequency distortion to less than 1%. Detrending, motion correction algorithms, and band-pass filtering were used to remove physiological noise, baseline drift, and motion artifacts from the fNIRS signal. A high fNIRS source switching frequency configuration above 100 Hz improves crosstalk suppression between fNIRS and EEG signals. The Stroop task was carried out to verify its performance; the patch can acquire event-related potentials and hemodynamic information associated with cognition in the prefrontal area.

Keywords: co-located; EEG-fNIRS; noise suppression; crosstalk suppression; acquisition module design; acquisition module mechanical design

1. Introduction

Electroencephalogram (EEG) and functional near-infrared spectroscopy (fNIRS) dual-modal synchronous brain signal monitoring systems can accurately and continuously measure the neuronal electrical signal of the surface area and hemodynamic activity of the brain deep area. It combines the advantages of the high spatial resolution of fNIRS and high temporal resolution of EEG to provide a comprehensive picture of brain function [1]. EEG-fNIRS systems have been applied across various fields of brain science. Clinically, EEG-fNIRS systems have been proven to provide important diagnostic information for the evaluation or treatment of stroke [2], seizure [3], and Alzheimer's disease [4], among other diseases [5,6]. In the field of brain–computer interfaces (BCIs) [7,8], the EEG-fNIRS system has been utilized to fabricate a hybrid BCI (hBCI) to improve classification accuracy [9,10]. To better study the spatiotemporal associations between the hemodynamic–electrical patterns of brain functions and further improve the classification and decoding accuracy of BCIs, co-located EEG-fNIRS signals attract attention because of their high spatial and temporal coupling and adaptation to tight time synchronization requirements [11].

In order to obtain functional imaging of EEG and fNIRS simultaneously, many discrete or integrated EEG-fNIRS systems or ICs have been developed, such as discrete commercial EEG systems and fNIRS systems and combined EEG-fNIRS system [12], NIRS/EEG monitoring of ASIC [13], and modular hybrid systems [14]. However, acquiring co-located EEG-fNIRS signals still remains a challenge due to the spatial interference between the EEG and fNIRS acquisition modules, signal crosstalk between EEG-fNIRS signals, and signal synchronization problems. Especially, as shown Figure 1, the prefrontal cortex region, which is related to cognition and emotions, needs to be monitored via simultaneous EEG and fNIRS signals in a limited area.

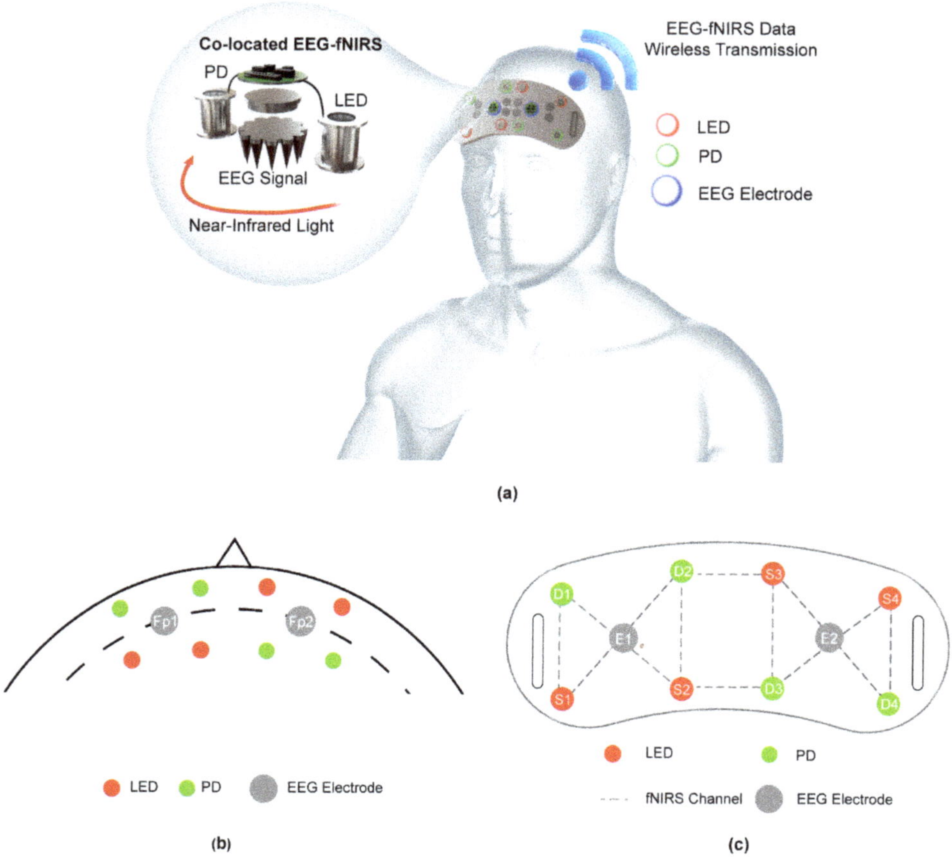

Figure 1. (**a**) Overall system architecture. (**b**) Layout of EEG and fNIRS sensors. (**c**) Positioning structure of EEG electrodes, LEDs, and PDs.

In this article, we report an integrated EEG-fNIRS patch with a novel circuit architecture and optimized acquisition module design, which can achieve two-channel EEG and ten-channel fNIRS measurements simultaneously. The patch achieves synchronized, low-noise, and low-crosstalk EEG-fNIRS acquisition by integrating the following features and structures.

- EEG-fNIRS acquisition module design and optimized mechanical design enables the acquisition module to obtain EEG and fNIRS signals at the same location and eliminates spatial interference, while increasing the scalability of the patch.

- EEG pre-amplifier design is utilized on the electrode side for EEG preprocessing, which can effectively improve weak EEG signal acquisition and noise suppression.
- ADS1299- and AFE4404-based analog front-end (AFE) architecture is designed, which achieves synchronous, high-resolution EEG and fNIRS signal measurements.
- Crosstalk between fNIRS signals and EEG signals is minimized through above 100 Hz high LED switching frequency configuration.

Several evaluation tests were performed to verify the co-located EEG-fNIRS hybrid data acquisition performance. We demonstrate that the patch performs with low input noise (0.9 V_{rms}), low frequency distortion (<1%), and low amplitude distortion (<2%). Based on these ideal properties, we show that the developed patch can acquire event-related potentials and hemodynamic information at prefrontal areas in the event-related Stroop task. Our approach provides a step towards highly coupled spatial and temporal EEG-fNIRS signal acquisition, laying the foundation for the comprehensive exploration of brain functional activity.

2. Materials and Methods

2.1. Overall System Architecture

The overall system architecture is shown in Figure 1a. This patch was used to support the co-located EEG-fNIRS signal acquisition in the forehead, and provides synchronous, low-noise, and low-crosstalk dual-mode signal acquisition while realizing integration and wireless data transmission. As shown in Figure 1b, according to the international 10–20 system, two EEG electrodes were placed at Fp1 and Fp2. Four optical sources and four optical detectors were located over the prefrontal area around Fp1, Fpz, and Fp2.

As shown in Figure 1c, in order to acquire neuronal activity from the same location, the EEG electrode was placed in the middle between the source (LED) and the detector (PD), so as to achieve the same channel configuration [15]. An LED was used as the light source because it can be directly attached to the scalp without fiber cables, which greatly increases the flexibility of the acquisition module layout. Each LED can provide 1 fNIRS channel, which has the same acquisition location as the EEG channel. And, 4 fNIRS channels were placed at the same acquisition location as the EEG channel. This patch can provide a total of 10 fNIRS channels and 2 EEG channels, in which 4 fNIRS channels are at the same acquisition location as the EEG channel. The patch can measure the EEG and fNIRS signals at Fp1 and Fp2 simultaneously while covering the active frontal brain regions as much as possible [16], which can support the monitoring needs of cerebral hemodynamic response and EEG response in depressive disorder, cognitive event classification, and other cognitive or emotional tasks [17,18].

2.2. System Design

EEG and fNIRS signals are highly sensitive to noise and prone to crosstalk. Therefore, the hardware architecture illustrated in Figure 2a has been designed to improve small-amplitude EEG signals acquisition, noise, and crosstalk suppression, which is in concordance with the system concept of "co-located EEG and fNIRS acquisition". As is shown in Figure 2a, EEG electrodes, LEDs, and detectors were integrated into separate EEG-fNIRS acquisition modules. This allows the monitoring range to be extended to the whole brain by simply adding EEG-fNIRS acquisition modules. The patch implements in this paper contains 4 EEG-fNIRS acquisition modules and 1 main board.

The acquired EEG signal was firstly processed by the EEG pre-circuit on the EEG-fNIRS acquisition module illustrated in Figure 2a. The EEG pre-circuit included a two-stage filter and amplifier circuit. High-frequency noise was filtered out using an OPA333-based active low-pass filter with a cutoff frequency of 50 Hz.

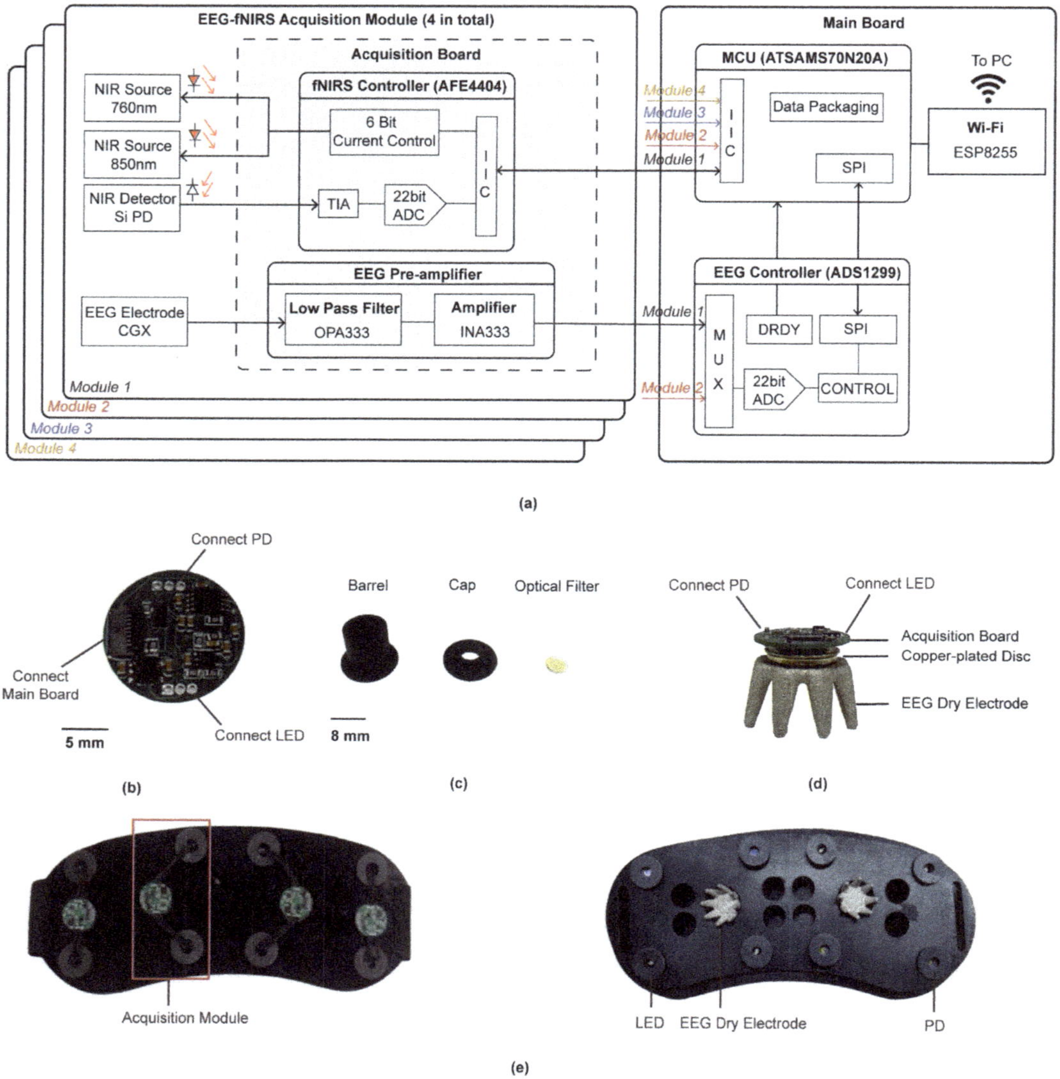

Figure 2. (**a**) The system circuit block diagram. (**b**) The proposed acquisition board. (**c**) The barrel, cap, and optical filter to fix the LED and PD. (**d**) The EEG-fNIRS acquisition module of the proposed patch. (**e**) Front and back view of the entire patch.

An INA333-based signal amplifier was employed to provide a voltage gain of 1000 v/v (60 dB), which was capable of improving the acquisition performance of small amplitude EEG signals and providing high input impedance (100 GΩ). EEG signals from multiple acquisition modules were fed into ADS1299 in parallel, and the multiplexer in ADS1299 allows low-crosstalk, multi-channel synchronous input without sampling and holding circuits, which improved the integration of the patch. Digitized by a 24-bit resolution ADC, the EEG signals were transmitted to MCU via an SPI bus. The module can acquire EEG signals at a sampling rate up to 16 kSPS.

The acquired bio-optical signal was input into AFE4404 on the acquisition module, converted into a voltage signal by an integrated transimpedance amplifier (TIA), and then digitized by an integrated 24-bit analog-to-digital converter (ADC). The high dynamic range (100 dB) enables an excellent signal to noise ratio (SNR), even for small amplitude bio-optical signals in the presence of large signal artifacts. The ADC data were subsequently transmitted to the micro controller unit (MCU) via an IIC bus. The module can acquire fNIRS signals at a sampling rate up to 100 Hz. The switching time between the two measured wavelengths was controlled by the "Data Ready" pin (DRDY) of ADS1299 to ensure that synchronization between EEG and bio-optical signals can be obtained even if there are errors in the reference clocks of the two AFEs.

As shown in Figure 2d, the LEDs and PDs were are connected to the acquisition board by wire, and a copper-plated disk was used to connect the EEG electrodes and the acquisition board to form an EEG-fNIRS acquisition module.

The whole system was embedded in a framework made up of an ATSAMS70N20A (Microchip) MCU on the main board. A detailed diagram of the signal processing workflow can be found in Figures S1 and S2. The MCU will send the packetized EEG and fNIRS data to the PC via the external ESP8285 module for further processing. Please see Note S1 for details of the data processing flow in the PC.

LEDs of 760 nm and 850 nm dual-wavelengths (Ushio epitex L760_850−04A) were used for fNIRS light sources. Each LED adopted wavelength time division multiplexing. Silicon photodiodes (Hamamatsu S5972) were used for fNIRS detectors. The PD exhibited high photoelectric sensitivity (>0.5 A/W) at both 760 nm and 850 nm while having the features of small size, low power dissipation, and a high level of noise suppression. As shown in Figure 2c, the fNIRS light sources and detectors were fixed using a probe. Each probe is consisted of a circular filter (LP900), a 3D-printed cap, and a 3D-printed barrel. The circular filter uses long-wave pass filter, which meets the high transmittance of emitted light at 760 nm and 850 nm while filtering out ambient light interference signals.

A claw-shaped dry electrode (CGX) was used for EEG acquisition [19]. The electrode was small in size, easy to install, and the surface was plated with a Ag/AgCl layer, which helped to realize miniaturization and high integration, overcoming the problem of signal quality degradation and the discomfort of the participants in continuous EEG acquisition based on traditional wet electrodes. The dry electrode can support continuous high-quality acquisition for a long time (>30 min) and provides high user comfort and reusability.

Considering the wearing comfortability and convenience of the participant, 3D printing was used to make the fixing belt shown in Figure 2e. The fixing belt was made of thermoplastic polyurethane (TPU), which has good flexibility and flexibility, and ensured that the EEG dry electrodes, LEDs, and PDs closely fit the skin on the forehead.

2.3. System Crosstalk Analysis and Suppression

The co-located dual-modal signal acquisition patch will introduce crosstalk between the dual-modal signals. In fact, for example, the instantaneously high current in fNIRS light source driving circuit can easily distort small-amplitude EEG and bio-optical signals [20]. A previous study also showed that switching of NIRS channels may cause high-amplitude noise in the same frequency of EEG, which would cause misjudgment of real neural activity [21]. Therefore, when designing an integrated EEG-fNIRS system, crosstalk between EEG signals and fNIRS signals must be taken into account. In our proposed patch, hardware architecture and software configuration were carefully designed to minimize crosstalk between the dual-modal signals.

To minimize crosstalk between fNIRS signals and EEG signals, first, the LED current switching frequency of the dual-wavelength LED current was configured to be >100 Hz, which far exceeds the EEG frequency band of interest (0–50 Hz), so the crosstalk related to the EEG signal could be clearly separated using a low-pass filter with a cutoff frequency of 50 Hz. Second, integrated EEG AFE circuits on the main board also provided higher crosstalk suppression performance for EEG signals by current path optimization and shielding optimization.

The crosstalk between the EEG signal and fNIRS signal was also minimized by a separate ground design on the acquisition board, ensuring electrical isolation of the EEG and fNIRS signals.

3. Evaluation and Experimental Procedure

3.1. Evaluation of EEG Acquisition Performance

We first evaluated the input-referred noise of the EEG acquisition circuit in the LED flashing condition and in the no-LED flashing condition. As shown in Figure 3a, it can be found that in the absence of LED flashing, the input-referred noise was 0.81 μV_{rms}. Even with the LED flashing condition, an input-referred noise of 0.89 μV_{rms} was measured and no fNIRS crosstalk component was observed in the spectrum in Figure 3b. These results show that the proposed patch has an excellent noise suppression performance of less than 0.9 μV_{rms}. In addition, we evaluated the amplitude distortion and frequency distortion of the acquired EEG signals. As shown in Figure 3c,d, the amplitude distortion and the frequency distortion were less than 2% and less than 1%, respectively. The results verify that the measured EEG signals have low frequency distortion and amplitude distortion. The EEG acquisition module is capable of obtaining high-quality EEG signals. More details about the evaluation experiment can be found in Note S2.

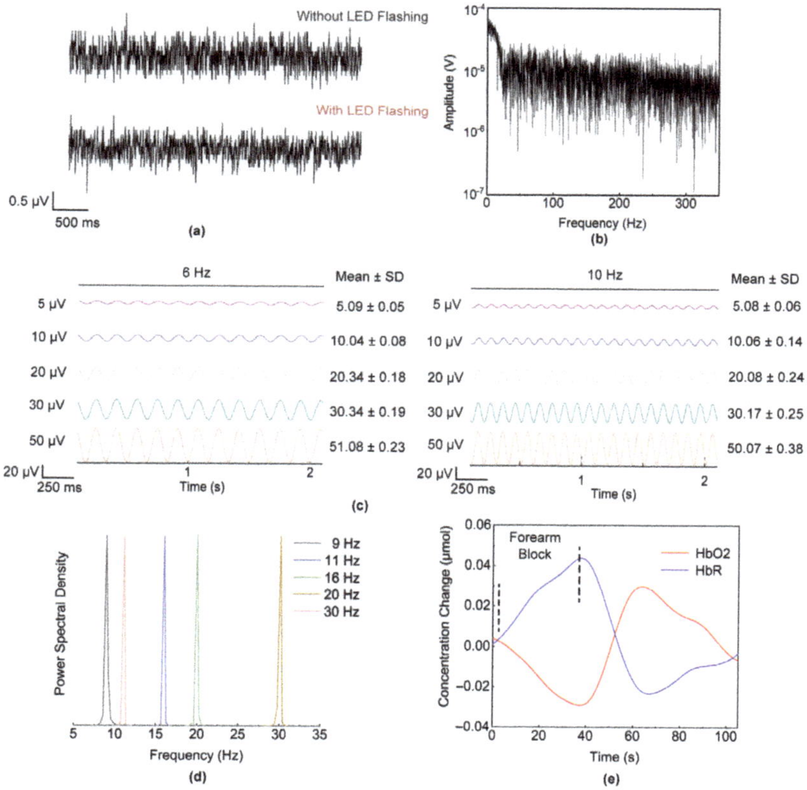

Figure 3. (**a**) EEG input-referred noise in no-LED flashing condition and LED flashing condition; (**b**) EEG input-referred noise spectrum in LED flashing condition; (**c**) EEG amplitude distortion measurement; (**d**) EEG frequency distortion measurement; and (**e**) ΔHbO_2, ΔHbR trend in forearm block experiment.

3.2. Evaluation of fNIRS Acquisition Performance

Referring to the experiment in [20,22], a forearm block experiment was performed to verify the performance of fNIRS acquisition. The experiment was carried out in a quiet laboratory with no strong light interference. The participants put their arm flat on the table with palm facing up and the wristband was tied to the participant's forearm. fNIRS light sources and detectors were attached to the participant's forearm.

We obtained the ΔHbO_2 and ΔHbR values by analyzing the fNIRS data and the results are plotted in Figure 3d. When the wristband sphygmomanometer was inflated, ΔHbO_2 dropped slowly and ΔHbR rose slowly due to blood blockage in the forearm. When the wristband sphygmomanometer was deflated and the forearm blood flow was released again, ΔHbO_2 and ΔHbR dramatically changed toward the baseline, overshooting occurred, and then they gradually converged to the baseline. The experimental results can be mutually verified with the results of the previous forearm blocking experiment [20], indicating that the patch can effectively collect changes in human hemodynamics.

3.3. Event-Related Stroop Task

To further validate the ability to acquire the co-located EEG-fNIRS signals, referring to the experiment in [22], an event-related Chinese character Stroop task was designed. The experimental paradigm was used to induce conflicts in cognitive psychology and the activation in participant's prefrontal cortex can be assessed by EEG and fNIRS signals.

As shown in Figure 4a, the stimuli consisted of a Chinese character with the same or different color and meaning. Under the interference of the meaning of the character, the participants were instructed to judge the color of the Chinese character and press the corresponding key on the keyboard with the right index finger within the time limit. Each task comprised 30 trials, with on-third of trials being congruent (the color and meaning coincided, e.g., the character means "Red" printed in the color red) and two-thirds of trials being incongruent (the word and color did not coincide, e.g., the character means "Red" printed in the color green). The congruent trial and incongruent trial were administered randomly. Each trial was displayed for 500 ms, with a randomly selected interval of 350–750 ms between trials. A detailed experimental design for the event-related Stroop task can be found in Note S3.

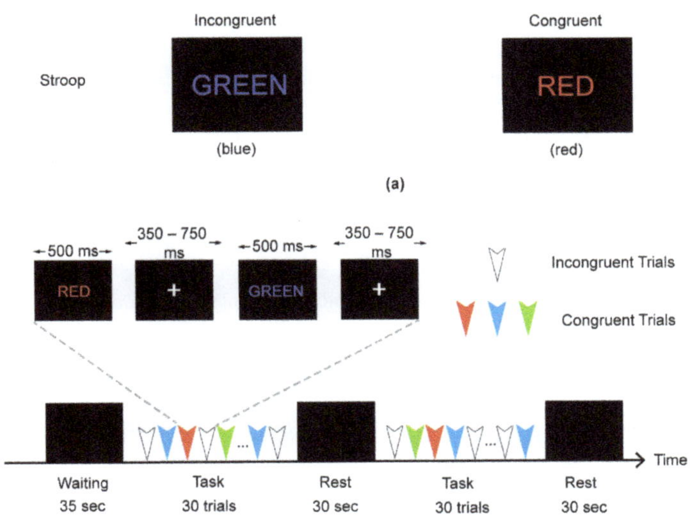

Figure 4. (**a**) Schematic diagram of incongruent and congruent trial. (**b**) Experimental paradigm for Stroop task.

The experimental paradigm flow used in this study is shown in Figure 4b. The experimental paradigm was divided into a waiting period, task period, and rest period. During the task period, participants were asked to perform the Stroop task. During the waiting period and rest period, the participants were asked to remain in a relaxed state.

Thirteen healthy volunteers (right-handed, native Chinese speakers, aged 20–29 years; four women and nine men) participated in this experiment. All participants had normal or corrected-to-normal vision, normal color vision, and normal cognitive function. Each participant was seated on an adjustable chair in a sound- and light-attenuated room. The PC monitor was placed 65 cm in front of the participant's eyes. As shown in Figure 1a, the acquisition module of the EEG-fNIRS patch was worn on the forehead of the participant to acquire EEG signals and fNIRS signals at Fp1 and Fp2. Prior to the formal experiment, participants were asked to run eight trials to make sure they were familiar with the experimental process and could respond correctly. During the experiment, the patch collected EEG signals and fNIRS signals at a sampling rate of 1 kHz and 100 Hz, respectively.

The original EEG signal was analyzed using MATLAB 2023a. Epochs were extracted ranging from −250 ms before to 750 ms after stimulus onset, and baseline signal from −250 ms to 0 ms were corrected. After that, the averaged event-related potentials (ERPs) were band-pass filtered with a cut-off frequency of 0.8 Hz to 17 Hz. On the basis of ERP data, three feature-based components, P450 (positive component from 400 to 450 ms), N500 (negative component from 450 to 550 ms), and P600 (positive component from 600 to 700 ms), were measured at Fp1 and Fp2.

Figure 5a shows the raw EEG data of Fp1 and Fp2. And, the ERP results from a trial are shown in Figure 5b. Figure 5c shows the average amplitude of three ERP components in Fp1 and Fp2 across all trials. The amplitude of P450 was -2.70 ± 0.14 and -2.63 ± 0.16 μV (Mean ± SD) in Fp1 and Fp2, respectively, while the amplitude of N500 component was -4.05 ± 0.20 and -4.37 ± 0.25 μV (Mean ± SD) in Fp1 and Fp2, respectively. And, the amplitude of P600 was -2.06 ± 0.27 and -1.67 ± 0.19 μV (Mean ± SD) in Fp1 and Fp2, respectively. Repeated measure analysis of variance (ANOVA) indicated statistically significant differences between the N500 component at the right prefrontal cortex and left prefrontal cortex ($p = 0.03 < 0.05$) and the P600 component at the right prefrontal cortex and left prefrontal cortex ($p = 0.042 < 0.05$). N500 had a stronger response at Fp2, and compared to right prefrontal cortex, P600 had a stronger response at Fp1. The P450 component at the right prefrontal cortex and left prefrontal cortex were not significantly different from each other ($p = 0.31 > 0.05$). The results shows that three ERP components activated in the forehead, which is consistent with the experimental phenomena in the previous literature obtained by the proposed patch [23].

Event-related fNIRS signals are highly susceptible to interference from physiological noise (e.g., 0.2–0.3 Hz respiration component, ~1 Hz heartbeat component, and ~0.1 Hz Mayer waves component) and motion artifacts [24]. Therefore, detrending, motion correction and band-pass filtering are used to remove physiological noise, baseline drift, and motion artifacts from the original fNIRS signal. As shown in Figure 5d, firstly, the modified Beer–Lambert law was utilized to calculate the concentration changes of oxygenated hemoglobin (HbO_2), deoxygenated hemoglobin (HbR), and total hemoglobin (HbT) according to the calculation method in previous studies [25]. Then, a first-order polynomial regression model was used to remove linear detrends and a temporal derivative distribution repair (TDDR)-based motion correction function was used to remove both spike artifacts and baseline shifts. Considering the hemodynamic response after neural activation embedded in 0.03–0.1 Hz [26], a third-order band-pass IIR filter with a cut-off frequency of 0.01 Hz to 0.08 Hz was applied to remove physiological noise components.

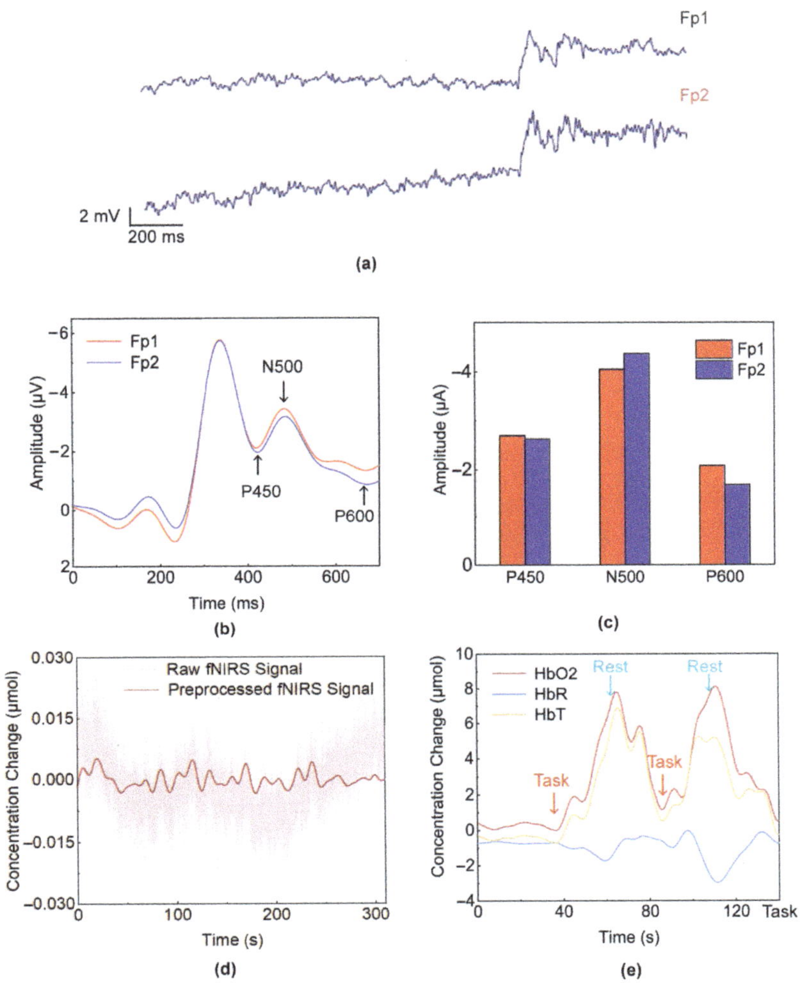

Figure 5. (**a**) Raw EEG data of Fp1 and Fp2; (**b**) ERP results in a trial; (**c**) average amplitude of three ERP components in Fp1 and Fp2; (**d**) comparison of original fNIRS signal and preprocessed fNIRS signal; and (**e**) the ΔHbO2, ΔHbR, and ΔHbT values of the brain Fp1 point in the Stroop task.

The ΔHbO_2, ΔHbR, and ΔHbT values of the brain Fp1 point and Fp2 point collected in fNIRS channels D1-S2 and D4-S3 (shown in Figure 1c), respectively, are shown in Figure 5e. During the waiting period, the concentrations of both HbO_2 and HbR remained stable. When the first Stoop task began, the HbO_2 concentration increased rapidly. At the cessation of the task and entry into the rest period, the HbO_2 concentration gradually returned to the baseline level. During this process, the concentration of HbR showed a roughly opposite trend to the change in the concentration of HbO_2, which is consistent with the analysis of the mechanism of neural–vascular coupling. It can also be found that the change in the concentration of HbR is smaller than the change in the concentration of HbO_2. From the perspective of brain activity, when the Stroop task starts, there is an increase in the oxygen demand of the prefrontal cortex involved in cognitive activity, which primarily leads to an increase in cerebral arterial blood flow and dominates the changes in local blood oxygen concentration, and this leads to an increase in HbT. In arterial blood, the proportion of HbO_2 is higher, which leads to a higher increase in the concentration of

HbO_2 than in the proportion of HbR. Additionally, Pearson correlation analysis showed that the peak amplitude of P600 at Fp1 had a strong correlation with the second peak value of ΔHbR (r = 0.752, $p = 0.009 < 0.01$). The peak amplitude of N500 at Fp1 also had a significant correlation with the first peak value of ΔHbR (r = 0.724, $p = 0.012$). However, peak amplitudes of P450 were not found to correlate with any peak of ΔHbR or ΔHbO_2. Therefore, a linear regression model can be established using the peak amplitude of P600 and N500 and peak values of ΔHbR to represent the hemodynamic–electrical patterns of brain functions. These conclusions are in good agreement with the findings in [23].

The co-located EEG and fNIRS signals in the Stroop task were effectively detected by our proposed patch, providing brain activation information such as the ERP response and trend in the ΔHbO_2, ΔHbR response. A conclusion can be drawn that the proposed EEG-fNIRS patch was capable of acquiring neuroelectric and hemodynamic responses at the same location.

4. Conclusions

In this study, a two-channel EEG and ten-channel fNIRS hybrid EEG-fNIRS brain monitoring patch has been proposed that can measure EEG and brain cerebral hemodynamic information at the same location. As shown in Table 1, compared with previous research, the proposed EEG-fNIRS acquisition module design and optimized acquisition module layout can acquire co-located EEG-fNIRS signals while eliminating spatial location interference, which can also easily extend the acquisition range to the whole brain. The EEG pre-amplifier on the electrode side effectively provided a high EEG signal noise suppression capability of less than 0.9 μV_{rms}, low-amplitude distortion to less than 2%, and low-frequency distortion to less than 1%. Moreover, high LED switching frequency configuration greatly reduces the high crosstalk between bio-optical signals and EEG signals. In addition, detrending, motion correction, and band-pass filter design effectively removed physiological noise, baseline drift, and motion artifacts, effectively improving the SNR. The forearm block experiment and Stroop task showed that the system is sufficiently capable for acquiring neuronal electrical signal and hemodynamic activity at the same location. The small size (about 78.54 mm^2) and lightweight (about 21.8 g) EEG-fNIRS acquisition module, EEG dry electrodes, and TPU flexible fixing belt can ensure long-term monitoring and wearing comfort to meet the co-located EEG-fNIRS acquisition needs of emotional or cognitive tasks or patients with mild cognitive impairment and major depressive disorder in the home or clinic. It is expected to provide new information and phenomena that cannot be detected when EEG and fNIRS are measured at separate locations, offering richer data for the comprehensive exploration of brain functional activities and introducing new signal acquisition methods for EEG-fNIRS research.

A limitation of our proposed system is that our EEG and fNIRS channels were limited and only covered the forehead, compared to discrete commercial EEG systems, fNIRS systems, and combined EEG-fNIRS system. Although our highly scalable acquisition module design can quickly extend the acquisition range to the whole brain, the low SNR caused by hair absorption and occlusion still limits its application in motor imagery, visual stimulation, and other clinical applications where hemodynamic measurements are required in parietal, occipital, or temporal lobe regions. In addition, a newly designed fixing belt is also needed to ensure that EEG measurements conform to the international 10–20 system. However, the current system has met our design goal of using a wearable, portable patch that allows high-quality acquisition of co-located EEG-fNIRS signals to support cognitive and emotional measurements at the prefrontal lobe. Therefore, our next steps should focus on how to reconstruct fNIRS signals impaired by extra-cranial confounds using both algorithms and hardware approaches to improve the usability of the system for brain–computer interfaces and brain research.

Table 1. Comparison of features between the proposed and previous EEG-fNIRS systems.

System	[13]	[14]	[20]	[27]	[28]	Our Work
EEG input-referred noise	1.21 μV_{rms}	1.39 μV_{pp}	0.14 μV_{rms}	29.9 μV_{rms}	0.44 μV_{rms}	0.89 μV_{rms}
EEG sampling rate	-	16 kSPS	250 Hz	250 SPS	2 kSPS	16 kSPS
fNIRS sampling rate	512 SPS	500 SPS	5 Hz	8 SPS	10 Hz	100 Hz
EEG resolution	15	24	24	24	12	24
fNIRS resolution	-	24	16	24	12	24
Dry EEG electrode	No	No	Yes	No	Yes	Yes
Co-located EEG/fNIRS acquisition	Yes	No	No	No	No	Yes
Crosstalk suppression	No	Yes	Yes	Yes	No	Yes
fNIRS physiological noise removal	16 Hz Low-pass filter	-	RC Low-pass filter	Low-pass filter	-	0.01–0.08 Hz Band-pass filter
fNIRS detrending	-	-	Baseline correction	-	-	First-order polynomial regression
fNIRS motion artifacts removal	-	-	-	-	-	TDDR

- This parameter is not provided in the reference.

Supplementary Materials: The following supporting information can be downloaded at: https://www.mdpi.com/article/10.3390/s24154847/s1, Figure S1: EEG signal processing workflow. Figure S2: fNIRS signal processing workflow. Note S1: EEG and fNIRS data processing process in PC. Note S2: EEG acquisition performance evaluation method. Note S3: Experimental design for the event-related Stroop task.

Author Contributions: Conceptualization, B.L. and J.X.; Data curation, B.L.; Formal analysis, B.L., M.L. and J.X.; Funding acquisition, H.J. and S.D.; Investigation, B.L.; Methodology, B.L., M.L. and J.X.; Project administration, H.J. and S.D.; Resources, B.L.; Software, B.L. and M.L.; Supervision, H.J., S.D. and J.L.; Validation, B.L. and M.L.; Visualization, B.L.; Writing—original draft, B.L.; Writing—review and editing, B.L., H.J., S.D. and J.L. All authors have read and agreed to the published version of the manuscript.

Funding: This research was funded by Zhejiang Province Key R & D programs (No. 2024C03001) and Zhejiang Province high-level talent special support plan (No.2022R52042).

Institutional Review Board Statement: This study was conducted in accordance with the Declaration of Helsinki and approved by the Ethics Committee of the Women's Hospital, School of Medicine, Zhejiang University, Hangzhou, China (protocol ID: No. 067 (2019)) for studies involving humans.

Informed Consent Statement: Informed consent was obtained from all participants involved in this study.

Data Availability Statement: The source data and source code for this article are available on GitHub. Please visit: https://github.com/Shirakami114514/Hybrid-integrated-wearable-patch-for-brain-EEG-fNIRS-monitoring (accessed on 22 July 2024).

Conflicts of Interest: The authors declare no conflicts of interest.

References

1. Han, C.-H.; Muller, K.-R.; Hwang, H.-J. Enhanced Performance of a Brain Switch by Simultaneous Use of EEG and NIRS Data for Asynchronous Brain-Computer Interface. *IEEE Trans. Neural Syst. Rehabil. Eng.* **2020**, *28*, 2102–2112. [CrossRef]
2. Li, R.; Li, S.; Roh, J.; Wang, C.; Zhang, Y. Multimodal Neuroimaging Using Concurrent EEG/fNIRS for Poststroke Recovery Assessment: An Exploratory Study. *Neurorehabil. Neural Repair.* **2020**, *34*, 1099–1110. [CrossRef]
3. Sirpal, P.; Kassab, A.; Pouliot, P.; Nguyen, D.K. fNIRS Improves Seizure Detection in Multimodal EEG-fNIRS Recordings. *J. Biomed. Opt.* **2019**, *24*, 1. [CrossRef] [PubMed]
4. Perpetuini, D.; Chiarelli, A.M.; Filippini, C.; Cardone, D.; Croce, P.; Rotunno, L.; Anzoletti, N.; Zito, M.; Zappasodi, F.; Merla, A. Working Memory Decline in Alzheimer's Disease Is Detected by Complexity Analysis of Multimodal EEG-fNIRS. *Entropy* **2020**, *22*, 1380. [CrossRef] [PubMed]
5. Khan, H.; Naseer, N.; Yazidi, A.; Eide, P.K.; Hassan, H.W.; Mirtaheri, P. Analysis of Human Gait Using Hybrid EEG-fNIRS-Based BCI System: A Review. *Front. Hum. Neurosci.* **2021**, *14*, 613254. [CrossRef] [PubMed]
6. Gentile, E.; Brunetti, A.; Ricci, K.; Delussi, M.; Bevilacqua, V.; De Tommaso, M. Mutual Interaction between Motor Cortex Activation and Pain in Fibromyalgia: EEG-fNIRS Study. *PLoS ONE* **2020**, *15*, e0228158. [CrossRef] [PubMed]

7. Maher, A.; Mian Qaisar, S.; Salankar, N.; Jiang, F.; Tadeusiewicz, R.; Pławiak, P.; Abd El-Latif, A.A.; Hammad, M. Hybrid EEG-fNIRS Brain-Computer Interface Based on the Non-Linear Features Extraction and Stacking Ensemble Learning. *Biocybern. Biomed. Eng.* **2023**, *43*, 463–475. [CrossRef]
8. Kwon, J.; Shin, J.; Im, C.-H. Toward a Compact Hybrid Brain-Computer Interface (BCI): Performance Evaluation of Multi-Class Hybrid EEG-fNIRS BCIs with Limited Number of Channels. *PLoS ONE* **2020**, *15*, e0230491. [CrossRef] [PubMed]
9. Khan, M.U.; Hasan, M.A.H. Hybrid EEG-fNIRS BCI Fusion Using Multi-Resolution Singular Value Decomposition (MSVD). *Front. Hum. Neurosci.* **2020**, *14*, 599802. [CrossRef]
10. Ghonchi, H.; Fateh, M.; Abolghasemi, V.; Ferdowsi, S.; Rezvani, M. Deep Recurrent–Convolutional Neural Network for Classification of Simultaneous EEG–fNIRS Signals. *IET Signal Process.* **2020**, *14*, 142–153. [CrossRef]
11. Casson, A.J. Wearable EEG and Beyond. *Biomed. Eng. Lett.* **2019**, *9*, 53–71. [CrossRef] [PubMed]
12. Cicalese, P.A.; Li, R.; Ahmadi, M.B.; Wang, C.; Francis, J.T.; Selvaraj, S.; Schulz, P.E.; Zhang, Y. An EEG-fNIRS Hybridization Technique in the Four-Class Classification of Alzheimer's Disease. *J. Neurosci. Methods* **2020**, *336*, 108618. [CrossRef]
13. Xu, J.; Konijnenburg, M.; Song, S.; Ha, H.; Van Wegberg, R.; Mazzillo, M.; Fallica, G.; Van Hoof, C.; De Raedt, W.; Van Helleputte, N. A 665 μW Silicon Photomultiplier-Based NIRS/EEG/EIT Monitoring ASIC for Wearable Functional Brain Imaging. *IEEE Trans. Biomed. Circuits Syst.* **2018**, *12*, 1267–1277. [CrossRef]
14. Von Luhmann, A.; Wabnitz, H.; Sander, T.; Muller, K.-R. M3BA: A Mobile, Modular, Multimodal Biosignal Acquisition Architecture for Miniaturized EEG-NIRS-Based Hybrid BCI and Monitoring. *IEEE Trans. Biomed. Eng.* **2017**, *64*, 1199–1210. [CrossRef] [PubMed]
15. Ahn, S.; Jun, S.C. Multi-Modal Integration of EEG-fNIRS for Brain-Computer Interfaces—Current Limitations and Future Directions. *Front. Hum. Neurosci.* **2017**, *11*, 503. [CrossRef]
16. Blum, S.; Emkes, R.; Minow, F.; Anlauff, J.; Finke, A.; Debener, S. Flex-Printed Forehead EEG Sensors (fEEGrid) for Long-Term EEG Acquisition. *J. Neural Eng.* **2020**, *17*, 034003. [CrossRef]
17. Yi, L.; Xie, G.; Li, Z.; Li, X.; Zhang, Y.; Wu, K.; Shao, G.; Lv, B.; Jing, H.; Zhang, C.; et al. Automatic Depression Diagnosis through Hybrid EEG and Near-Infrared Spectroscopy Features Using Support Vector Machine. *Front. Neurosci.* **2023**, *17*, 1205931. [CrossRef] [PubMed]
18. Chen, J.; Xia, Y.; Zhou, X.; Vidal Rosas, E.; Thomas, A.; Loureiro, R.; Cooper, R.J.; Carlson, T.; Zhao, H. fNIRS-EEG BCIs for Motor Rehabilitation: A Review. *Bioengineering* **2023**, *10*, 1393. [CrossRef] [PubMed]
19. Lin, S.; Jiang, J.; Huang, K.; Li, L.; He, X.; Du, P.; Wu, Y.; Liu, J.; Li, X.; Huang, Z.; et al. Advanced Electrode Technologies for Noninvasive Brain–Computer Interfaces. *ACS Nano* **2023**, *17*, 24487–24513. [CrossRef]
20. Lee, S.; Shin, Y.; Kumar, A.; Kim, M.; Lee, H.-N. Dry Electrode-Based Fully Isolated EEG/fNIRS Hybrid Brain-Monitoring System. *IEEE Trans. Biomed. Eng.* **2019**, *66*, 1055–1068. [CrossRef]
21. Von Luhmann, A.; Muller, K.-R. Why Build an Integrated EEG-NIRS? About the Advantages of Hybrid Bio-Acquisition Hardware. In Proceedings of the 2017 39th Annual International Conference of the IEEE Engineering in Medicine and Biology Society (EMBC), Jeju, Republic of Korea, 11–15 July 2017; IEEE: Jeju, Republic of Korea, 2017; pp. 4475–4478.
22. Lei, H.; Yi, J.; Wang, H.; Zhang, X.; Dong, J.; Zhou, C.; Fan, J.; Zhong, M.; Zhu, X. Inhibitory Deficit in Semantic Conflict in Obsessive–Compulsive Disorder: An Event-Related Potential Study. *Neurosci. Lett.* **2013**, *552*, 162–167. [CrossRef]
23. Zhai, J.; Li, T.; Zhang, Z.; Gong, H. Hemodynamic and Electrophysiological Signals of Conflict Processing in the Chinese-Character Stroop Task: A Simultaneous near-Infrared Spectroscopy and Event-Related Potential Study. *J. Biomed. Opt.* **2009**, *14*, 054022. [CrossRef]
24. Nguyen, H.-D.; Yoo, S.-H.; Bhutta, M.R.; Hong, K.-S. Adaptive Filtering of Physiological Noises in fNIRS Data. *Biomed. Eng. Online* **2018**, *17*, 180. [CrossRef]
25. Kocsis, L.; Herman, P.; Eke, A. The Modified Beer–Lambert Law Revisited. *Phys. Med. Biol.* **2006**, *51*, N91–N98. [CrossRef]
26. Rahman, M.A.; Rashid, M.A.; Ahmad, M. Selecting the Optimal Conditions of Savitzky–Golay Filter for fNIRS Signal. *Biocybern. Biomed. Eng.* **2019**, *39*, 624–637. [CrossRef]
27. Mohamed, M.; Jo, E.; Mohamed, N.; Kim, M.; Yun, J.; Kim, J.G. Development of an Integrated EEG/fNIRS Brain Function Monitoring System. *Sensors* **2021**, *21*, 7703. [CrossRef]
28. Ha, U.; Lee, J.; Kim, M.; Roh, T.; Choi, S.; Yoo, H.-J. An EEG-NIRS Multimodal SoC for Accurate Anesthesia Depth Monitoring. *IEEE J. Solid-State Circuits* **2018**, *53*, 1830–1843. [CrossRef]

sensors

MDPI

Article

Assessment of Physiological Signals from Photoplethysmography Sensors Compared to an Electrocardiogram Sensor: A Validation Study in Daily Life

Rana Zia Ur Rehman [1], Meenakshi Chatterjee [2,*], Nikolay V. Manyakov [3], Melina Daans [3], Amanda Jackson [4], Andrea O'Brisky [5], Tacie Telesky [5], Sophie Smets [3], Pieter-Jan Berghmans [3], Dongyan Yang [4], Elena Reynoso [6], Molly V. Lucas [6], Yanran Huo [7], Vasanth T. Thirugnanam [8], Tommaso Mansi [7] and Mark Morris [6]

1 Janssen Research & Development, Buckinghamshire HP12 4EG, UK
2 Janssen Research & Development, Cambridge, MA 02142, USA
3 Janssen Research & Development, 2340 Beerse, Belgium
4 Janssen Research & Development, LLC, San Diego, CA 92121, USA
5 Janssen Research & Development, Raritan, NJ 08869, USA
6 Janssen Research & Development, Spring House, PA 19477, USA
7 Janssen Research & Development, Titusville, NJ 08560, USA
8 Janssen Research & Development, Brisbane, CA 94005, USA
* Correspondence: mchatte4@its.jnj.com

Abstract: Wearables with photoplethysmography (PPG) sensors are being increasingly used in clinical research as a non-invasive, inexpensive method for remote monitoring of physiological health. Ensuring the accuracy and reliability of PPG-derived measurements is critical, as inaccuracies can impact research findings and clinical decisions. This paper systematically compares heart rate (HR) and heart rate variability (HRV) measures from PPG against an electrocardiogram (ECG) monitor in free-living settings. Two devices with PPG and one device with an ECG sensor were worn by 25 healthy volunteers for 10 days. PPG-derived HR and HRV showed reasonable accuracy and reliability, particularly during sleep, with mean absolute error < 1 beat for HR and 6–15 ms for HRV. The relative error of HRV estimated from PPG varied with activity type and was higher than during the resting state by 14–51%. The accuracy of HR/HRV was impacted by the proportion of usable data, body posture, and epoch length. The multi-scale peak and trough detection algorithm demonstrated superior performance in detecting beats from PPG signals, with an F1 score of 89% during sleep. The study demonstrates the trade-offs of utilizing PPG measurements for remote monitoring in daily life and identifies optimal use conditions by recommending enhancements.

Keywords: wearables; ECG; PPG; heart rate; heart rate variability; pulse rate; pulse rate variability; autonomic nervous system; remote monitoring; beat detection; multi-scale peak and trough detection algorithm

1. Introduction

The continuous assessment of heart rate (HR) and heart rate variability (HRV) in daily life is crucial for pre-emptive health monitoring and management of chronic diseases [1,2]. Diseases such as inflammatory bowel disease, including Crohn's disease and ulcerative colitis, are linked to complex interactions between the autonomic nervous system and gut inflammation, with stress exacerbating the condition [3]. HRV, as a reliable indicator of autonomic nervous system balance, can reflect physical and emotional stress and is predictive of cardiovascular morbidity and mortality [4]. Continuous HR monitoring assists in detecting arrhythmias and other heart conditions that may go unnoticed in episodic clinical tests [5,6]. Thus, daily life variability in HR and HRV can provide a more accurate picture of an individual's health. Wearable PPG based devices are increasingly being used in continuous monitoring of HR and HRV. PPG devices use optical sensors to detect blood volume changes in tissue and are convenient for a variety of settings, including personal health applications. The PPG sensors, however, do not technically measure HR but rather specifically measure the pulse rate (PR) from the blood volume change. Therefore, they do not measure HRV, but they do technically measure pulse rate variability (PRV). However, for the purpose of simplicity, we will use the terms HR and HRV for both ECG- and PPG-derived measurements but specifically note if they have been derived from a PPG or ECG sensor. Various studies [7–9] have validated the utility of PPG in different contexts, including resting, post-exercise, and field conditions, demonstrating its versatility and effectiveness.

Despite their promise, the utilization of PPG-based devices in clinical research presents several limitations that must be first understood and addressed before deploying them in clinical trials. A key issue is the impact of individual differences, such as skin tone, age, and gender, on PPG readings [10–14]. Physiological aspects like respiration, venous pulsation, and body temperature can introduce noise in PPG signals [15–18]. Additionally, external factors such as motion artifacts, ambient light, and pressure applied to the skin can affect the accuracy of PPG devices [19–23]. Since this can negatively impact the quality of the data, careful consideration is necessary in the selection and use of PPG devices for health monitoring.

PPG-based devices can provide a plethora of features primarily categorized into HR and HRV. HRV features can be further categorized into time domain, frequency domain, and non-linear domain features [4]. The previous studies validating physiological measures from PPG devices have been primarily conducted in controlled environments, which do not represent the challenges encountered in data quality, compliance, and reliability when used in free-living settings. Furthermore, the results reporting accuracy of PPG-derived HRV vary in literature, and there is a paucity of studies evaluating HRV features in free-living conditions. For example, Polar H10 reported good agreement with an ECG-based device for interbeat intervals (R-R intervals) and HR; however, results were not reported for any HRV feature [24]. Polar V800 showed weak absolute agreement (intra class correlation (ICC) < 0.3) with an ECG-based device for time domain HRV features such as root mean square of successive differences (RMSSD) and standard deviation of normal RR (NN) intervals (SDNN) [25]. In another study [26], six wearable devices were evaluated in sleep lab settings, where good agreement was found for HR and poor agreement for RMSSD. The validation of PPG-derived R-R intervals and HR was performed in [27], where analysis was conducted under a resting state and over a very short recording time of 45 s. Another study validated the Samsung smartwatch during awake and asleep state against an ECG-based device using an epoch length of 5-min, showing weak to moderate correlation for HR and HRV during awake state and moderate to strong correlation during asleep state [28].

For precise heartbeat detection, especially under varying cardiac conditions, it is crucial to collect and analyze raw PPG data [29]. Innovative algorithms play a pivotal role in this context. For example, a study employed a peak detection algorithm for smartwatch PPG signals, resulting in significantly enhanced heart rate estimation accuracy in scenarios including atrial fibrillation [30]. A bidirectional recurrent denoising auto-encoder method demonstrated effectiveness in denoising and accentuating PPG waveform features, thereby improving signal quality and heart rate detection [31]. Additionally, the implementation of a novel hybrid motion artifact detection-reduction method using support vector machines has been shown to improve the accuracy of motion artifact detection, which is crucial for real-time vital sign monitoring [32]. However, before application of such complex algorithms, there is a need to first understand the baseline performance of traditional algorithms [33].

In this study, we address the gap in the existing research by performing a rigorous validation of PPG-derived physiological measures. Specifically, the objectives are as follows:

(1) Assessment of the feasibility of collecting continuous data from PPG devices and their usability in daily life settings.

(2) Validation of the HR and HRV derived from PPG devices during awake, asleep, or the full day period compared to that of an ECG sensor.
(3) Investigation of impact of data quality, body posture, activity types, epoch length for HRV estimation, use of dominant vs. non-dominant hand on estimation of HR and HRV from PPG devices.
(4) Assessment of the test–retest reliability of PPG-derived HR and HRV features in the daily life settings under awake, asleep, and full day periods.
(5) Investigation of the performance of seven algorithms to detect beats from the raw PPG waveform signal to identify potentially superior approaches to analyze noisy sensor data in the daily life.

2. Methods

2.1. Study Participants

Twenty-five healthy volunteers participated in this non-interventional exploratory study. The clinical study was performed at a single clinical pharmacology unit in Belgium during November 2022 to March 2023. The individuals were 18 years of age or older and determined to be healthy based on physical examination, medical history, and vital signs recorded during screening. The participants were required to comply with study instructions: wear two PPG devices and an ECG sensor simultaneously for two consecutive five-day periods and complete daily morning questionnaires and an end-of-study survey. The participants were excluded from the study if they had current or prior medical conditions, concomitant therapies, and current or prior participation in a clinical study within 28 days of the start of this study. Furthermore, they were also excluded if they had any constraints on sleep schedule, exposure to high frequency equipment during monitoring period, or tattoos on their wrist or torso potentially interfering with PPG/ECG measurements. They were not allowed to perform intensive exercise nor activities submerging devices in water during the monitoring period. The study received approval from the ethics committee of UZA/UAntwerp (3738-BUN B3002022000126). All participants provided written informed consent. This study followed the procedure according to the Declaration of Helsinki.

2.2. Measurement Setup

Two PPG-based devices (the Whoop 4.0 [34] and the Corsano CardioWatch 287-1B [35]) and one ECG device (Vital Patch [36]) were used in this study. The Corsano CardioWatch 287-1B (manufacturer: Corsano Healthcare BV, Den Haag, The Netherlands) is a wrist-worn research-based home monitoring device and consists of an accelerometer, PPG sensors, and a battery. The bracelet connects via Bluetooth to a mobile app and then to Corsano's secure cloud. It sampled acceleration and PPG signals at 25 Hz and used firmware version 4.13. In addition the to raw data, it also provides the following readings: heart rate, R-R intervals, heart rate variability (e.g., RMSSD), respiration rate, activity count, activity type, steps, energy expenditure, and sleep stages.

The Whoop 4.0 (manufacturer: Whoop, Boston, MA, USA) is a wrist worn commercial device and captures continuous data from its accelerometer and PPG sensors. The Whoop strap containing the actual measuring device connects via Bluetooth to a mobile app and then to secure cloud storage. The firmware version 41.9.2-11.5 was used for Whoop. The device measures the following: sleep duration, sleep staging, sleep disturbances, sleep efficiency, resting heart rate, heart rate variability (RMSSD), respiratory rate, SpO2, heart rate, R-R intervals, and skin temperature.

The Vital Patch device (manufacturer: VitalConnect Inc, San Jose, CA, USA) is adhered to the chest and provides high quality single-lead ECG readings of heart rate and heart rate variability. The VitalConnect device wirelessly transmits data from the Vital Patch sensor to a smartphone and then to the PhysIQ (manufacturer: PhysIQ, Chicago, IL, USA) cloud for storage and analysis [2]. The firmware version used for PhysIQ was 3.5.1.4. The patch is equipped with ECG and accelerometer sensors to measure various physiological parameters such as heart rate, R-R intervals, respiratory rate, body temperature, skin temperature, fall detection, activity (including step count), posture (body position relative to gravity), and sleep stages.

2.3. Study Design

This study included two periods of data collection (Figure 1) from daily life for passive home-based remote monitoring. The first data collection period included Day 1 through Day 6. The second data collection period included Day 8 through Day 13. On Day 1, the participants began wearing all three devices (Whoop 4, Corsano Cardiowatch 287-1B, Vital Patch) simultaneously. During the first data collection period, the Vital Patch was worn on the chest. The Whoop 4 was worn on the participant's non-dominant hand, while the Corsano Cardiowatch 287-1B was worn on their dominant hand. The devices were worn for 5 consecutive days and nights, which included at least 1 weekend night. On Day 8, the participants began the second data collection period wearing all three devices. The Vital Patch was worn in the designated location on the chest as indicated during the site visit. The Corsano Cardiowatch 287-1B was worn on the participant's non-dominant hand, while the Whoop 4 was worn on their dominant hand. The devices were worn for an additional 5 consecutive days and nights, which included at least 1 weekend night. During the whole data collection period, on every third day participants were instructed to charge the devices for at least three hours in the evening.

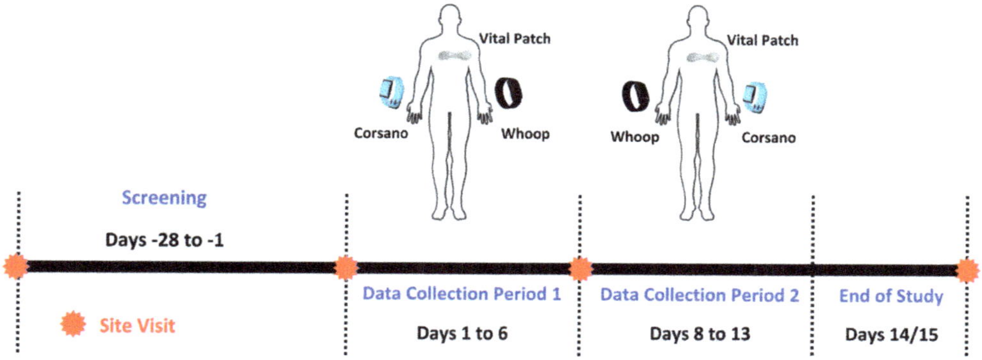

Figure 1. Study design, device attachments, and continuous data collection periods.

Participants completed a daily morning questionnaire, prompted at 9 a.m., which asked two questions: the time at which the participant went to bed the previous night and the time at which the participant woke up that day. Responses from the morning questionnaire were collected on Day 2–Day 6 and Day 9–Day 13. A participant was considered to have completed the study if the participant had completed the two data collection periods of five consecutive days and nights, daily device assessments, and the end of study survey.

2.4. Device Usability Assessment

An end-of-study survey was used to evaluate the usability of each device in daily life. The following usability aspects of each device were assessed on a Likert scale from 1–5 (1 indicates strongly disagree to 5 indicates strongly agree) based on the modified version of the standardized questionnaire for the system usability scale [37].

(1) I thought it was easy putting the device on and taking it off
(2) I experienced discomfort wearing the device
(3) I experienced trouble sleeping due to the device
(4) My device stayed in place
(5) I would like to use the device frequently

(6) I found the device easy to use
(7) I needed support of a technical person to be able to use the device
(8) I experienced restrictions in my daily activities due to device
(9) I felt confident wearing the device
(10) I needed to learn a lot of things before I could get going with the device
(11) I found various functions of the device were well integrated (wearing, charging, application features, etc.)
(12) I found the device very cumbersome to use
(13) I experienced skin irritability wearing the device

3. Data Analysis

3.1. Coverage Assessment

To assess the feasibility of the PPG devices to be used for daily continuous monitoring, coverage of each PPG device data was calculated in two different ways. The first assessment focused on the collection of continuous raw PPG/Acceleration data in daily life, and the second assessment concentrated on the ability of the devices to be used for continuous beat detection in daily life. For the first assessment, the raw data coverage of each device was calculated on an hourly basis as a percentage of the available sample data points in a particular hour to the intended number of samples in this hour. Hourly coverage was further aggregated into full day (across 24 h) and different parts of the day (midnight to 8 a.m., 8 a.m. to 8 p.m., and 8 p.m. to midnight) for reporting. To assess the feasibility of the PPG devices for continuous beat detection in daily life, R-R intervals obtained from the devices were utilized. For simplicity, we use R-R intervals to refer to beat-to-beat intervals for PPG and R-R intervals for ECG. For coverage estimation, a 5-min epoch length was considered for the analysis. The data coverage within this epoch was calculated first, and if there were at least 40% of the data present, this epoch was considered valid. Further, the processed data hourly coverage was estimated by counting the valid epochs within an hour divided by the intended possible number of 5-min epochs in that hour. The hourly coverage was further aggregated into full-day periods (24 h) and specific time intervals for reporting: midnight to 8 a.m., 8 a.m. to 8 p.m., and 8 p.m. to midnight. The charging times of the devices were not adjusted in the coverage calculation to simulate real-world daily life scenarios.

3.2. PPG/ECG Device Data (R-R Intervals) Processing

From each device, valid 5-min epoch R-R interval data were further processed before feature engineering. The R-R interval data provided by each device were processed first by sorting it based on the timestamps and removing any duplicates. The R-R intervals were then cleaned by removing the outliers based on unrealistic physiological values and ectopic beats to extract the cleaned normal-to-normal (N-N) intervals for robust feature engineering [38]. The procedure for computing normal-to-normal (N-N) intervals from R-R intervals consisted of several sequential steps. Initially, R-R interval outliers, defined as the ones outside of the 300–2000 ms range [4,39], were identified and replaced with NaN values to clean the data. Subsequently, any NaN values in between the reliable R-R interval values were interpolated using a linear interpolation. This step ensures continuity in the data by filling gaps with interpolated values. Following this, ectopic beats, or abnormal heartbeats, were removed from the interpolated R-R intervals using the Malik method (where the consecutive interval deviation is more than 20% from the previous one) [40]. This generated a series of N-N intervals representing the time intervals between consecutive normal heartbeats. However, the ectopic beat removal may introduce new NaN values, necessitating a second interpolation step. The same interpolation method applied earlier was utilized again to fill in any remaining NaN values within the N-N intervals. Due to the validation nature of this work in daily life, the same interpolation technique was used for all features instead of considering different interpolation techniques for each HRV feature [41]. The result is a list of interpolated N-N intervals, where physiological unrealistic and ectopic beats have been systematically removed, and missing values have been filled in. This comprehensive pre-processing approach ensures a robust and adaptable foundation for further heart rate variability (HRV) analysis. However, an ablation study was also conducted to compare the impact of the current interpolation technique with that of no interpolation of HRV features (Appendix B).

3.3. Feature Engineering

Cleaned epochs of 5-min N-N intervals from each device were further used to extract HRV features related to time, frequency, and non-linear domains along with the mean value of heart rate and N-N intervals. For the further validation analysis, only representative features from each domain were considered and described in Table 1. More information regarding feature definitions can be found in the work by Shaffer and Ginsberg [4].

Table 1. List of HR and HRV features, along with their definitions, used in the validation analysis. HRV features were extracted from 5-min epochs of N-N intervals.

Feature (Units)	Domain	Definition
Mean HR (BPM)	Time	The average heart rate.
Std HR (BPM)	Time	Standard deviation of heart rate
Mean N-N (ms)	Time	The mean of the N-N intervals, which are the normal-to-normal intervals or the time between successive normal heartbeats.
SDNN (ms)	Time	The standard deviation of the N-N intervals, indicating overall HRV.
SDSD (ms)	Time	The standard deviation of successive differences between adjacent N-N intervals, emphasizing short-term variations.
RMSSD (ms)	Time	The square root of the mean of the sum of the squares of differences between adjacent N-N intervals.
CVSD	Time	Coefficient of variation of successive differences between adjacent N-N intervals.
CVNN	Time	Coefficient of variation equal to the ratio of SDNN divided by Mean N-N intervals
LF (ms^2)	Frequency	Low-frequency power spectral density (0.04 to 0.15 Hz)
HF (ms^2)	Frequency	High-frequency power spectral density (0.15 to 0.40 Hz)
LF/HF	Frequency	A ratio of LF to HF
Sample Entropy	Non-linear	A non-linear measure that quantifies the complexity or irregularity of the HRV signal

3.4. Factors Affecting the PPG Device Performance

In addition to measuring HR and HRV throughout the full day (from midnight to next midnight for each day), it is crucial to consider the influence of the body's circadian rhythm. This natural rhythm can cause HR/HRV features to vary between day and night, subsequently affecting their accuracy. Particularly during periods of sleep with minimal wrist movement, HRV features tend to be more accurate compared to wakeful periods when daily activities are performed. Morning questionnaire responses were used to crop the data based on subjective asleep and awake timings for each day.

Moreover, there are several other factors, including data coverage within epochs used for HRV estimation, postural transitions, activity types, walking vs. non-walking, epoch length, and device position, which can impact the estimation of PPG derived HR/HRV features.

Coverage within a 5-min epoch used for HRV estimation: Continuous detection of beats from PPG raw data without gaps is key for reliable HRV feature calculation. The impact of R-R data coverage within 5-min epochs was investigated by increasing the coverage threshold from 40% to 100% with increments of 10%.

Postural transitions: Body posture in daily life can also impact the PPG data reliability. Postural information obtained from Vital Patch, such as upright, reclined, lying right, lying left, prone, and supine information, was used to label each 5-min epoch of data used for HR/HRV estimation. A specific posture label was assigned based on its dominance within the 5-min epoch of data in case the participant changed a posture with this 5-min time interval.

Activity type: Performance of the PPG devices was also assessed under various daily living activities such as cycling, rest, walking, and running provided by the Corsano device after processing the accelerometer data.

Walking vs. *non-walking:* Specifically, walking detected by the chest-worn device (Vital Patch), which can be more reliable compared to wrist-worn devices, was also used to check the performance of the PPG devices.

Epoch length: The impact of epoch length on the error rate of HRV estimation during asleep, awake, and full day periods was explored by using epoch lengths of 10, 30, and 60 min. Apart from these epoch lengths, whole asleep and awake periods were also investigated.

Dominant vs. *non-dominant hand:* Five complete days of data from each collection period from each subject were used to investigate the impact of wearing the PPG devices on dominant vs. non-dominant hands during the asleep, awake, and full day periods.

3.5. Data Consideration for Reliability Assessment of HRV Features

Reliability of the HRV features was further explored. For reliability assessment, as shown in Figure 2, the data were considered separately when the device was attached to the dominant and non-dominant hand. Within each period of device attachment, two separate full days (24 h) were considered. To compute reliability, the spearman correlation was performed between HRV estimates obtained from synchronized 5-min epochs between day 1 and day 2. Similarly, a reliability assessment was performed during the first day awake/asleep period with the second day awake/asleep period based on the synchronized 5-min epochs of the HRV features.

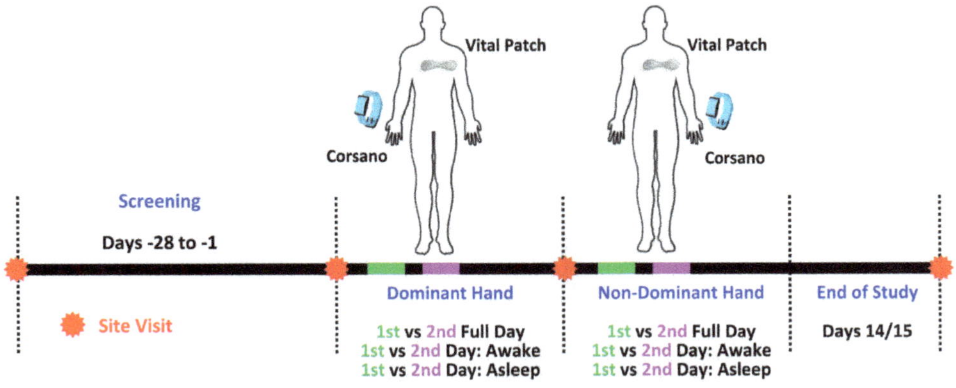

Figure 2. Data consideration for the reliability assessment of the HR and HRV features.

3.6. Algorithms for Beat Detection from Raw PPG and ECG Data

Only Corsano provided raw PPG data at 25 Hz frequency. Seven open-source algorithms, which performed well on PPG data in a previous study [33], were employed to detect beats from the raw PPG data. A short description of each algorithm is provided in Table 2. The methodology for beat detection from raw PPG data methodology was adopted from the prior work [42]. Briefly, raw PPG green signals were subjected to band-pass filtration to remove extraneous cardiac frequencies. Beats were identified over specific length PPG intervals with certain overlap. Redundant detections from overlaps were excluded. Segments with a continuous flat signal exceeding 0.2 s, often due to sensor disengagement or saturation, were discarded. For validation, the beat (R peaks) detected from the simultaneously recorded ECG signal by two different beat detectors were used as reference following the previous work [33]. The two beat detectors utilized were the 'jqrs', which employ the Pan and Tompkins technique [43,44], and Clifford's 'rpeakdetect' ECG beat detector [42]. Outputs from these two algorithms were aligned and then merged, with 'correct' beats in the merged signal being those identified by both within a 150 ms interval. Any 20-s segments without consensus between the two detectors were omitted from the analysis.

Table 2. Brief description of the beat detection algorithms used during validation analysis.

Algorithm Name	Description
1. Automatic Beat Detection (ABD) by [45]	This algorithm computes a Fourier-based power spectral density (PSD) to isolate the signal's primary energy bands. Subsequently, the signal undergoes band-pass filtering, emphasizing distinct heart rate frequencies. This is complemented by derivative-based filtering, which makes rapid signal transitions prominent. A modification is made to the percentile threshold, initially set around the 90th percentile in the original algorithm but later modified to the 75th percentile, to detect peaks in the derivative (75th percentile used in this work). After filtering, the algorithm identifies pulse peaks. To enhance accuracy, it corrects potential peak location errors, removes false positives based on interbeat intervals and median heart rate thresholds, and integrates missing peaks to account for false negatives.
2. Automatic Multi-Scale Peak Detection (AMPD) by [46]	The PPG signal is first detrended and then segmented into overlapping windows of 6 s in duration with 20% overall. Within these windows, the algorithm constructs a local maxima scalogram (LMS) matrix. Rows of the LMS corresponded to scales, spanning from a single sample up to half of the window's duration, while columns represent individual PPG samples. The algorithm updates specific LMS matrix entries to zero when a PPG sample surpasses its neighboring values at a given scale, indicating a local maximum. By analyzing the LMS, the algorithm determines the optimal scale (lambda), which represents the scale capturing the most local maxima. The LMS matrix is then truncated to retain only scales smaller than this optimal lambda. The final beat detection step identifies beats as those PPG samples that are recognized as local maxima across all the retained scales in the truncated LMS.
3. Event-Related Moving Averages (ERMA) by [47]	The algorithm processes the PPG signal with a Butterworth bandpass filter, limiting the frequency range to 0.5 Hz to 8 Hz. The filtered signal was subsequently squared, ensuring non-negative values. Two specific moving averages are then applied: the first, with a 111 ms duration, is designed to emphasize systolic peaks, while the second, spanning 667 ms, makes individual beats prominent. A threshold is computed as 2% of the squared signal's mean. Within 111 ms windows, beats are pinpointed when the first moving average exceeds the sum of the second moving average and the defined threshold.
4. HeartPy by [48]	This algorithm starts by processing the PPG signal through multiple iterations of squaring and normalization, emphasizing its peaks. Following this, the signal is subjected to a rolling mean over a 0.75-s duration. A sliding window approach then segments the signal, with each window's size being the product of the window duration and the sampling rate. For acceptable peak detection, constraints are set with a beats per minute (BPM) range of 40 to 180, and peak-to-peak (PP) intervals were of particular focus. A PP range is established around the mean PP interval, using either a fixed 300 milliseconds or 30% of this mean to define the upper and lower thresholds. These thresholds are crucial for discerning acceptable PP intervals, facilitating the identification of significant peaks. Furthermore, signal segments with more than three unreliable detections within 10 beats are discarded to ensure the reliability of the detected peaks.
5. Multi-Scale Peak and Trough Detection (MSPTD) by [49]	This algorithm operates by segmenting the PPG signal into overlapping windows, each spanning 6 s with a 20% overlap. Within each window, the algorithm employs the modified AMPD algorithm. This algorithm initiates by detrending the signal and computing local maxima and minima scalograms. These scalograms are matrices indicating the presence of local maxima and minima at varying scales. The method then determines the scales with the most local maxima and minima and truncates the scalograms accordingly. Peaks and onsets are identified based on these processed scalograms. After this pulse peak and pulse onset detection, the algorithm refines the peak and onset indices by searching within a 5% tolerance of the sampling frequency around the detected positions to pinpoint the exact maxima (for peaks) or minima (for onsets). After processing all windows, the detected peaks and onsets are ordered chronologically, with redundant detections discarded to ensure a unique set of pulse events.

Table 2. *Cont.*

Algorithm Name	Description
6. Adapted Onset Detector (qppgfast) by [50]	The algorithm employs a slope sampling approach over a defined window size of 170 ms to compute the signal's slope. For peak identification, dynamic thresholds are set. One threshold is adjusted based on a running peak value observed in the current processing interval, with this peak value being incremented by one-tenth of its difference from the threshold. A secondary threshold is established as one-third of the primary threshold. After a peak is detected, a specific lockout interval (340 ms) is applied, preventing the detection of subsequent beats for a set duration. Additionally, if no pulse was detected over an extended period, the primary threshold is reduced, provided it exceeds a minimum limit, to capture potential low-amplitude beats.
7. Symmetric Projection Attractor (SPAR) by [51,52]	This algorithm first segments the PPG data into windows, each spanning 20 s. Within each window, the average cycle length is derived using autocorrelation, due to the periodic nature of the PPG signal. This technique is bound by an HR range of 40 to 200 BPM, ensuring that the detected cycle lengths were physiologically plausible. The derived average cycle length subsequently informs the time delay parameter, which is integral to the symmetric projection attractor reconstruction (SPAR) method. This method maps the signal into two values, based on delay coordinates and specific mathematical projections. After a rotation using an optimal angle, beats are detected by pinpointing crossings of a particular line in the rotated coordinates. To ensure thorough beat detection, the algorithm adjusted for potential mismatches between windows and incorporated mechanisms to handle missed or extra beats.

The alignment between PPG and ECG detected beats is not always exact. Therefore, we used the methodology proposed by Charlton et al. [33]. Briefly, to synchronize the PPG beats with ECG, the time discrepancy between each ECG beat and its nearest PPG counterpart was computed. If this difference was less than 150 ms, the beat was deemed accurately identified. In increments of 20 ms for shifting either PPG or ECG beat sequence, this alignment procedure was repeated while offsetting the beats by lags ranging from −10 to 10 s. The offset yielding the most accurate beat identifications was taken as the genuine lag and utilized to harmonize beat timings.

3.7. Validation Approach and Statistical Analysis

The validation workflow is shown in Figure 3, where the performance of the devices was assessed based on the provided R-R intervals. Each PPG device feature extracted from N-N intervals was compared with the ECG-derived features during the same time interval. All the devices were synchronized based on local UTC time. During this validation analysis, depending on the coverage and pre-processing of the R-R intervals, HRV features from various domains were calculated (Table 1). To assess the accuracy of measurements, the relative error and absolute error were quantified. The relative agreement between HRV features of the PPG device and ECG was assessed with correlation coefficient. Absolute agreement between the devices was calculated with the ICC coefficient. The relationship between the PPG and ECG features was further visualized through the scatter plots. In addition, to analyze the difference between devices (PPG vs. ECG), Bland–Altman plots were used, and other validation metrics such as bias (mean error) and 95% limit of agreements were calculated. The reliability of the HRV features was assessed with the ICC coefficient within each data collection period for the dominant and non-dominant hands during asleep, awake, and full day periods. The feasibility of continuous remote data collection in home settings was assessed by an evaluation of the coverage and usability of devices. Average values of the coverage and usability along with the standard deviation were reported as bar plots.

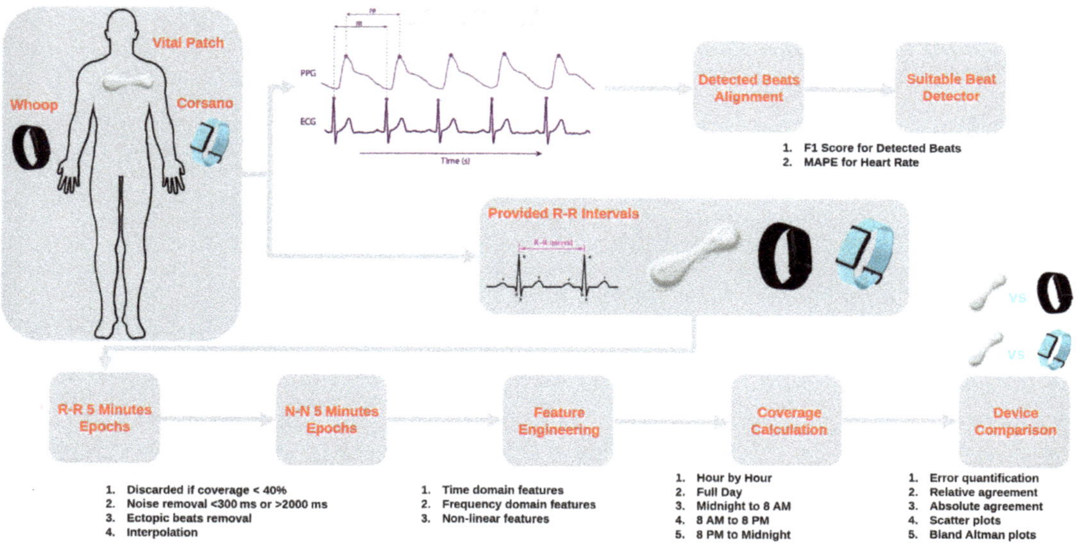

Figure 3. Validation workflow of wearable PPG-based devices for HR and HRV.

The performance of the beat detectors on the raw PPG data was assessed by comparing the detected beats with the reference ECG beats. A tolerance window of ±150 ms as described in Section 3.6 was used for assessing the correctness of beat detection between PPG and ECG. For example, if the detected beat from the PPG data is present within this window of the reference ECG beat, then it is considered to be correctly identified. For full day, asleep, and awake periods, the numbers of correct beats, reference beats, and PPG beats were identified to calculate the sensitivity and positive predictive value (PPV). The harmonic mean of PPV and sensitivity, as well as the F1 score, was used to identify the best performing beat detectors. Furthermore, for time points corresponding to each beat, the HR was using the preceding 8 s interval [33]. The performance of HR estimation for different beat detectors was assessed as mean absolute percentage error (MAPE). All the performance metrics for the evaluation of beat detectors are reported as median values along with 95% confidence intervals.

A mathematical formulation of the evaluation metrics is given below.

Mean Absolute Error (MAE): MAE is the average of the absolute differences between measured (PPG) and true values (ECG), calculated as

$$\mathrm{MAE} = \frac{1}{n}\sum_{i=1}^{n}\left|x_{measurement,\ i} - x_{true,i}\right|$$

where

- $x_{measurement,i}$ is the i-th measured value of the epoch,
- $x_{true,i}$ is the i-th true value of the epoch,
- n is the total number of measurements.

Mean Relative Error (MRE): MRE measures the average relative error as a percentage of the true value:

$$\mathrm{MRE} = \frac{1}{n}\sum_{i=1}^{n}\frac{\left|x_{measurement,\ i} - x_{true,i}\right|}{x_{true,i}} \times 100$$

Spearman Correlation: This correlation coefficient (ρ) assesses the rank-order relationship between two variables, which is non-parametric and useful when there is a non-linear relationship between the variables:

$$\rho = 1 - \frac{6 \sum d_i^2}{n(n^2 - 1)}$$

where

- d_i is the difference between the ranks of $x_{measurement,i}$ and $x_{true,i}$
- n is the total number of measurements.

Intra-Class Correlation (ICC): ICC 2,1 (two-way random effects, single measurement) quantifies the degree of agreement between two sets of measurements, considering both individual variability and systematic differences:

$$ICC(2,1) = \frac{MSR - MSE}{MSR + (k-1)MSE + \frac{k(MSC - MSR)}{n}}$$

where

- MSR is the mean square of rows (subjects)
- MSE is the mean square error (residual)
- MSC is the mean square for columns (devices)
- k is the number of devices
- n is the number of subjects

Sensitivity: The proportion of true positives (TP) correctly identified by the algorithm to TP and FN (false negative):

$$Sensitivity = \frac{TP}{TP + FN}$$

Positive Predictive Value (PPV): The proportion of predicted positives that are true positives to TP and FP (false positive):

$$PPV = \frac{TP}{TP + FP}$$

F1 Score: The F1 score is the harmonic mean of precision (PPV) and sensitivity:

$$F1 = 2 \times \frac{PPV \times Sensitivity}{PPV + Sensitivity}$$

4. Results

The demographic characteristics for the participating subjects collected at screening are shown in Table 3. The average age of participants was 46.9 years, with majority (n = 17) being female (F). Participants had a body mass index in the range of 24.68 ± 3.10 kg/m^2.

Table 3. Demographic characteristics of 25 study participants collected at screening.

Demographic Characteristics	Total Participants (n = 25) (Mean ± Standard Deviation)
M/F (n)	8/17
Age (years)	46.92 ± 16.61
Height (cm)	168.72 ± 10.07
Weight (kg)	70.54 ± 12.40
BMI (kg/m^2)	24.68 ± 3.10
Race	White (n = 24) American Indian or Alaska Native (n = 1)

4.1. *Feasibility of PPG Devices in Daily Life*

The feasibility analysis is divided into (1) the coverage analysis of the raw PPG and the R-R interval data processed by the device and (2) the usability analysis of the PPG device deployment in daily life.

4.1.1. A Coverage Analysis

The coverage for raw ECG/PPG/Acceleration data and processed R-R interval data is presented as median value along with min and max values in Table 4. Additionally, the coverage of the processed R-R intervals is also shown in Figure 4 as average values along with a 95% confidence interval. Vital Patch provided 100% coverage of the raw ECG data during most of the study days whenever it was attached to the body. Corsano had similar coverage for the raw PPG data. However, the Whoop device had slightly less coverage each day when compared to Corsano.

Table 4. Raw data coverage from all devices—where min, max, and median values are based on the coverage across all subjects.

Day Timings	Vital Patch Median [min, max]		Corsano Median [min, max]		Whoop Median [min, max]
	Raw ECG	R-R	Raw PPG	R-R	R-R
Full Day	100 [1, 100]	98 [0, 100]	100 [33, 100]	52 [0, 94]	44 [0, 79]
Midnight to 8 a.m.	100 [1, 100]	100 [0, 100]	100 [33, 100]	88 [0, 100]	77 [0, 100]
8 a.m. to 8 p.m.	100 [1, 100]	98 [0, 100]	100 [39, 100]	31 [0, 93]	19 [0, 68]
8 p.m. to midnight	100 [3, 100]	100 [0, 100]	100 [33, 100]	75 [0, 100]	68 [0, 100]

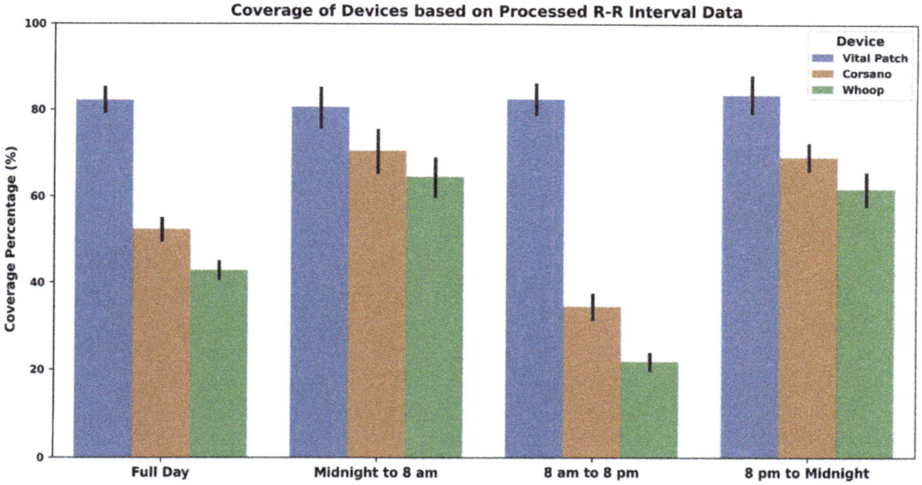

Figure 4. R-R interval data coverage—where the height of the bars indicates the average coverage values while the whiskers correspond to 95% confidence intervals.

As demonstrated in Figure 4 and Table 4, it is clear that the ECG-based device detected more beats in the data and had better coverage than PPG devices. PPG devices detected fewer beats during the daytime as compared to night. Therefore, the median coverage varied from 44–52% during a full day period to 77–88% only during the night. Overall, Corsano has better coverage for the processed R-R interval data as compared to Whoop.

4.1.2. Usability Analysis

The second aspect of the feasibility assessment was to investigate the usability of the wearables. A 13-item questionnaire (Section 2.4) was answered by each participant at the end of the study, and their responses are shown in Figure 5. The results indicated that all devices were easy to use, they stayed in place, had low discomfort when wearing, were not cumbersome, and functioned well. However, for Whoop, participants indicated a slight need to learn more before one could get going with the device and a need for more technical support when compared to Corsano. Furthermore, Vital Patch had higher skin irritation, followed by Whoop and then Corsano.

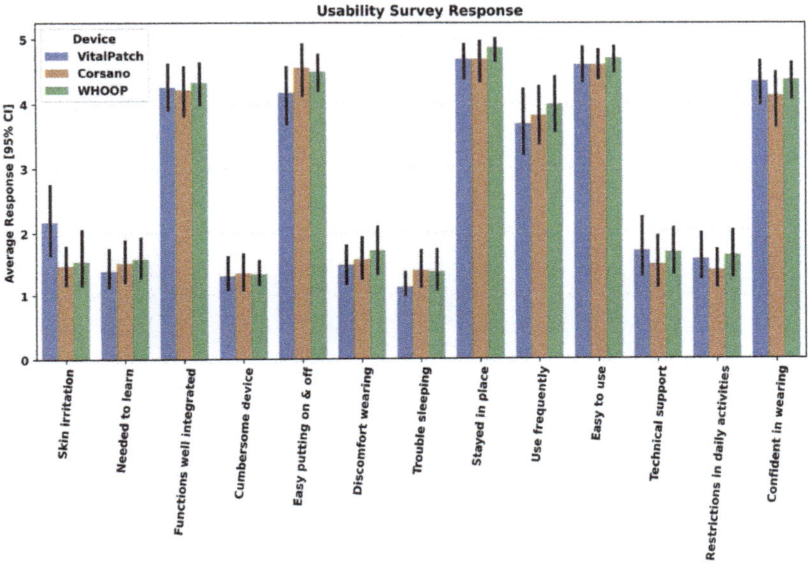

Figure 5. Usability evaluation of devices. Participants completed an end-of-study survey comprising a 13-item questionnaire assessing the usability of each device. Figure here shows abbreviated versions of the questions described in Section 2.4.

4.2. Mutual Data for Validation

Based on coverage analysis in Section 4.1.1, Vital Patch had more processed R-R interval data each day when compared to the Corsano and Whoop. Therefore, it is critical to understand when the majority of the data are available for the validation. Since validation could be performed only using data from such epochs, which are considered valid for both devices under comparison, we computed the number of such mutually valid epochs for different times a day for Corsano–Vital Patch and Whoop–Vital Patch pairs. Figure 6 shows the comparison for both Corsano and Whoop with Vital Patch, where each bar corresponds to the matched number of valid 5-min epochs between an ECG- and PPG-based device across all participants and days. Figure 6 is further divided into the night, day, and evening. During night and evening, both devices had more matched data when compared to daytime for the validation.

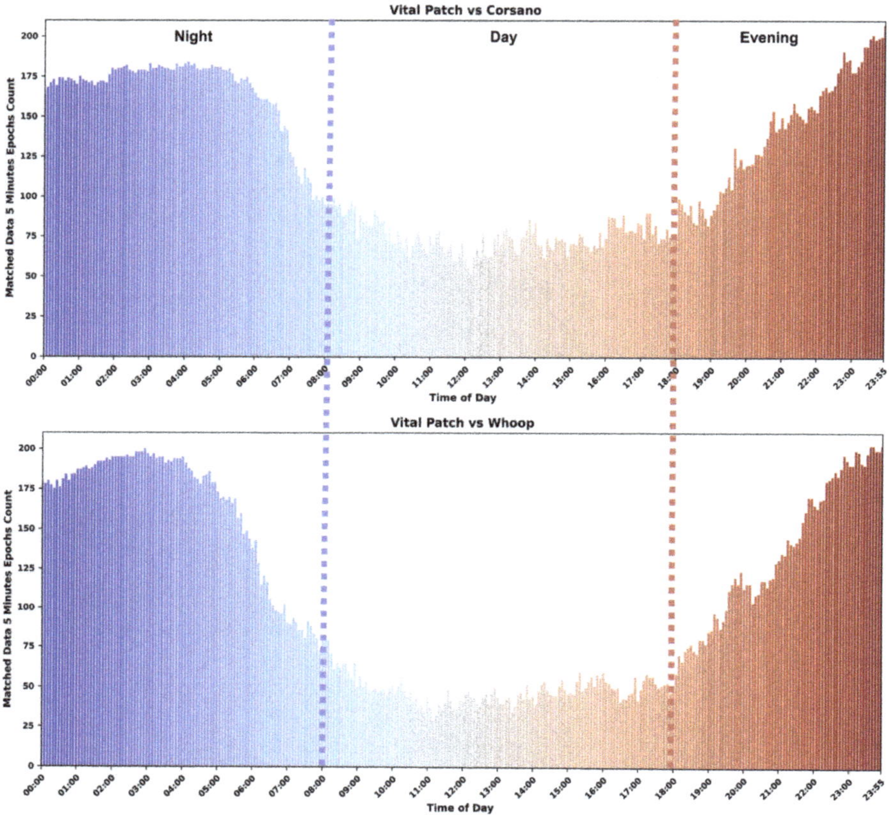

Figure 6. Bar plot showing the availability of 5-min epochs, which are valid for both devices, across days and participants.

4.3. Performance of the PPG Devices

The results of the comparison of HR/HRV features obtained from PPG devices to the same features derived from ECG device are shown in Table 5. The performance comparison is reported based on three time intervals: when participants were asleep, awake, and during the full day. Scatter plots and Bland–Altman plots showing alignment between the N-N interval and heart rate are shown in Figure 7.

During the full day period, Whoop had higher error in N-N intervals and HR compared to Corsano. However, both PPG devices had good relative and absolute agreement in N-N intervals and HR with the ECG device. For time domain HRV features like RMSSD, and SDNN, both devices performed similarly in terms of their agreements with ECG. In the frequency domain, both devices had a high error rate during the full day and low absolute agreement.

The error rate during asleep time was lower than awake time for all HR/HRV features. The mean error for HR during asleep time was less than one beat and for N-N intervals was less than 10 ms. However, both devices overestimated the N-N intervals during both awake and asleep periods when compared to the ECG device. Time domain HRV during asleep time had errors in a range of 6–10 ms for Corsano, while Whoop had errors in a range of 7–15 ms. For frequency domain features, the error rate was drastically lower during the asleep time compared to awake time for both devices, the reduction being more in the case of Corsano than Whoop. Both PPG devices had a lower error rate and good agreement with the ECG device during asleep time as compared to awake time.

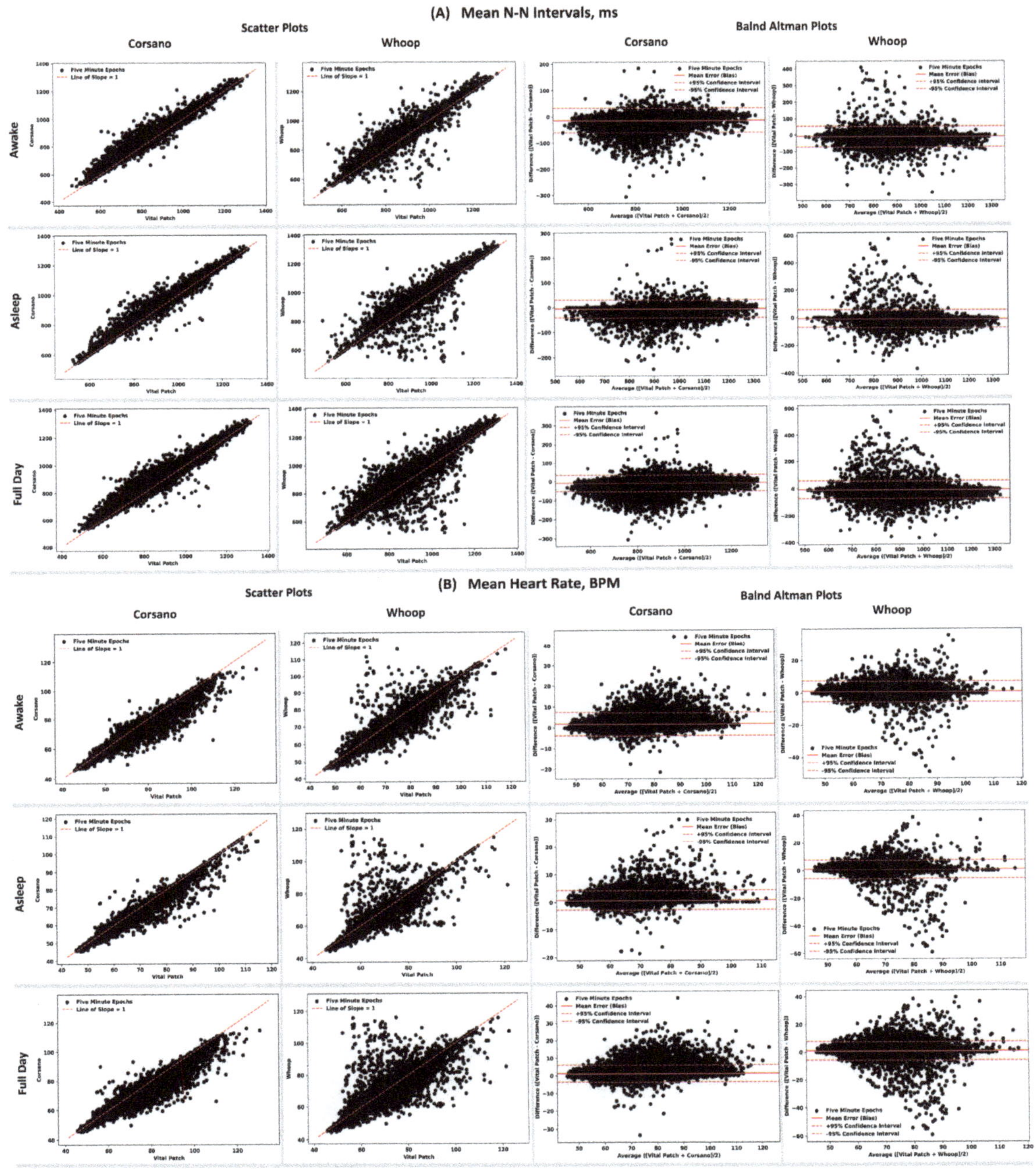

Figure 7. Scatter and Bland–Altman plots showing the performance of the PPG devices compared to ECG device for (**A**) mean N-N intervals (top) and (**B**) HR (bottom) across 5-min epochs.

Table 5. Performance of PPG-based devices compared to ECG for HR and HRV features. Accuracy between PPG- and ECG-derived measurements was quantified with mean absolute error. Agreement between PPG- and ECG-derived measurements was quantified with the spearman correlation coefficient, ICC coefficient, and Bland–Altman analysis. Bold text for each feature indicates the best performing device for the specific part of the day.

Time	Device	Mean Absolute Error	Spearman Correlation ρ (*p*-Value)	ICC (*p*-Value)	Mean Error (Bias)	Bland–Altman Limits of Agreement CI 95% (+, −)
			Heart Rate, BPM			
Full Day	Corsano	1.36	0.98 (<0.001)	0.97 (<0.001)	1.14	[5.99, −3.71]
	Whoop	1.50	0.96 (<0.001)	0.93 (<0.001)	0.80	[7.47, −5.86]
Awake	Corsano	1.84	0.96 (<0.001)	0.95 (<0.001)	1.59	[7.17, −3.98]
	Whoop	1.71	0.95 (<0.001)	0.94 (<0.001)	0.90	[7.37, −5.58]
Asleep	**Corsano**	**0.85**	**0.98 (<0.001)**	**0.98 (<0.001)**	**0.65**	**[4.2, −2.9]**
	Whoop	1.31	0.96 (<0.001)	0.92 (<0.001)	0.71	[7.38, −5.96]
			Variability in Heart Rate (SD of HR), BPM			
Full Day	Corsano	1.65	0.73 (<0.001)	0.44 (<0.001)	0.93	[7.03, −5.18]
	Whoop	1.92	0.65 (<0.001)	0.35 (<0.001)	0.68	[7.74, −6.38]
Awake	Corsano	1.98	0.56 (<0.001)	0.31 (<0.001)	0.80	[7.6, −6]
	Whoop	2.12	0.54 (<0.001)	0.33 (<0.001)	0.16	[7.42, −7.1]
Asleep	**Corsano**	**1.27**	**0.87 (<0.001)**	**0.57 (<0.001)**	**1.04**	**[6.02, −3.95]**
	Whoop	1.72	0.75 (<0.001)	0.38 (<0.001)	1.13	[7.74, −5.48]
			N−N Intervals, ms (Mean of the N-N intervals)			
Full Day	Corsano	13.20	0.98 (<0.001)	0.98 (<0.001)	−10.38	[32.33, −53.08]
	Whoop	16.04	0.97 (<0.001)	0.96 (<0.001)	−9.49	[54.94, −73.92]
Awake	Corsano	17.10	0.97 (<0.001)	0.97 (<0.001)	−14.70	[31.88, −61.28]
	Whoop	17.93	0.96 (<0.001)	0.96 (<0.001)	−10.74	[52.78, −74.26]
Asleep	**Corsano**	**9.04**	**0.99 (<0.001)**	**0.99 (<0.001)**	**−5.83**	**[29.6, −41.26]**
	Whoop	14.28	0.97 (<0.001)	0.96 (<0.001)	−8.33	[56.12, −72.79]
			SDNN, ms (SD of the N−N intervals)			
Full Day	Corsano	13.89	0.78 (<0.001)	0.69 (<0.001)	4.41	[50.67, −41.85]
	Whoop	17.31	0.72 (<0.001)	0.57 (<0.001)	3.18	[64.11, −57.75]
Awake	Corsano	16.47	0.62 (<0.001)	0.55 (<0.001)	1.08	[52.28, −50.12]
	Whoop	19.71	0.62 (<0.001)	0.48 (<0.001)	−3.01	[62.55, −68.57]
Asleep	**Corsano**	**10.92**	**0.91 (<0.001)**	**0.8 (<0.001)**	**7.91**	**[45.7, −29.89]**
	Whoop	15.06	0.82 (<0.001)	0.66 (<0.001)	8.79	[62.11, −44.53]
			SDSD, ms (SD of successive differences between adjacent N-N intervals)			
Full Day	Corsano	12.52	0.7 (<0.001)	0.65 (<0.001)	−9.43	[22.77, −41.64]
	Whoop	9.42	0.76 (<0.001)	0.75 (<0.001)	−2.96	[26.07, −31.99]
Awake	Corsano	17.99	0.58 (<0.001)	0.43 (<0.001)	−15.43	[20.04, −50.9]
	Whoop	11.86	0.67 (<0.001)	0.63 (<0.001)	−6.45	[24.4, −37.3]
Asleep	**Corsano**	**6.89**	**0.89 (<0.001)**	**0.87 (<0.001)**	**−3.57**	**[18.27, −25.4]**
	Whoop	7.14	0.86 (<0.001)	0.84 (<0.001)	0.13	[25.46, −25.19]

Table 5. *Cont.*

Time	Device	Mean Absolute Error	Spearman Correlation ρ (*p*-Value)	ICC (*p*-Value)	Mean Error (Bias)	Bland–Altman Limits of Agreement CI 95% (+, −)
RMSSD, ms (Square root of mean of the sum of squares of differences between adjacent N-N intervals)						
Full Day	Corsano	12.53	0.7 (<0.001)	0.65 (<0.001)	−9.43	[22.78, −41.64]
	Whoop	9.42	0.76 (<0.001)	0.75 (<0.001)	−2.96	[26.07, −31.99]
Awake	Corsano	17.99	0.58 (<0.001)	0.43 (<0.001)	−15.43	[20.04, −50.91]
	Whoop	11.86	0.67 (<0.001)	0.63 (<0.001)	−6.45	[24.4, −37.3]
Asleep	**Corsano**	**6.89**	**0.89 (<0.001)**	**0.87 (<0.001)**	**−3.57**	**[18.27, −25.4]**
	Whoop	7.14	0.86 (<0.001)	0.84 (<0.001)	0.13	[25.46, −25.19]
CVSD (Coefficient of variation of successive differences between adjacent N-N intervals)						
Full Day	Corsano	0.01	0.66 (<0.001)	0.53 (<0.001)	−0.01	[0.03, −0.05]
	Whoop	0.01	0.71 (<0.001)	0.66 (<0.001)	0.00	[0.03, −0.04]
Awake	Corsano	0.02	0.49 (<0.001)	0.32 (<0.001)	−0.02	[0.03, −0.06]
	Whoop	0.01	0.6 (<0.001)	0.54 (<0.001)	−0.01	[0.03, −0.05]
Asleep	**Corsano**	**0.01**	**0.87 (<0.001)**	**0.82 (<0.001)**	**0.00**	**[0.02, −0.03]**
	Whoop	0.01	0.82 (<0.001)	0.76 (<0.001)	0.00	[0.03, −0.03]
CVNN (Coefficient of variation equal to the ratio of SDNN divided by Mean N-N intervals)						
Full Day	Corsano	0.02	0.74 (<0.001)	0.59 (<0.001)	0.01	[0.06, −0.05]
	Whoop	0.02	0.68 (<0.001)	0.48 (<0.001)	0.00	[0.08, −0.07]
Awake	Corsano	0.02	0.56 (<0.001)	0.42 (<0.001)	0.00	[0.07, −0.06]
	Whoop	0.02	0.57 (<0.001)	0.4 (<0.001)	0.00	[0.08, −0.08]
Asleep	**Corsano**	**0.01**	**0.9 (<0.001)**	**0.75 (<0.001)**	**0.01**	**[0.05, −0.03]**
	Whoop	0.02	0.8 (<0.001)	0.57 (<0.001)	0.01	[0.07, −0.05]
LF: variance (power) in HRV in the low Frequency (0.04 to 0.15 Hz), ms^2						
Full Day	Corsano	392.70	0.76 (<0.001)	0.45 (<0.001)	21.02	[1906.22, −1864.18]
	Whoop	427.39	0.7 (<0.001)	0.33 (<0.001)	119.11	[2195.07, −1956.84]
Awake	Corsano	479.81	0.62 (<0.001)	0.34 (<0.001)	−41.58	[2002.9, −2086.06]
	Whoop	464.56	0.61 (<0.001)	0.32 (<0.001)	44.94	[2069.97, −1980.09]
Asleep	**Corsano**	**282.50**	**0.89 (<0.001)**	**0.61 (<0.001)**	**75.75**	**[1627.54, −1476.04]**
	Whoop	386.94	0.78 (<0.001)	0.35 (<0.001)	182.01	[2218.12, −1854.1]
HF: variance (power) in HRV in the High Frequency (0.15 to 0.40 Hz), ms^2						
Full Day	Corsano	312.58	0.66 (<0.001)	0.29 (<0.001)	−49.69	[1519.79, −1619.16]
	Whoop	268.87	0.68 (<0.001)	0.25 (<0.001)	63.74	[1769.18, −1641.71]
Awake	Corsano	404.71	0.56 (<0.001)	0.21 (<0.001)	−142.96	[1525.31, −1811.23]
	Whoop	298.56	0.6 (<0.001)	0.22 (<0.001)	4.81	[1591.43, −1581.81]
Asleep	**Corsano**	**202.24**	**0.84 (<0.001)**	**0.43 (<0.001)**	**34.86**	**[1351.93, −1282.2]**
	Whoop	236.42	0.78 (<0.001)	0.28 (<0.001)	112.07	[1845.99, −1621.85]

Table 5. *Cont.*

Time	Device	Mean Absolute Error	Spearman Correlation ρ (p-Value)	ICC (p-Value)	Mean Error (Bias)	Bland–Altman Limits of Agreement CI 95% (+, −)
			Ratio: LF/HF			
Full Day	Corsano	1.62	0.65 (<0.001)	0.51 (<0.001)	1.24	[6.17, −3.7]
	Whoop	1.34	0.69 (<0.001)	0.59 (<0.001)	0.80	[5.24, −3.65]
Awake	Corsano	2.16	0.55 (<0.001)	0.29 (<0.001)	1.93	[7.6, −3.74]
	Whoop	1.58	0.57 (<0.001)	0.44 (<0.001)	1.15	[6.03, −3.72]
Asleep	**Corsano**	**1.13**	**0.8 (<0.001)**	**0.73 (<0.001)**	**0.60**	**[4.46, −3.26]**
	Whoop	1.17	0.78 (<0.001)	0.69 (<0.001)	0.51	[4.57, −3.55]
			Sample Entropy			
Full Day	Corsano	0.41	0.45 (<0.001)	0.4 (<0.001)	−0.23	[0.69, −1.15]
	Whoop	0.45	0.45 (<0.001)	0.4 (<0.001)	0.21	[1.3, −0.87]
Awake	Corsano	0.46	0.32 (<0.001)	0.26 (<0.001)	−0.30	[0.7, −1.29]
	Whoop	0.59	0.32 (<0.001)	0.25 (<0.001)	0.41	[1.62, −0.8]
Asleep	Corsano	0.36	0.58 (<0.001)	0.53 (<0.001)	−0.17	[0.67, −1.01]
	Whoop	**0.33**	**0.65 (<0.001)**	**0.61 (<0.001)**	**0.05**	**[0.88, −0.79]**

4.4. Factors Impacting the Performance of a PPG-Based Device

The impact of coverage within epoch, body posture, daily life activities, epoch length, dominant vs. non-dominant hands, on the performance of the PPG-based device was explored only for the Corsano device, which provided the raw PPG data. While exploring the impact of these factors, a relative error in percentage is reported for the representative HR/HRV features.

We hypothesized that increasing the threshold for quantifying a valid epoch will lead to a more accurate estimation of HR/HRV features. Therefore, we experimented with the coverage threshold for a 5-min epoch from 40% to 100% and investigated its impact on the performance of HR/HRV features as shown in Figure 8. The relative error decreased for all the HR/HRV features on increasing the coverage. The error rate for RMSSD and SDNN reduced by approximately around 20% and 10%, respectively. Similar trends were observed for frequency and non-linear domain HRV features.

The impact of a variety of body postures, such as upright, reclined, lying left and right, prone, and supine positions, on PPG-derived HR/HRV features was investigated and presented in Figure 9. In all HR/HRV features, a higher error was observed during the upright and reclined positions. Specific lying positions played a critical role, such as lying face down in the prone position, which had a higher error rate compared to the supine position for the HR/HRV features. Similarly, lying on the right side has higher error than lying on the left side. The most appropriate position for PPG HRV features engineering was the lying position and especially lying on the left side. Various repetitive and cyclic daily living activities such as cycling, walking, and running resulted in a higher error rate in all the HR/HRV features, as shown in Figure 10. The lowest relative error was observed during rest, where the SDNN has a relatively lower error than RMSSD. Mobility, here, walking vs. non-walking, influenced the accuracy of PPG features, as shown in Figure 11. During walking, the relative error was higher than non-walking for all the HR/HRV features. The difference in the relative error between the two activities was 10% for SDNN and 15% for RMSSD. This difference increased further for the frequency and non-linear features as shown in Figure 11. Wearing the device on the dominant or non-dominant hand did not exhibit any significant difference (Appendix A).

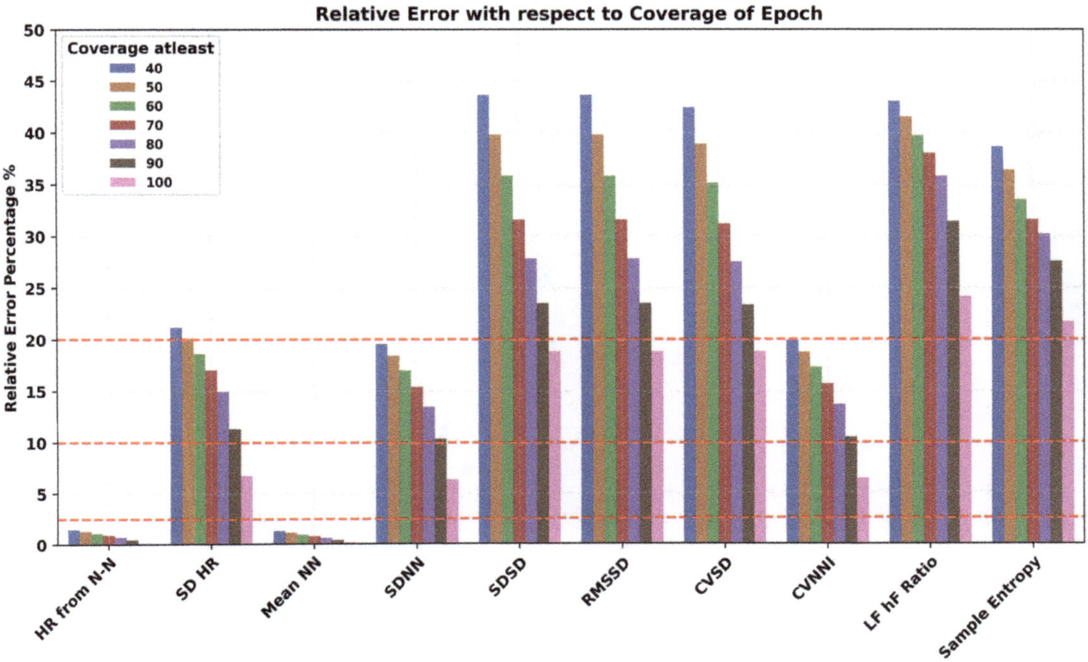

Figure 8. Impact of coverage within a 5-min epoch on the accuracy of PPG-derived HR and HRV features.

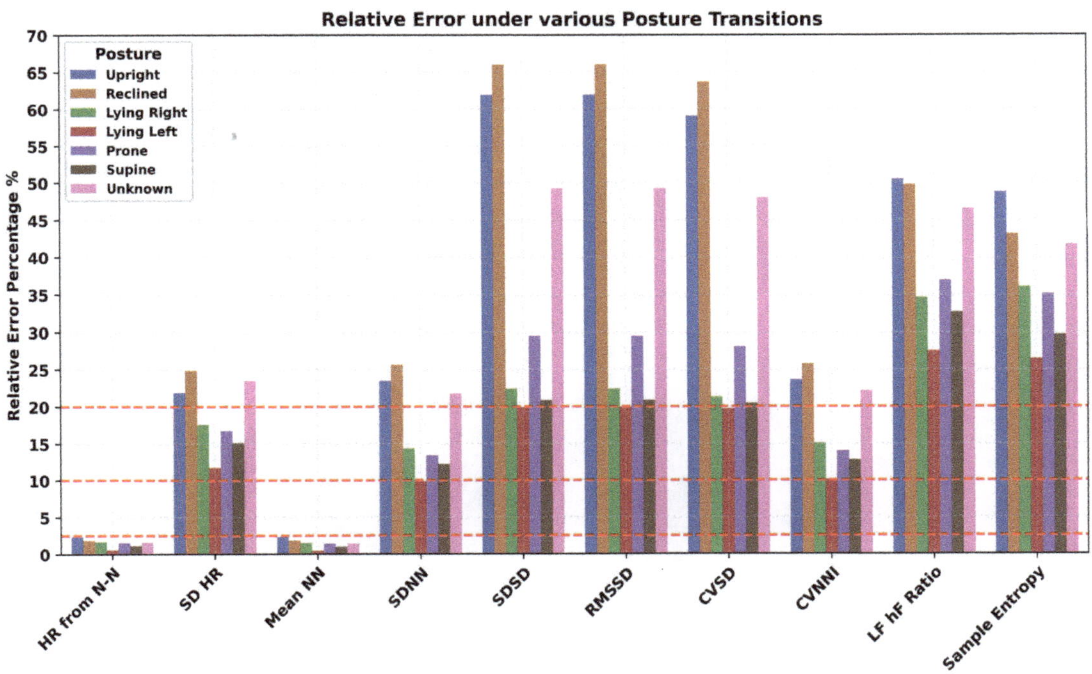

Figure 9. Impact of body posture on accuracy of PPG-derived HR and HRV features.

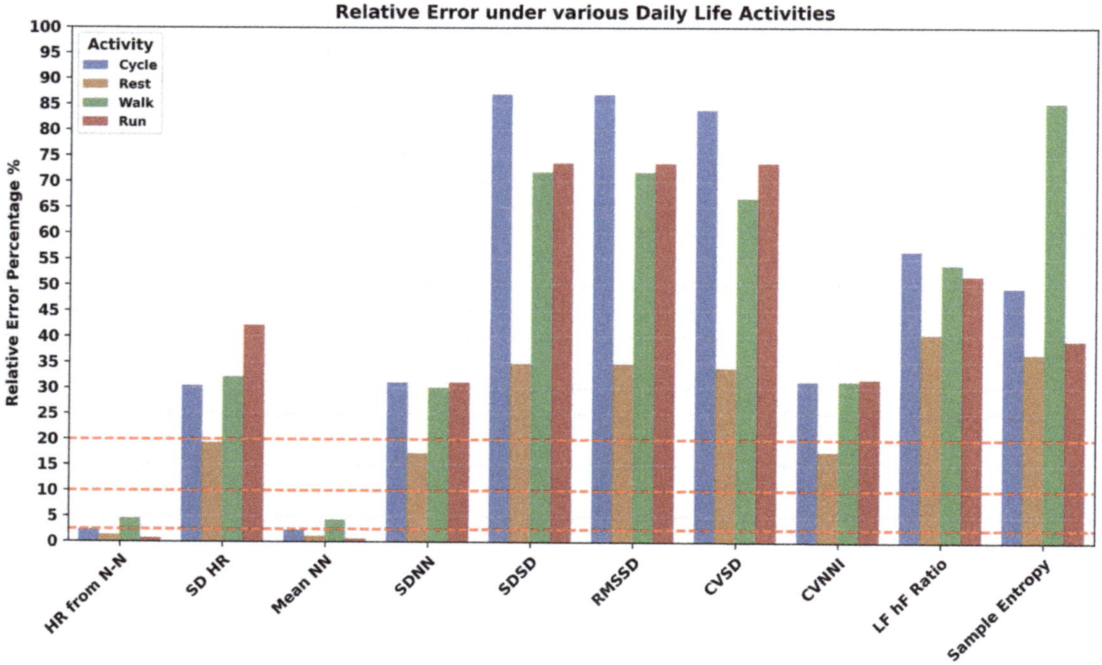

Figure 10. Impact of daily life activities on accuracy of PPG-derived HR and HRV features.

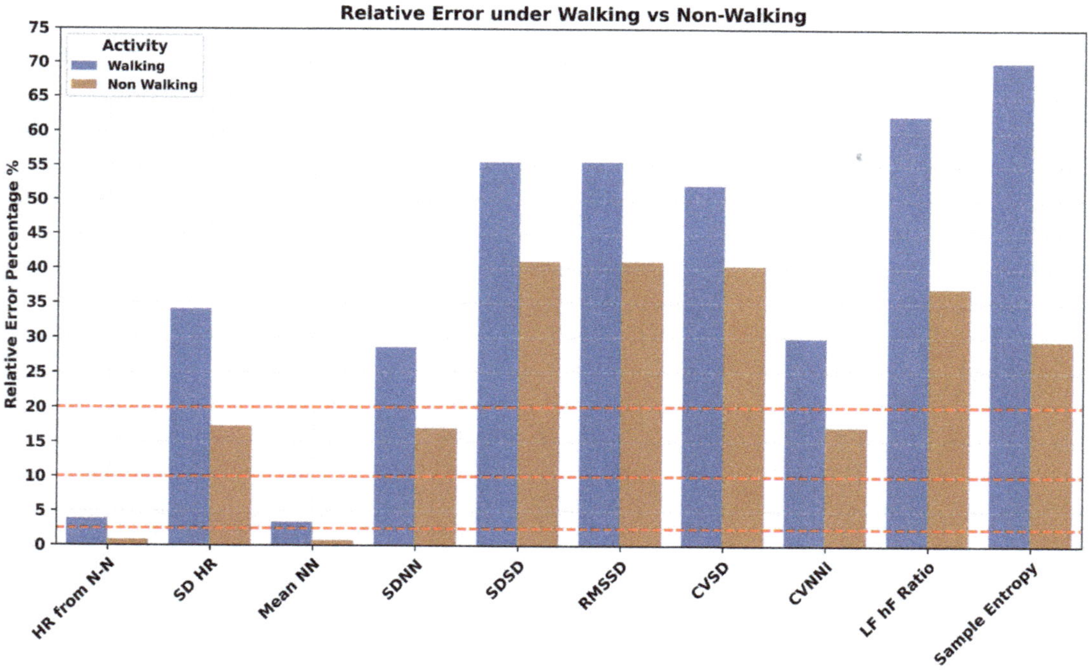

Figure 11. Impact of mobility on accuracy of PPG-derived HR and HRV features.

The impact of epoch length was explored under the awake (Figure 12A), asleep (Figure 12B), and full day periods (Figure 12C). Various epoch lengths, such as the default 5 min, 10 min, 30 min, and 60 min, whole awake time during the day, and whole asleep time during the night for all HR and HRV features estimation, were investigated. Interestingly, the correspondence of different PPG-derived HR and HRV features to ECG-derived ones behaves differently under various epoch lengths. The relative error rate increased for the mean HR and mean N-N intervals under both asleep and awake conditions while increasing the epoch length from 5 to 60 min. In contrast, for the majority of the time domain HRV features, the error rate reduced while increasing the epoch lengths. However, the relative error increased for the SDNN during the asleep period and did not follow the same trend as during the awake period. Similarly, the frequency domain HRV features also resulted in a lower error rate while increasing the epoch length. For non-linear features such as the sample entropy, the relative error went up with the increase in the epoch length. The asleep period resulted in the lowest relative error for the RMSSD. Again, SDNN behaved differently than RMSSD, where the SDNN performed well during the awake period compared to the asleep period.

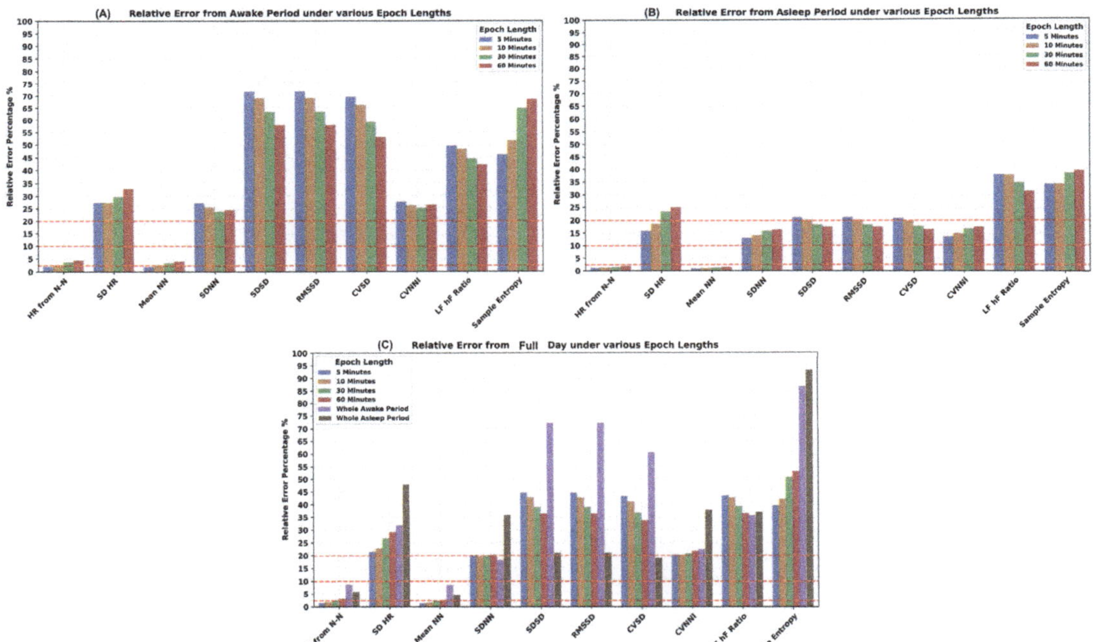

Figure 12. Impact of epoch length on accuracy of PPG-derived HR and HRV features.

4.5. Test–Retest Reliability of the HR and HRV Features in Daily Life

The test–retest reliability of the HRV features obtained from Corsano is shown in Table 6. Scatter plots for alignment of N-N intervals and HR estimated at the same time at two different adjacent days are provided in Figure 13 for both dominant and non-dominant hands. The dominant hand had higher reliability than non-dominant hands under awake, asleep, and full day periods. For all time domain HRV features, test–retest reliability was higher during the asleep periods compared to the awake periods. Frequency domain features also showed higher reliability during the asleep period compared to the awake period, except the LF/HF ratio, which had higher reliability during the awake period. Among all features, RMSSD from time domain HRV and HF from the frequency domain HRV had better reliability.

Table 6. Reliability assessment of HR and HRV features in daily life. Values in the table indicate the magnitude of intraclass correlation between Day 1 and Day 2 and their corresponding *p*-values in parenthesis.

Feature	Timings of the Day					
	Full Day		Awake		Asleep	
	Dominant	Non-Dominant	Dominant	Non-Dominant	Dominant	Non-Dominant
Heart Rate	0.72 (<0.001)	0.66 (<0.001)	0.65 (<0.001)	0.47 (<0.001)	0.68 (<0.001)	0.66 (<0.001)
SD HR	0.26 (<0.001)	0.33 (<0.001)	0.25 (<0.001)	0.20 (<0.001)	0.33 (<0.001)	0.35 (<0.001)
Mean N-N	0.76 (<0.001)	0.70 (<0.001)	0.71 (<0.001)	0.55 (<0.001)	0.67 (<0.001)	0.69 (<0.001)
SDNN	0.44 (<0.001)	0.42 (<0.001)	0.31 (<0.001)	0.26 (<0.001)	0.47 (<0.001)	0.42 (<0.001)
SDSD	0.70 (<0.001)	0.61 (<0.001)	0.30 (<0.001)	0.38 (<0.001)	0.77 (<0.001)	0.68 (<0.001)
RMSSD	0.70 (<0.001)	0.61 (<0.001)	0.30 (<0.001)	0.38 (<0.001)	0.77 (<0.001)	0.68 (<0.001)
CVSD	0.63 (<0.001)	0.59 (<0.001)	0.21 (<0.001)	0.31 (<0.001)	0.73 (<0.001)	0.66 (<0.001)
CVNN	0.32 (<0.001)	0.35 (<0.001)	0.20 (<0.001)	0.19 (<0.001)	0.41 (<0.001)	0.41 (<0.001)
LF	0.33 (<0.001)	0.31 (<0.001)	0.22 (<0.001)	0.09 (0.015)	0.34 (<0.001)	0.27 (<0.001)
HF	0.62 (<0.001)	0.59 (<0.001)	0.40 (<0.001)	0.33 (<0.001)	0.65 (<0.001)	0.60 (<0.001)
Ratio: LF/HF	0.39 (<0.001)	0.30 (<0.001)	0.69 (<0.001)	0.50 (<0.001)	0.28 (<0.001)	0.20 (<0.001)
Sample Entropy	0.11 (<0.001)	0.09 (<0.001)	0.05 (0.151)	0.08 (0.035)	0.20 (<0.001)	0.09 (0.001)

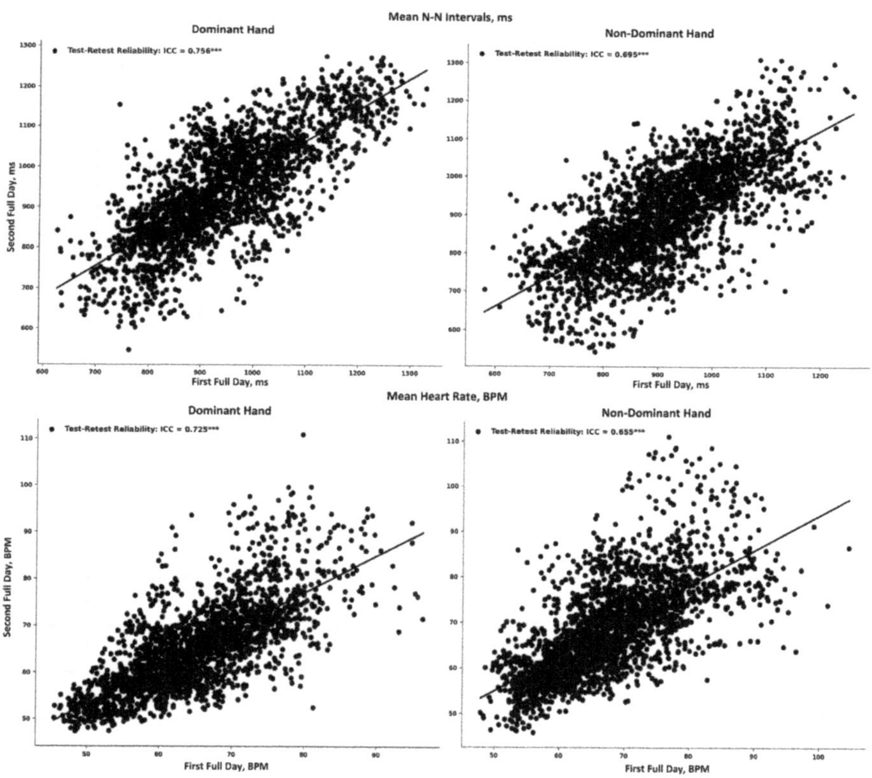

Figure 13. Test–retest reliability of mean N-N intervals (top row) and HR (bottom row) from dominant (left column) and non-dominant (right column) hands. Each black dot represents a synchronized 5-min epoch. *** indicates *p*-value is <0.001.

4.6. Performance of Beat Detection Algorithms on the Noisy PPG Sensor Data

A suite of seven beat detection algorithms was investigated to evaluate their performance in analyzing raw PPG signals collected in daily life settings. The performance of each algorithm to detect beat and mean absolute percentage error (MAPE) for HR estimation is shown in Figure 14A,B and Table 7. Considering all the recorded data, the performance of the algorithms for the beat detection assessed via F1 score appeared to be similar (Figure 14A). When the performance was evaluated using MAPE for HR estimation, differences between algorithm performance emerged, with only three algorithms, MSPDT, ERMA, and AMPD, having MAPE lower than 10%. The beat detection F1 score performance of these algorithms was around 62% with a 95% CI in the range of 44% to 87%. The median sensitivity was 59–61% with a 95% CI in the range of 42% to 95%. The positive predictive value (PPV) was 63–64%. For HR estimation, apart from MAPE, the mean absolute error (MAE) for three top-performing algorithms was 7 BPM with a negative bias of around 2–3 beats. For the interbeat interval estimation, the MAE error for the top performing algorithms ranged in between 249 ms and 337 ms (Table 7).

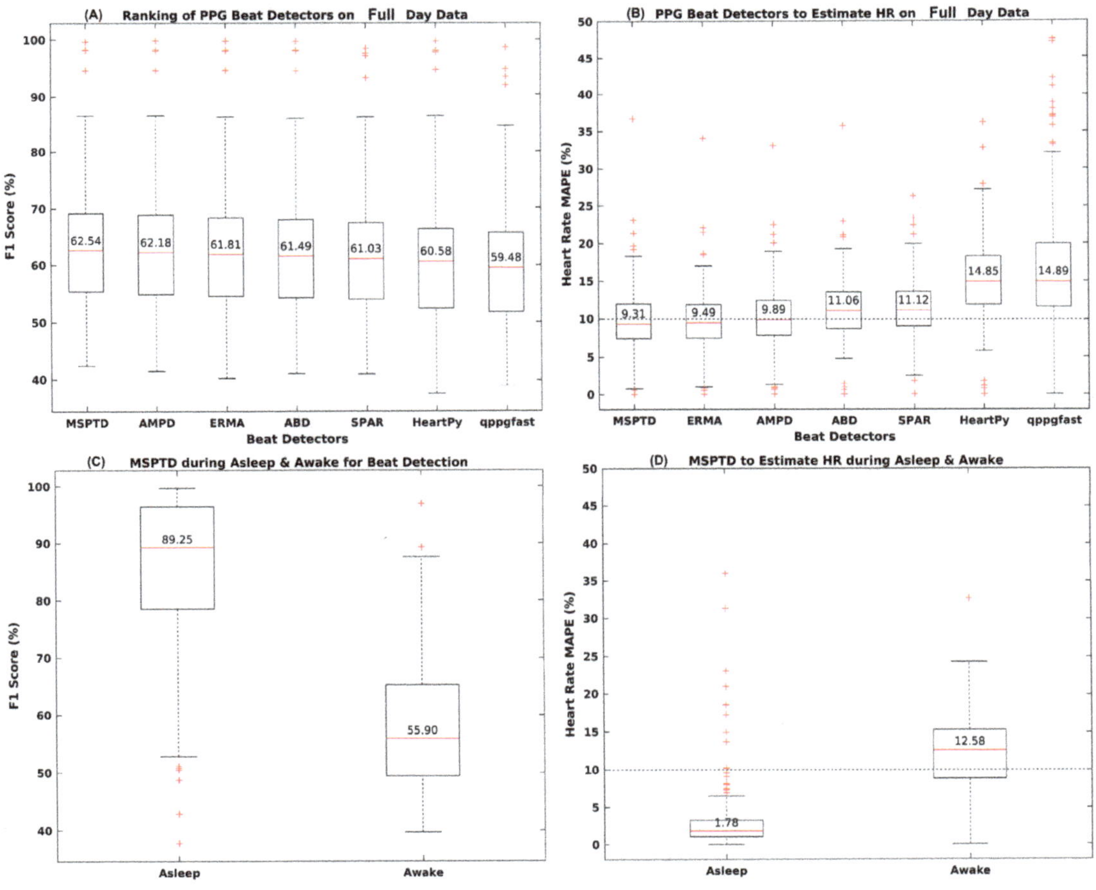

Figure 14. Performance of various beat detectors on the noisy PPG data compared to R-peak detected from ECG in daily life recordings.

Table 7. Performance metric of PPG beat detectors compared to R-peak detected from ECG in daily life recordings. All the performance metrics are reported as median values along with 95% confidence intervals.

Task	Metric	Beat Detector Selection on the Full Day PPG Data						
		MSPTD	**AMPD**	**ERMA**	**ABD**	**SPAR**	**HeartPy**	**qppgfast**
Beat Detection	F1 Score	62.54 [45.10, 86.95]	62.18 [44.70, 86.89]	61.81 [44.68, 86.61]	61.49 [44.32, 86.28]	61.03 [44.13, 86.37]	60.58 [42.29, 86.60]	59.48 [43.05, 84.78]
	Sensitivity	61.66 [44.48, 94.78]	60.67 [43.60, 89.90]	59.85 [42.91, 86.55]	59.93 [43.07, 86.03]	58.92 [42.51, 85.70]	55.68 [37.23, 84.74]	57.61 [38.82, 84.35]
	PPV	63.03 [44.33, 89.79]	63.83 [44.80, 90.02]	64.16 [45.14, 89.29]	63.56 [44.80, 89.19]	64.11 [45.09, 88.79]	66.21 [45.74, 90.51]	61.35 [44.66, 85.20]
HR Estimation, BPM	MAPE	9.31 [1.18, 19.26]	9.89 [1.27, 20.04]	9.49 [1.26, 18.48]	11.06 [1.38, 19.35]	11.12 [3.31, 20.03]	14.85 [1.73, 27.06]	14.89 [6.87, 38.95]
	MAE	7.27 [2.31, 15.87]	7.59 [2.33, 18.02]	7.24 [2.38, 16.11]	8.44 [2.99, 17.74]	8.89 [2.86, 19.29]	11.28 [3.51, 23.48]	11.57 [4.83, 25.78]
	Bias	−1.91 [−9.83, 3.58]	−3.58 [−12.96, 1.00]	−3.46 [−14.35, 1.48]	−3.78 [−13.00, 2.24]	−5.63 [−16.08, −0.79]	−8.61 [−20.71, −0.78]	−1.91 [−11.15, 15.63]
	LOA	[12.29, 57.37]	[12.27, 52.21]	[11.96, 38.47]	[13.89, 42.02]	[12.55, 44.79]	[16.68, 50.11]	[19.77, 60.13]
Inter Beat Interval, ms	MAE	249.68 [118.52, 439.18]	269.88 [133.50, 461.53]	337.57 [139.99, 895.76]	355.39 [182.3, 644.1]	309.57 [174.3, 516.9]	637.15 [286.8, 2143.03]	951.21 [259.5, 2949.68]
	Bias	−54.27 [−249.82, 61.42]	−23.79 [−232.97, 97.49]	25.84 [−168.32, 651.07]	42.92 [−229.3, 342.66]	21.54 [−207.3, 165.29]	328.71 [−23.4, 1938.50]	564.21 [−19.66, 2621.57]
	LOA	[620.64, 3228.51]	[664.93, 3276.37]	[792.02, 10956.50]	[844.73, 7507.64]	[815.26, 3363.01]	[1413.30, 13,584.81]	[2692.00, 27,274.76]

The top-performing algorithm, MSPDT, which is a modified version of the AMPD algorithm, was explored further on a subset of data corresponding to the asleep and awake periods separately. The results are shown in Figure 14C,D and Table 8. The F1 score for beat detection with MSPTD went up from 55% during the awake period to 89% during the asleep period. The sensitivity of the MSPTD during asleep was 89% and 54% during the awake period. Furthermore, the PPV was also 89% during the asleep and 57% during the awake period (Figure 14C). The MAPE for HR estimation significantly reduced from 12.58% during the awake period to 1.78% during the asleep period (Figure 14D). The MAE for HR estimation was around 1 beat during asleep and 10 beats during the awake period. Additionally, MSPTD MAE for the interbeat intervals was also significantly reduced to 54 ms during the asleep period compared to 220 ms during the awake period.

Table 8. Top performing PPG beat detector (MSPTD) performance under awake and asleep periods. All the performance metrics are reported as median values along with 95% confidence intervals.

Task	Metric	MSPTD Performance During Awake and Asleep Period	
		Awake	Asleep
Beat Detection	F1 Score	55.90 [43.26, 83.75]	89.25 [50.91, 99.37]
	Sensitivity	54.76 [43.79, 86.48]	89.94 [50.85, 99.46]
	PPV	57.62 [41.18, 86.27]	89.45 [50.98, 99.34]
HR Estimation, BPM	MAPE	12.58 [3.17, 22.91]	1.78 [0.65, 18.60]
	MAE	10.01 [3.67, 20.84]	1.12 [0.41, 14.47]
	Bias	−3.44 [−15.47, 3.29]	0.03 [−4.39, 7.66]
	LOA	[14.64, 59.31]	[2.44, 75.21]
Inter Beat Interval, ms	MAE	219.99 [107.23, 421.95]	53.80 [25.94, 205.58]
	Bias	67.29 [−243.54, 189.07]	−4.50 [−58.29, 65.19]
	LOA	[450.25, 2534.76]	[129.31, 1457.40]

5. Discussion

In this paper, we performed a systematic validation of physiological measures derived from PPG devices collected over multiple days in free living settings, which, to the best of our knowledge, is the first of its kind. Specifically, we investigated the feasibility of the remote collection of physiological measures from PPG devices in daily life, the usability of such devices, and the accuracy of derived features at different time intervals of day: awake, asleep, or throughout the day. We examined the impact of body posture, mobility, and data coverage on the accuracy of the features and evaluated their test–retest reliability. Furthermore, we quantified the performance of various algorithms to detect heartbeats from noisy raw PPG signals.

5.1. Feasibility of PPG Data Collection and Device Performance

Our results showed that users found PPG devices comfortable and easy to use, resulting in positive usability ratings. While the ECG data yielded 100% coverage for most days and consistent beat detection throughout the day, PPG devices showed variability in coverage and detected fewer beats at daytime compared to nighttime. The prior work has shown coverage rates ranging from 70% to 90% for estimating heart rate and 50% to 90% for estimating pulse arrival time (PAT) or pulse amplitude variability (PAV), with variations based on sensor location and quality [53].

Corsano generally had a lower error in estimating N-N intervals and HR compared to Whoop. Both devices showed good relative and absolute agreement with ECG-derived features and performed similarly for time-domain HRV features like RMSSD and SDNN. In the frequency domain, both devices showed higher error rates and lower absolute agreement. This is in line with the previous work, which showed that the frequency-domain HRV features explored previously in elderly vascular patients, especially those associated with high-frequency content, were systematically overestimated [54]. This overestimation resulted in a relatively large bias, indicating that care should be taken in interpreting these parameters when derived from wrist-worn wearable devices. The error rates in our work were lower during asleep than awake periods for all HRV features. Corsano demonstrated superior performance, particularly during asleep periods, with mean errors for heart rate and N-N intervals being minimal. This finding from Corsano and Whoop aligns with the general observation that wearable PPG devices tend to perform better in situations with minimal motion, such as during sleep [28,55]. However, these conclusions cannot be generalized to all PPG devices without further comparative evaluations. Both devices, however, tended to overestimate N-N intervals across all conditions. This is due to the inherent limitations of PPG technology in accurately capturing beat-to-beat intervals under varying conditions. Motion artifacts, diverse skin types, and signal crossover, among others, could contribute to such potential inaccuracies in PPG-derived measurements [56].

5.2. Factors Impacting the Performance of PPG-Based Devices and Derived Features

The performance of PPG devices was influenced by several factors. The coverage within a 5-min epoch significantly impacted the accuracy of HR/HRV features. Increasing the epoch coverage from 40% to 100% decreased the relative error in HR/HRV features, with a 20% reduction in error rate for RMSSD and over 10% for SDNN. The estimation of SDNN showed small biases when compared with the ECG reference, while RMSSD exhibited systematic overestimation in the range of 10%. This indicates that the accuracy and reliability of HRV measurements from PPG can significantly vary based on the quality and coverage of the data [54].

Human body posture during daily life activities influenced the estimation of PPG-derived features. Higher error rates in HR/HRV features were observed in upright and reclined positions compared to specific lying positions. The prone position showed a higher error rate than the supine position. Lying on the right side resulted in higher errors than lying on the left side, irrespective of whether the device was on the right or left hand. The most suitable position for PPG HRV features engineering was the lying position, particularly on the left side. It is likely that during upright positions, there is more movement in the upper body and hands compared to lying positions. Daily life activities like cycling, walking, and running resulted in higher error rates in all PPG HR/HRV features. The difference in relative error between walking and non-walking was significant, nearly 10% for SDNN and 15% for RMSSD. This difference increased further for frequency and non-linear HRV features, suggesting that PPG data should ideally be recorded during non-walking activities for more accurate results. According to a prior study, absolute error across wearable devices was 30% higher on average during motion than during rest for HR/HRV [56]. Another study showed that wearable devices can detect heart rates accurately under resting conditions; however, daily life physical activities impact the performance of these PPG-based devices [57].

Different epoch lengths (5, 10, 30, 60 min) for HR and HRV feature estimation were analyzed. There was an increase in error for mean HR and N-N intervals with longer epochs and a decrease in error for most time domain HRV features. For frequency domain and non-linear features, error generally increased with longer epochs. The lowest error for RMSSD was noted during the asleep period. Short-term spectral HRV analysis, typically conducted over a few minutes, is useful for tracking rapid changes in cardiac autonomic function. In contrast, long-term spectral HRV analysis, ranging from an hour to a full day, provides a more stable assessment of autonomic function, capturing longer fluctuations and better predicting prognosis. However, long-term analyses are more resource-intensive and susceptible to noise and variability due to environmental factors and daily activities [58]. Furthermore, HRV indices vary significantly across distinct sleep epochs, challenging the practice of aggregating HRV indices across these epochs from the whole asleep period.

The previous work [59] found that both rapid eye movement (REM) and non-REM stage 2 (N2) sleep epochs showed a change in HRV indices throughout the night. This variability suggests that aggregating HRV indices across sleep stages could obscure important transient effects.

5.3. Reliability of the PPG-Based Assessments in Daily Life

Different levels of reliability based on hand dominance and state of consciousness (awake/asleep) were observed in this study. Generally, the features extracted from a signal recorded from the dominant hand showed higher reliability across all periods. Time domain HRV features exhibited greater test–retest reliability during asleep periods than awake periods. Similarly, frequency domain HRV features, except the LF/HF ratio, showed better reliability during asleep periods. In contrast, the LF/HF ratio had improved reliability during awake periods. Non-linear HRV features displayed better reliability with the dominant hand during asleep periods. In the context of HRV reliability during repetitive low-intensity activities, a study found that the time interval between repeated measurements did not influence the HRV values, indicating HRV's reliability under different low intensity activities [60]. Furthermore, the previous work [61] also showed HRV's potential as a reliable measure in varying states of consciousness, supporting our observed findings of varying levels of HRV reliability based on the state of consciousness (awake/asleep).

5.4. Algorithms for Beat Detection from Noisy PPG Sensor Data During Daily Life

In the evaluation of algorithms for processing noisy PPG data, three out of seven algorithms—MSPDT, ERMA, and AMPD—stood out by achieving heart rate estimation accuracy with a MAPE below 10%. Furthermore, MSPDT showed significantly better performance during asleep than when awake, with improvements in beat detection and a substantial reduction in both MAPE and MAE for inter-beat intervals. In terms of algorithmic logic, the AMPD algorithm's [46] strength lies in its local maxima scalogram matrix, which identifies optimal scales for capturing the most local maxima in a PPG signal. This scale-based approach allows for more precise beat detection amidst variable signal quality. ERMA [47] uses Butterworth bandpass filtering and applies specific moving averages to emphasize systolic peaks and individual beats. This method enhances the signal's features relevant for accurate beat detection, even in the presence of noise. MSPDT [49] employs a modified version of the AMPD algorithm, optimizing the detection of local maxima and minima in PPG signals. This approach is particularly effective in differentiating true signal peaks from noise, which is crucial in noisy environments. The previous work also highlights the importance of choosing the right PPG beat detector algorithm, noting that algorithms like MSPDT show complementary performance characteristics in different conditions, such as rest and exercise, and in different patient demographics [33,62]. More details on the MSPDT algorithm and their implementation can be found in a prior work [63].

5.5. Key Insights and Recommendations

This study provides crucial insights into the use of PPG devices for HRV monitoring in daily life settings. It reveals that while PPG devices like the Corsano and Whoop show reasonable accuracy in comparison to ECG data, especially during sleep, their performance is affected by various factors such as data coverage, body posture, activity types, and epoch length. Time domain HRV features exhibit higher reliability during asleep periods. Frequency domain features, except for the LF/HF ratio, show better agreement during asleep periods. Additionally, algorithms like MSPDT, ERMA, and AMPD are effective in processing noisy PPG data, with MSPDT being particularly effective during asleep periods.

Based on these insights, several recommendations are proposed. There is a need for manufacturers to enhance data coverage and optimize algorithms to improve PPG device accuracy, particularly during daytime activities. Emphasis should be placed on design aspects like sensor placement and stability to minimize motion artifacts. Users and clinicians should be informed of the optimal conditions for PPG device use, understanding their limitations, especially during high-intensity activities. Future research should focus on reducing the impact of motion artifacts and other external factors on PPG data quality and developing more robust algorithms for various real-life conditions. Finally, while PPG devices offer a convenient means for HRV monitoring, caution is advised in interpreting data for clinical decisions, especially in scenarios where high precision is required. These recommendations highlight the potential of PPG devices in HRV monitoring while acknowledging the necessity for further improvements in technology and usage guidelines.

5.6. Study Limitations

The study presents several limitations. It focused on healthy individuals, limiting its assessment to the patient population. The scope of this work has been limited to two PPG devices, and future work should explore a broader range of PPG technologies, such as those worn on fingers. Future work should also include heterogenous demographics to assess the impact of skin tone, which has not been investigated in this work. In this study, the impact of charging on data coverage has not been explored, which may be investigated in future studies through the collection of self-reported questionnaires on participant's charging times or duration throughout the study. Moreover, the use of signal-processing-based beat detectors, while reliable, highlights the necessity for the development of novel algorithms. These new algorithms would be instrumental in enhancing beat detection accuracy in challenging scenarios, marking a key direction for future advancements in wearable health technology.

6. Conclusions

This work evaluated the performance of wearable PPG devices for HR and HRV monitoring in daily life settings, thus enhancing the applicability of our findings to real-world scenarios, which is vital for both consumer and clinical applications. Our results showed that, overall, PPG-based devices showed promise in monitoring physiological features. The data coverage of PPG devices was lower during active daytime hours, and beat detection capability was noticeably diminished during the day. Data coverage and beat detection accuracy were high, especially when the users were sleeping. Agreement varied by coverage threshold, epoch length, body posture, and activity type. Users found the devices comfortable and user-friendly, resulting in good positive usability ratings. A MSPDT algorithm performed best in detecting beats from noisy raw PPG signals. The study recommends optimal PPG data collection strategy and analysis methodologies that should be employed in a clinical trial where such devices may be used for remote health monitoring to minimize estimation error of HR and HRV and thus aid in accurate clinical decision making.

Author Contributions: Conceptualization, M.C., M.M. and N.V.M.; design of study and wearable data, M.C. and M.M.; formal analysis plan and implementation, R.Z.U.R., M.C. and N.V.M.; data compliance monitoring, R.Z.U.R., A.O., T.T. and Y.H.; vendor management, M.M., M.D., A.O. and T.T.; trial data transfer, Y.H. and V.T.T.; trial data collection, M.D., A.J., S.S. and P.-J.B.; project feedback, T.M., M.V.L., E.R. and D.Y.; manuscript preparation, R.Z.U.R. and M.C.; manuscript review, all authors; supervision, M.C. and M.M. All authors have read and agreed to the published version of the manuscript.

Funding: This research received no external funding.

Institutional Review Board Statement: All subjects gave their informed consent for inclusion before they participated in the study. The study was conducted in accordance with the Declaration of Helsinki, and the protocol was approved by the Ethics Committee of UZA/UAntwerp (3738-BUN B3002022000126).

Informed Consent Statement: Written informed consent was obtained from all participants involved in the study.

Data Availability Statement: The data sharing policy of Janssen Pharmaceutical Companies of Johnson and Johnson is available at https://www.janssen.com/clinical-trials/transparency (accessed on 21 October 2024). Requests for access to the study data can be submitted through Yale Open Data Access (YODA) project site at http://yoda.yale.edu (accessed on 21 October 2024).

Acknowledgments: The authors are thankful to the study participants who contributed to the data collection.

Conflicts of Interest: All authors are employed by Janssen R&D and may own company stock.

Appendix A. Impact of Dominant vs. Non-Dominant Hand on PPG Device Performance

Impact of the dominant vs. non-dominant hand wearing position on the accuracy of PPG derived HR/HRV features was explored during awake (Figure A1A), asleep (Figure A1B), and full day periods (Figure A1C). Overall, for all the HR/HRV features, the difference between the dominant and non-dominant hands was not significant. During the awake period, the dominant hand had slightly higher error for time domain HRV compared to the non-dominant hand. However, during the asleep period, the non-dominant hand had a slightly higher error compared to the dominant hand for all HRV features. During the full day period, the difference between the dominant and non-dominant hand was negligible.

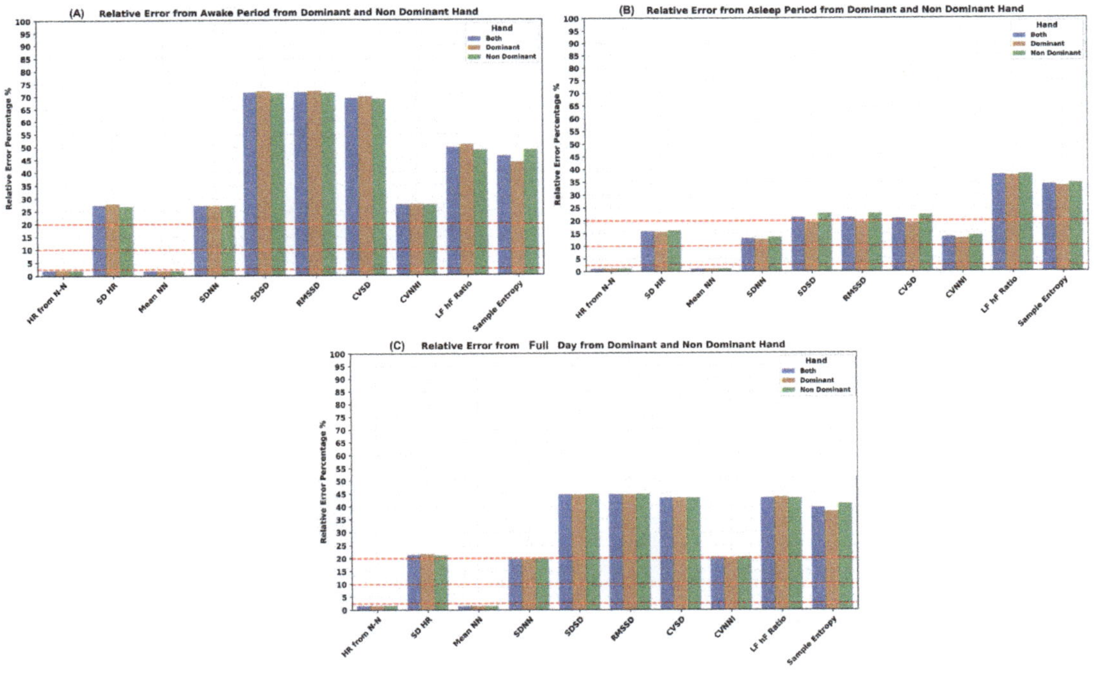

Figure A1. Impact of dominant vs. non-dominant wrist on accuracy of PPG-derived HR and HRV features.

Appendix B. Impact of Interpolation and No-Interpolation Within the 5-min Epoch of N-N Intervals on the Accuracy of the HRV Features (e.g., SDNN, RMSSD)

This topic of signal preprocessing and its impact on heart rate variability (HRV) metrics has already been investigated in greater detail, particularly in a study such as "Effects of Missing Data on Heart Rate Variability Metrics" by [41]. According to this paper, "*The optimal correction methodology for HRV metrics varies: correction without gap filling is superior for SDNN, RMSSD, and Poincaré plot metrics when missing beats occur predominantly in bursts, while gap-filling methods are advantageous for instances of sporadic missing beats. Gap-filling methodologies achieved optimal performance regarding frequency-domain parameters"*. There are mixed results in terms of which features to interpolate. This study [41] highlights that different interpolation techniques (including linear interpolation) have varying effects on HRV metrics, depending on the nature of the missing data. For example, while linear interpolation works well for scattered missing beats, other approaches may be more suitable for burst-type data loss. However, to simplify the preprocessing for our validation study, we opted to use linear interpolation for all HRV features rather than adopting different interpolation strategies for each feature. We prioritized the practical application in real-world settings, allowing for typical interruptions like motion artifacts or signal dropouts, with a 40% data presence threshold per epoch to ensure robustness. Additionally, an ablation study comparing SDNN and RMSSD metrics, with and without interpolation, showed improved results with longer epoch coverage, as seen in Table A1.

Table A1. Impact of interpolation and no-interpolation on the performance of the HRV features (e.g., SDNN, RMSSD) when extracted from a PPG-based device and compared with an ECG-based device.

Time	Interpolation/ No-Interpolation	Mean Absolute Error	Spearman Correlation ρ (*p*-Value)	ICC (*p*-Value)	Mean Error (Bias)	Bland–Altman Limits of Agreement CI 95% (+, −)
			SDNN, ms (SD of the N-N intervals)			
Full Day	Interpolation	13.89	0.78 (<0.001)	0.69 (<0.001)	4.41	[50.67, −41.85]
	No-Interpolation	12.67	0.80 (<0.001)	0.72 (<0.001)	4.36	[46.60, −37.87]
Awake	Interpolation	16.47	0.62 (<0.001)	0.55 (<0.001)	1.08	[52.28, −50.12]
	No-Interpolation	14.92	0.66 (<0.001)	0.59 (<0.001)	1.53	[48.22, −45.15]
Asleep	Interpolation	10.92	0.91 (<0.001)	0.80 (<0.001)	7.91	[45.7, −29.89]
	No-Interpolation	10.09	0.92 (<0.001)	0.82 (<0.001)	7.34	[42.07, −27.37]
			RMSSD, ms (Square root of mean of the sum of squares of differences between adjacent N-N intervals)			
Full Day	Interpolation	12.53	0.7 (<0.001)	0.65 (<0.001)	−9.43	[22.78, −41.64]
	No-Interpolation	16.76	0.65 (<0.001)	0.53 (<0.001)	−10.97	[38.31, −60.25]
Awake	Interpolation	17.99	0.58 (<0.001)	0.43 (<0.001)	−15.43	[20.04, −50.91]
	No-Interpolation	23.98	0.50 (<0.001)	0.32 (<0.001)	−18.92	[35.92, −73.75]
Asleep	Interpolation	6.89	0.89 (<0.001)	0.87 (<0.001)	−3.57	[18.27, −25.4]
	No-Interpolation	9.13	0.85 (<0.001)	0.79 (<0.001)	−3.16	[30.86, −37.18]

The ablation study in Table A1 shows that for SDNN, no-interpolation slightly improves performance, especially during awake periods, while RMSSD performs better with interpolation, particularly when handling larger data gaps. These findings confirm our methodology's robustness, suggesting that no-interpolation may be beneficial for SDNN, but linear interpolation helps manage RMSSD variability due to missing data.

References

1. Antikainen, E.; Njoum, H.; Kudelka, J.; Branco, D.; Rehman, R.Z.U.; Macrae, V.; Davies, K.; Hildesheim, H.; Emmert, K.; Reilmann, R.; et al. Assessing Fatigue and Sleep in Chronic Diseases Using Physiological Signals from Wearables: A Pilot Study. *Front. Physiol.* **2022**, *13*, 968185. [CrossRef] [PubMed]
2. Avey, S.; Chatterjee, M.; Manyakov, N.V.; Cooper, P.; Sabins, N.; Mosca, K.; Mori, S.; Baribaud, F.; Morris, M.; Lehar, J.; et al. Using a Wearable Patch to Develop a Digital Monitoring Biomarker of Inflammation in Response to LPS Challenge. *Clin. Transl. Sci.* **2024**, *17*, e13734. [CrossRef] [PubMed]
3. Kim, K.-N.; Yao, Y.; Ju, S.-Y. Heart Rate Variability and Inflammatory Bowel Disease in Humans. *Medicine* **2020**, *99*, e23430. [CrossRef] [PubMed]
4. Shaffer, F.; Ginsberg, J.P. An Overview of Heart Rate Variability Metrics and Norms. *Front. Public Health* **2017**, *5*, 258. [CrossRef]
5. Nitulescu, A.; Crisan-Vida, M.; Stoicu-Tivadar, L. Continuous Monitoring and Statistical Modelling of Heart Rate Variability. *Stud. Health Technol. Inf.* **2020**, *270*, 128–132. [CrossRef]

6. Monfredi, O.J.; Moore, C.C.; Sullivan, B.A.; Keim-Malpass, J.; Fairchild, K.D.; Loftus, T.J.; Bihorac, A.; Krahn, K.N.; Dubrawski, A.; Lake, D.E.; et al. Continuous ECG Monitoring Should Be the Heart of Bedside AI-Based Predictive Analytics Monitoring for Early Detection of Clinical Deterioration. *J. Electrocardiol.* **2023**, *76*, 35–38. [CrossRef]
7. Pinheiro, N.; Couceiro, R.; Henriques, J.; Muehlsteff, J.; Quintal, I.; Goncalves, L.; Carvalho, P. Can PPG Be Used for HRV Analysis? *Annu. Int. Conf. IEEE Eng. Med. Biol. Soc.* **2016**, *2016*, 2945–2949. [CrossRef]
8. Plews, D.J.; Scott, B.; Altini, M.; Wood, M.; Kilding, A.E.; Laursen, P.B. Comparison of Heart-Rate-Variability Recording With Smartphone Photoplethysmography, Polar H7 Chest Strap, and Electrocardiography. *Int. J. Sports Physiol. Perform.* **2017**, *12*, 1324–1328. [CrossRef]
9. Martín Gómez, R.; Allevard, E.; Kamstra, H.; Cotter, J.; Lamb, P. Validity and Reliability of Movesense HR+ ECG Measurements for High-Intensity Running and Cycling. *Sensors* **2024**, *24*, 5713. [CrossRef]
10. Leveque, J.L.; Corcuff, P.; de Rigal, J.; Agache, P. In Vivo Studies of the Evolution of Physical Properties of the Human Skin with Age. *Int. J. Dermatol.* **1984**, *23*, 322–329. [CrossRef]
11. Dao, H.; Kazin, R.A. Gender Differences in Skin: A Review of the Literature. *Gend. Med.* **2007**, *4*, 308–328. [CrossRef] [PubMed]
12. Preejith, S.P.; Alex, A.; Joseph, J.; Sivaprakasam, M. Design, Development and Clinical Validation of a Wrist-Based Optical Heart Rate Monitor. In Proceedings of the 2016 IEEE International Symposium on Medical Measurements and Applications (MeMeA), Benevento, Italy, 15–18 May 2016; pp. 1–6.
13. Ahn, J.M. New Aging Index Using Signal Features of Both Photoplethysmograms and Acceleration Plethysmograms. *Health Inf. Res.* **2017**, *23*, 53–59. [CrossRef] [PubMed]
14. Phuong, C.; Maibach, H.I. Gender Differences in Skin. In *Textbook of Aging Skin*; Farage, M.A., Miller, K.W., Maibach, H.I., Eds.; Springer: Berlin/Heidelberg, Germany, 2017; pp. 1729–1755. ISBN 978-3-662-47398-6.
15. Allen, J. Photoplethysmography and Its Application in Clinical Physiological Measurement. *Physiol. Meas.* **2007**, *28*, R1. [CrossRef]
16. Meredith, D.J.; Clifton, D.; Charlton, P.; Brooks, J.; Pugh, C.W.; Tarassenko, L. Photoplethysmographic Derivation of Respiratory Rate: A Review of Relevant Physiology. *J. Med. Eng. Technol.* **2012**, *36*, 1–7. [CrossRef]
17. Khan, M.; Pretty, C.G.; Amies, A.C.; Elliott, R.; Shaw, G.M.; Chase, J.G. Investigating the Effects of Temperature on Photoplethysmography. *IFAC-PapersOnLine* **2015**, *48*, 360–365. [CrossRef]
18. Charlton, P.H.; Bonnici, T.; Tarassenko, L.; Clifton, D.A.; Beale, R.; Watkinson, P.J. An Assessment of Algorithms to Estimate Respiratory Rate from the Electrocardiogram and Photoplethysmogram. *Physiol. Meas.* **2016**, *37*, 610. [CrossRef]
19. Teng, X.-F.; Zhang, Y.-T. Theoretical Study on the Effect of Sensor Contact Force on Pulse Transit Time. *IEEE Trans. Biomed. Eng.* **2007**, *54*, 1490–1498. [CrossRef]
20. Kim, J.; Lee, T.; Kim, J.; Ko, H. Ambient Light Cancellation in Photoplethysmogram Application Using Alternating Sampling and Charge Redistribution Technique. In Proceedings of the 2015 37th Annual International Conference of the IEEE Engineering in Medicine and Biology Society (EMBC), Milan, Italy, 25–29 August 2015; pp. 6441–6444.
21. Zong, C.; Jafari, R. Robust Heart Rate Estimation Using Wrist-Based PPG Signals in the Presence of Intense Physical Activities. In Proceedings of the 2015 37th Annual International Conference of the IEEE Engineering in Medicine and Biology Society (EMBC), Milan, Italy, 25–29 August 2015; pp. 8078–8082.
22. Stahl, S.E.; An, H.-S.; Dinkel, D.M.; Noble, J.M.; Lee, J.-M. How Accurate Are the Wrist-Based Heart Rate Monitors during Walking and Running Activities? Are They Accurate Enough? *BMJ Open Sport Exerc. Med.* **2016**, *2*, e000106. [CrossRef]
23. Dooley, E.E.; Golaszewski, N.M.; Bartholomew, J.B. Estimating Accuracy at Exercise Intensities: A Comparative Study of Self-Monitoring Heart Rate and Physical Activity Wearable Devices. *JMIR Mhealth Uhealth* **2017**, *5*, e7043. [CrossRef]
24. Schaffarczyk, M.; Rogers, B.; Reer, R.; Gronwald, T. Validity of the Polar H10 Sensor for Heart Rate Variability Analysis during Resting State and Incremental Exercise in Recreational Men and Women. *Sensors* **2022**, *22*, 6536. [CrossRef]
25. Cilhoroz, B.; Giles, D.; Zaleski, A.; Taylor, B.; Fernhall, B.; Pescatello, L. Validation of the Polar V800 Heart Rate Monitor and Comparison of Artifact Correction Methods among Adults with Hypertension. *PLoS ONE* **2020**, *15*, e0240220. [CrossRef] [PubMed]
26. Miller, D.J.; Sargent, C.; Roach, G.D. A Validation of Six Wearable Devices for Estimating Sleep, Heart Rate and Heart Rate Variability in Healthy Adults. *Sensors* **2022**, *22*, 6317. [CrossRef] [PubMed]
27. Blok, S.; Piek, M.A.; Tulevski, I.I.; Somsen, G.A.; Winter, M.M. The Accuracy of Heartbeat Detection Using Photoplethysmography Technology in Cardiac Patients. *J. Electrocardiol.* **2021**, *67*, 148–157. [CrossRef]
28. Sarhaddi, F.; Kazemi, K.; Azimi, I.; Cao, R.; Niela-Vilén, H.; Axelin, A.; Liljeberg, P.; Rahmani, A.M. A Comprehensive Accuracy Assessment of Samsung Smartwatch Heart Rate and Heart Rate Variability. *PLoS ONE* **2022**, *17*, e0268361. [CrossRef]
29. Charlton, P.H.; Pilt, K.; Kyriacou, P.A. Establishing Best Practices in Photoplethysmography Signal Acquisition and Processing. *Physiol. Meas.* **2022**, *43*, 050301. [CrossRef]
30. Han, D.; Bashar, S.K.; Lázaro, J.; Mohagheghian, F.; Peitzsch, A.; Nishita, N.; Ding, E.; Dickson, E.L.; DiMezza, D.; Scott, J.; et al. A Real-Time PPG Peak Detection Method for Accurate Determination of Heart Rate during Sinus Rhythm and Cardiac Arrhythmia. *Biosensors* **2022**, *12*, 82. [CrossRef]
31. Lee, J.; Sun, S.; Yang, S.M.; Sohn, J.J.; Park, J.; Lee, S.; Kim, H.C. Bidirectional Recurrent Auto-Encoder for Photoplethysmogram Denoising. *IEEE J. Biomed. Health Inf.* **2019**, *23*, 2375–2385. [CrossRef]

32. Chong, J.W.; Dao, D.K.; Salehizadeh, S.M.A.; McManus, D.D.; Darling, C.E.; Chon, K.H.; Mendelson, Y. Photoplethysmograph Signal Reconstruction Based on a Novel Hybrid Motion Artifact Detection-Reduction Approach. Part I: Motion and Noise Artifact Detection. *Ann. Biomed. Eng* **2014**, *42*, 2238–2250. [CrossRef]
33. Charlton, P.H.; Kotzen, K.; Mejía-Mejía, E.; Aston, P.J.; Budidha, K.; Mant, J.; Pettit, C.; Behar, J.A.; Kyriacou, P.A. Detecting Beats in the Photoplethysmogram: Benchmarking Open-Source Algorithms. *Physiol. Meas.* **2022**, *43*, 085007. [CrossRef]
34. Whoop®. Available online: https://www.whoop.com/gb/en/thelocker/developing-4-0-product-validation-whoop-labs (accessed on 26 April 2024).
35. Corsano®. Available online: https://corsano.com/products/bracelet-2/ (accessed on 26 April 2024).
36. VitalConnect®. Available online: https://vitalconnect.com/newsroom/resources/publications/ (accessed on 26 April 2024).
37. Brooke, J. SUS: A Retrospective. *J. Usability Stud.* **2013**, *8*, 29–40.
38. Peltola, M.A. Role of Editing of R-R Intervals in the Analysis of Heart Rate Variability. *Front. Physiol.* **2012**, *3*, 148. [CrossRef] [PubMed]
39. Tanaka, H.; Monahan, K.D.; Seals, D.R. Age-Predicted Maximal Heart Rate Revisited. *J. Am. Coll. Cardiol.* **2001**, *37*, 153–156. [CrossRef] [PubMed]
40. Malik, M.; Camm, A.J. Heart Rate Variability. *Clin. Cardiol.* **1990**, *13*, 570–576. [CrossRef] [PubMed]
41. Cajal, D.; Hernando, D.; Lázaro, J.; Laguna, P.; Gil, E.; Bailón, R. Effects of Missing Data on Heart Rate Variability Metrics. *Sensors* **2022**, *22*, 5774. [CrossRef] [PubMed]
42. Charlton, P.H. Peterhcharlton/Ppg-Beats: V.1.0.0 Accompanying Beat Detection Paper 2022. Available online: https://zenodo.org/records/6975501 (accessed on 26 April 2024).
43. Behar, J.; Johnson, A.; Clifford, G.D.; Oster, J. A Comparison of Single Channel Fetal ECG Extraction Methods. *Ann. Biomed. Eng.* **2014**, *42*, 1340–1353. [CrossRef]
44. Johnson, A.E.; Behar, J.; Andreotti, F.; Clifford, G.D.; Oster, J. R-Peak Estimation Using Multimodal Lead Switching. In Proceedings of the Computing in Cardiology 2014, Cambridge, MA, USA, 7–10 September 2014; pp. 281–284.
45. Aboy, M.; McNames, J.; Thong, T.; Tsunami, D.; Ellenby, M.S.; Goldstein, B. An Automatic Beat Detection Algorithm for Pressure Signals. *IEEE Trans. Biomed. Eng.* **2005**, *52*, 1662–1670. [CrossRef]
46. Scholkmann, F.; Boss, J.; Wolf, M. An Efficient Algorithm for Automatic Peak Detection in Noisy Periodic and Quasi-Periodic Signals. *Algorithms* **2012**, *5*, 588–603. [CrossRef]
47. Elgendi, M.; Norton, I.; Brearley, M.; Abbott, D.; Schuurmans, D. Systolic Peak Detection in Acceleration Photoplethysmograms Measured from Emergency Responders in Tropical Conditions. *PLoS ONE* **2013**, *8*, e76585. [CrossRef]
48. van Gent, P.; Farah, H.; van Nes, N.; van Arem, B. HeartPy: A Novel Heart Rate Algorithm for the Analysis of Noisy Signals. *Transp. Res. Part F Traffic Psychol. Behav.* **2019**, *66*, 368–378. [CrossRef]
49. Bishop, S.M.; Ercole, A. Multi-Scale Peak and Trough Detection Optimised for Periodic and Quasi-Periodic Neuroscience Data. In *Intracranial Pressure & Neuromonitoring XVI*; Heldt, T., Ed.; Springer International Publishing: Cham, Switzerland, 2018; pp. 189–195.
50. Vest, A.N.; Poian, G.D.; Li, Q.; Liu, C.; Nemati, S.; Shah, A.J.; Clifford, G.D. An Open Source Benchmarked Toolbox for Cardiovascular Waveform and Interval Analysis. *Physiol. Meas.* **2018**, *39*, 105004. [CrossRef]
51. Aston, P.J.; Christie, M.I.; Huang, Y.H.; Nandi, M. Beyond HRV: Attractor Reconstruction Using the Entire Cardiovascular Waveform Data for Novel Feature Extraction. *Physiol. Meas.* **2018**, *39*, 024001. [CrossRef] [PubMed]
52. Lyle, J.V.; Aston, P.J. Symmetric Projection Attractor Reconstruction: Embedding in Higher Dimensions. *Chaos Interdiscip. J. Nonlinear Sci.* **2021**, *31*, 113135. [CrossRef] [PubMed]
53. Armañac-Julián, P.; Kontaxis, S.; Rapalis, A.; Marozas, V.; Laguna, P.; Bailón, R.; Gil, E.; Lázaro, J. Reliability of Pulse Photoplethysmography Sensors: Coverage Using Different Setups and Body Locations. *Front. Electron.* **2022**, *3*, 906324. [CrossRef]
54. Hoog Antink, C.; Mai, Y.; Peltokangas, M.; Leonhardt, S.; Oksala, N.; Vehkaoja, A. Accuracy of Heart Rate Variability Estimated with Reflective Wrist-PPG in Elderly Vascular Patients. *Sci. Rep.* **2021**, *11*, 8123. [CrossRef] [PubMed]
55. Antikainen, E.; Ur Rehman, R.Z.; Ahmaniemi, T.; Chatterjee, M. Predicting Daytime Sleepiness from Electrocardiography Based Respiratory Rate Using Deep Learning. In Proceedings of the 2022 Computing in Cardiology (CinC), Tampere, Finland, 4–7 September 2022; Volume 498, pp. 1–4.
56. Bent, B.; Goldstein, B.A.; Kibbe, W.A.; Dunn, J.P. Investigating Sources of Inaccuracy in Wearable Optical Heart Rate Sensors. *NPJ Digit. Med.* **2020**, *3*, 18. [CrossRef]
57. Alfonso, C.; Garcia-Gonzalez, M.A.; Parrado, E.; Gil-Rojas, J.; Ramos-Castro, J.; Capdevila, L. Agreement between Two Photoplethysmography-Based Wearable Devices for Monitoring Heart Rate during Different Physical Activity Situations: A New Analysis Methodology. *Sci. Rep.* **2022**, *12*, 15448. [CrossRef]
58. Li, K.; Rüdiger, H.; Ziemssen, T. Spectral Analysis of Heart Rate Variability: Time Window Matters. *Front. Neurol.* **2019**, *10*, 545. [CrossRef]
59. Eddie, D.; Bentley, K.H.; Bernard, R.; Mischoulon, D.; Winkelman, J.W. Aggregating Heart Rate Variability Indices across Sleep Stage Epochs Ignores Significant Variance through the Night. *Sleep Med.* **2022**, *90*, 262–266. [CrossRef]
60. Hallman, D.M.; Srinivasan, D.; Mathiassen, S.E. Short- and Long-Term Reliability of Heart Rate Variability Indices during Repetitive Low-Force Work. *Eur. J. Appl. Physiol.* **2015**, *115*, 803–812. [CrossRef]
61. Stein, P.K.; Pu, Y. Heart Rate Variability, Sleep and Sleep Disorders. *Sleep Med. Rev.* **2012**, *16*, 47–66. [CrossRef]

62. Bizzego, A.; Esposito, G. Performance Assessment of Heartbeat Detection Algorithms on Photoplethysmograph and Functional NearInfrared Spectroscopy Signals. *Sensors* **2023**, *23*, 3668. [CrossRef]
63. Charlton, P.H.; Argüello-Prada, E.J.; Mant, J.; Kyriacou, P.A. The MSPTDfast Photoplethysmography Beat Detection Algorithm: Design, Benchmarking, and Open-Source Distribution. *medRxiv* **2024**. [CrossRef]

sensors

MDPI

Article

Correlation Between Pain Intensity and Trunk Sway in Seated Posture Among Office Workers with Chronic Spinal Pain: A Pilot Field-Based Study

Eduarda Oliosi [1,2,*], Afonso Caetano Júlio [1], Luís Silva [1], Phillip Probst [1], João Paulo Vilas-Boas [3], Ana Rita Pinheiro [4] and Hugo Gamboa [1]

1 Laboratory for Instrumentation, Biomedical Engineering and Radiation Physics (LIBPhys), NOVA School of Science & Technology, NOVA University Lisbon, 2829-516 Caparica, Portugal; afonso.caetano93@gmail.com (A.C.J.); lmd.silva@fct.unl.pt (L.S.); p.probst@campus.fct.unl.pt (P.P.); hgamboa@fct.unl.pt (H.G.)

2 Research Centre in Physical Activity, Health, and Leisure (CIAFEL), Faculty of Sports, University of Porto, 4099-002 Porto, Portugal

3 Centre for Research, Education, Innovation, and Intervention in Sport (CIFI2D) and Porto Biomechanics Laboratory (LABIOMEP), Faculty of Sports, University of Porto, 4200-450 Porto, Portugal; jpvb@fade.up.pt

4 Institute of Biomedicine (iBiMED), School of Health Sciences, University of Aveiro, 3810-193 Aveiro, Portugal; anaritapinheiro@ua.pt

* Correspondence: up202002726@up.pt

Abstract: This pilot study examines the relationship between pain intensity and trunk sitting postural control in 10 office workers with chronic spinal pain, using field-based real-time inertial sensors. Pain intensity was assessed with the Numeric Pain Rating Scale (NPRS) before and after work across three non-consecutive workdays, while postural control was evaluated through estimated center of pressure (COP) displacements. Linear and nonlinear metrics, including sway range, velocity, the Hurst exponent, and sample entropy, were derived from the estimated COP time series. Pearson correlation coefficients (r) and corresponding p-values were used to analyze the relationship between pain intensity and postural control. Significant correlations, though limited to specific metrics, were found ($r = -0.860$ to 0.855; $p < 0.05$), suggesting that higher pain intensity may be correlated with reduced postural variability. These findings provide preliminary insights into the potential link between pain intensity and postural control. Understanding trunk posture dynamics could inform the development of targeted ergonomic interventions to reduce musculoskeletal stress and improve sitting comfort in office environments.

Keywords: musculoskeletal disorders; chronic pain; pain intensity; postural control; variability; inertial sensors

1. Introduction

Musculoskeletal disorders (MSDs), particularly chronic spinal conditions such as neck and lower back pain, represent a significant global occupational health challenge. By 2050, low back pain is projected to affect 843 million people, up from 619 million in 2020 [1], while neck pain, which impacted 203 million in 2020, is expected to rise to 269 million [2]. The increasing prevalence of sedentary office work, combined with aging populations and obesity rates, is expected to exacerbate this problem [1,3,4]. Office workers are especially vulnerable due to prolonged sitting, highlighting the urgent need for ergonomic strategies to mitigate the impacts of MSDs [5–8].

Addressing this issue requires innovative approaches, such as those proposed within the framework of Industry 4.0 and 5.0. These paradigms introduce opportunities to improve workplace health through technology integration and human-centered design. While Industry 4.0 emphasizes automation and digital transformation, Industry 5.0 prioritizes worker well-being and sustainable ergonomics [9–11]. In this context, addressing the health risks of prolonged sitting is essential. For example, nearly 40% of EU workers report sitting for excessive durations [5], prompting the EU-OSHA to recommend limiting sitting to less than half of the workday [5].

Movement variability and variation in posture represent complementary ergonomic principles that are particularly relevant in this regard. Movement variability refers to the natural, inherent fluctuations in motor performance across task repetitions [12]. This intrinsic property of biological systems [12,13] facilitates the redistribution of muscle activity, reducing localized fatigue, and improving activation patterns [14]. In contrast, variation in posture and movement involves intentional changes in body position, such as alternating between sitting and standing [15]. These postural adjustments are linked to enhancing comfort and productivity by up to 6.5% [16].

Recent reviews reinforce the benefits of these principles in workplace settings. Standing interventions have been shown to effectively reduce sedentary behavior without compromising productivity [17], while active breaks incorporating postural changes can alleviate pain and discomfort [18]. Advances in technologies, such as inertial measurement units (IMUs), further support ergonomic interventions by enabling the detailed analysis of movement and postural behaviors [19–23]. Together, these findings highlight the critical importance of movement variability as a central component of strategies to reduce back pain and improve workplace well-being.

Despite this growing recognition of the role of movement variability in reducing musculoskeletal discomfort, there remains a limited understanding of how specific aspects, such as trunk posture variability, influence pain intensity. Inconsistencies in kinematic data and a lack of focused studies hinder a comprehensive understanding of the role of movement in the management of chronic spinal pain [24,25].

This study aims to address these gaps by investigating the relationship between motor variability—measured through linear and nonlinear postural sway metrics derived from the estimated center of pressure (COP) time series—and pain intensity in office workers with chronic spinal pain, particularly those in tax authorities engaged in computer-based tasks while seated. By utilizing IMUs integrated into smartphones, this research seeks to advance our understanding of motor patterns and contribute to the development of interventions and digital health solutions tailored to this population. Based on the existing literature, the following is hypothesized:

1. Higher pain intensity is associated with reduced variability and complexity in trunk sway (e.g., lower entropy), reflecting increased trunk stiffness and a shift towards a more rigid and predictable postural control strategy. These adaptations likely serve as a compensatory mechanism to minimize movement-related stress and protect the spine during prolonged sitting [26–29].

2. Work-related activities modulate postural control and pain perception, leading to increased pain intensity and reduced movement variability in the post-work period (PM) compared to the pre-work period (AM). This effect may be attributed to cumulative biomechanical strain and fatigue associated with sustained "static" postures during prolonged occupational sitting [28,30].

2. Materials and Methods

2.1. Study Design

This cross-sectional study, part of the PrevOccupAI Project (Prevention of Occupational Disorders in Public Administrations using Artificial Intelligence), was conducted at offices of the Portuguese Tax and Customs Authority (AT) located in the Lisbon Metropolitan Area. A multidisciplinary team accomplished risk assessments for randomly selected tax enforcement professionals from the AT's Human Resources department. As an incentive to participate in this study, evidence-based recommendations were developed to improve resilience and address occupational health challenges, informed by sources such as the ILO [31], the EU-OSHA [5], and Slater et al. [32]. Ethical approval was granted by NOVA University Lisbon (No. CE/FCT/005/2022) in accordance with the Declaration of Helsinki and GDPR. Informed consent was obtained from all participants.

2.2. Participants

A total of 10 workers were eligible to participate in this study. All participants were adults aged 18 years or older, with no history of neurological, orthopedic, rheumatic, oncological, or cardiorespiratory conditions; pregnant women were excluded. To meet the eligibility criteria, participants were required to have a history of non-specific spinal pain lasting at least three months, as defined by the International Association for the Study of Pain (IASP) and the International Classification of Diseases, 11th Revision (ICD-11) [33].

2.3. Procedures

A standardized data collection protocol was implemented using a dedicated cross-platform application developed within the PrevOccupAI project. This application enabled the acquisition of multimodal biosignals and self-reported questionnaire responses via smartphone and computer interfaces. Data collection spanned one workweek, adhering to protocols established in prior studies [34]. Each workday began with participants reporting to a designated workplace room for device setup. They first completed a daily pain questionnaire before the recording schedule was configured in the PrevOccupAI application. A smartphone, securely positioned on the chest, continuously recorded inertial sensor data and ambient noise throughout the workday, ensuring the uninterrupted monitoring of postural sway and movement patterns in a real-world occupational setting. Participants engaged in their regular work tasks while the smartphone passively captured movement-related data. At the end of the workday, participants returned for device removal and disinfection, followed by a second pain questionnaire to assess changes in pain perception. This methodology facilitated a comprehensive, ecologically valid evaluation of postural sway dynamics, leveraging smartphone-based sensing for continuous and unobtrusive monitoring.

2.3.1. Demographics

Demographic data, including age, gender, height, and body mass, were captured using an integrated questionnaire module. The Body Mass Index (BMI) was calculated based on the standard formula BMI = mass (kg) / height $(m)^2$. Data regarding work (years of work experience, weekly work schedule in hours) were also collected. Subjective assessments were conducted using validated instruments to assess physical activity levels, psychosocial risks, and chronic pain experiences.

2.3.2. Pain Experience

In 2020, the IASP [35] revised its definition of pain to include both physical and emotional dimensions. Accordingly, pain perception was evaluated along three dimensions: intensity, distress, and interference [33].

Pain intensity was assessed daily using the Numerical Pain Rating Scale (NPRS), where participants reported their pain levels at the beginning and end of each workday, ranging from 0 ("no pain") to 10 ("worst pain imaginable"). Pain-related distress, representing the emotional impact of persistent or recurrent pain, was measured weekly on an 11-point numerical scale, with 0 indicating "no distress" and 10 indicating "extreme pain-related distress". Pain-related interference, quantifying the extent to which pain disrupted daily activities, was self-reported on a scale from 0 (no interference) to 10 (complete inability to perform activities) [33].

To optimize pain assessment, this project's app integrated a body map tool, which allowed participants to precisely localize pain and quantify symptom distribution (Figure 1). Unmarked regions were assigned a pain intensity value of 0, ensuring a comprehensive and personalized representation of pain across anatomical regions.

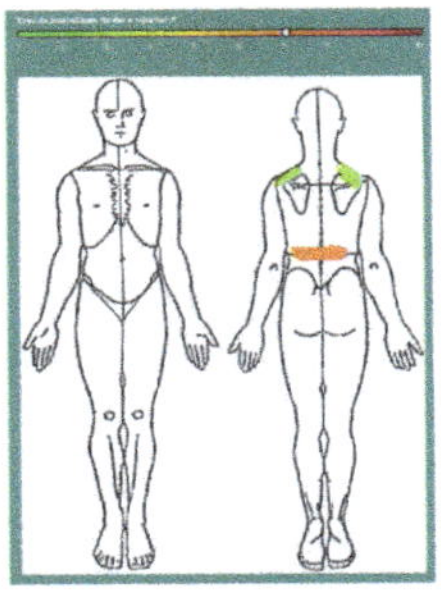

Figure 1. Interface for assessing pain location and intensity.

2.3.3. Physical Activity Levels

The European Portuguese version of the Short-Form International Physical Activity Questionnaire (IPAQ-SF) assessed physical activity, categorizing participants' weekly activity as low, moderate, or high based on metabolic equivalents. This tool, validated for adults aged 18–65, captures vigorous, moderate, walking, and sitting activities over a past week [36].

2.3.4. Psychosocial Risks

Workplace psychosocial risks were evaluated using the Portuguese version of the Copenhagen Psychosocial Questionnaire II (COPSOQ II) [37], covering multimodal domains such as work demands, interpersonal relations, and health and well-being [38]. This tool includes 76 items rated on a 5-point Likert scale. Results were grouped into their domains, expressed as percentages, and used to descriptively characterize the sample population, with input from occupational health stakeholders, management, and worker representatives [37].

2.3.5. Data Collection and Analysis

Data acquisition was performed using a Xiaomi Redmi Note 9 smartphone, which captured signals from the accelerometer (ACC), gyroscope (GYR), magnetometer (MAG), and rotation vector (RV). Sampling rates were constrained by the Android OS, with the ACC, GYR, and RV recorded at 100 Hz and MAG at 50 Hz. Motor biosignals were collected using these integrated sensors within the smartphone, which was securely fixed on the sternum with straps. The COP displacement time series represented an estimated COP derived from smartphone inertial sensor data. The collected data were represented in the orthogonal components of the anteroposterior (AP) and mediolateral (ML) directions, reflecting forward–backward (AP) and side-to-side (ML) trunk sway (see Figure 2). This approach provides a reliable method for quantifying postural sway, as supported by previous studies using force plates and smartphone-based inertial sensors to assess postural stability with demonstrated accuracy and consistency [39–44].

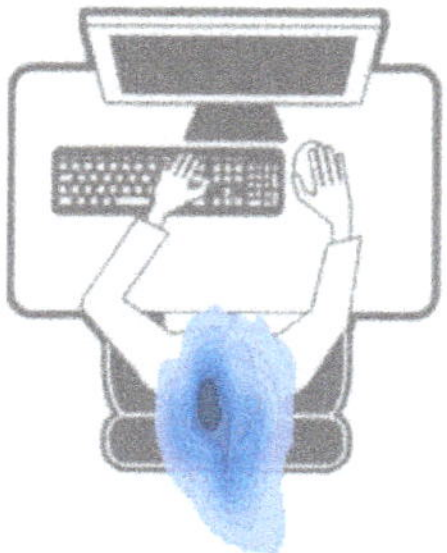

Figure 2. Illustration of COP sway during seated posture.

Linear measures of postural sway were computed from the COP time series. Key metrics included mean acceleration (in m/s^2), standard deviation (SD) (in m/s^2), sway range (in mm), sway area (in mm), sway path (in mm), and sway velocity (in mm/s). Sway range and area represent the maximum COP displacement in the resultant (overall) or AP and ML directions, sway path reflects the total COP distance traveled, and sway velocity indicates the rate of COP movement, offering insights into postural adjustment speed and variability [45–47]. These measures are indicators of centrality, describing magnitude and variability around a central point, and thus characterize movement quantity in data [48,49].

Nonlinear metrics, including Sample Entropy (SaEn) and Multifractal Detrended Fluctuation Analysis (MF-DFA), were used to assess postural control complexity (i.e., to describe the structure within the time series) [47]. SaEn quantifies sway regularity, where higher values indicate more complex and adaptable movement strategies. It also reflects how physiological health influences postural regulation by identifying signals under stationary conditions, such as reduced variability in less adaptable postural states. The Hurst exponent, derived from DFA, measures the long-term persistence and fractality of sway behavior. DFA analyzes time series by removing short-term fluctuations (detrending) to reveal long-term correlations, highlighting complex patterns in postural sway. DFA is assessed across different q-orders, which provide varying levels of detail: higher q-orders focus on fine-grained fluctuations, while lower q-orders capture broader trends. This multiscale analysis offers deeper insights into the dynamics and adaptability of postural control across different time scales [47,50–53].

The combination of these features was selected due to their widespread use in studies on seated posture, particularly in ergonomic and occupational contexts [54–57].

2.3.6. Data Processing

All acquired signals were synchronized using timestamp alignment and resampled to a uniform frequency of 100 Hz to ensure consistency across modalities. The preprocessing pipeline for the ACC and RV data followed validated methodologies from previous studies [58]. The ACC data underwent a multi-step processing approach to remove noise and extract movement-related features. A low-pass filter with a 10 Hz cutoff was applied to suppress high-frequency noise and sensor artifacts. The gravitational acceleration component was then removed using an adaptive filtering technique to isolate dynamic movement. Systematic biases were corrected through detrending by subtracting the mean acceleration value from each sample, and a 150-sample moving average filter was used to smooth signal fluctuations. Similarly, RV signals were processed using a 5-sample moving average filter to minimize transient sensor noise and improve orientation stability. Given the extended duration of data collection (approximately 5 h per day), segmentation was performed using a 15-minute windowing approach to facilitate analysis. Data segments were classified into morning (AM1–AMx), lunch, and afternoon (PM1–PMx) periods.

To ensure that only seated postural sway data were analyzed, an algorithm was implemented to detect and exclude non-seated intervals based on acceleration magnitude thresholds. The magnitude of acceleration (mag) was computed as $mag = \sqrt{x_{acc}^2 + y_{acc}^2 + z_{acc}^2}$, with a threshold of 2 m/s^2 derived from biomechanical analyses and metabolic equivalent (MET) calculations [59,60]. This threshold effectively distinguished seated from non-seated activities, ensuring that only relevant data were retained.

Postural sway was quantified by estimating the COP displacement from inertial sensor data. The RV signal was converted into quaternions and transformed into Euler angles to derive COP projections in the AP and ML directions. To ensure alignment across participants, the median of each Euler angle was subtracted to establish a reference position at the origin (0,0). The chest-mounted smartphone's orientation was used to project Euler angles into the xz-plane, mapping postural movements throughout the workday (Figure 3). To standardize postural sway analysis, an elliptical boundary was applied based on prior research [61], with an AP radius of 25 mm and an ML radius of 18 mm. Data outside this predefined region were excluded to maintain consistency in postural sway assessment [58].

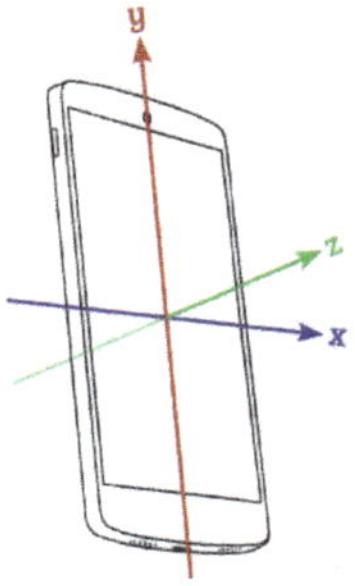

Figure 3. Coordinate system for smartphone-assisted postural analysis.

2.4. *Previous Reporting on This Dataset*

Previous analyses utilizing this dataset have examined how chronic spinal pain influences trunk movement patterns and postural dynamics in office settings. Ref. [58] applied a mixed ANOVA to analyze trunk sway, revealing that pain-free participants displayed distinct trunk movement characteristics in certain features compared to those with chronic spinal pain, particularly regarding fine motor adjustments. In another analysis, ref. [62] assessed postural variability among 40 office workers throughout the workday without segmenting by pain status or utilizing nonlinear metrics. The results indicated increased posture variability from morning to afternoon, with a notable rise in positional adjustments later in the day. This paper presents novel analyses focused on the relationship between postural dynamics and pain intensity, specifically within the cohort experiencing chronic spinal pain.

2.5. Statistical Analysis

Descriptive and inferential statistics were performed using SPSS 29. Sample demographics and questionnaire scores were used to characterize the participants. For continuous variables, normally distributed data were summarized with the mean and SD, while non-normally distributed data were described using the median and interquartile range (IQR). Categorical variables were reported as counts and proportions. Parametric assumptions were verified for normality using the Shapiro–Wilk test. To examine changes in pain intensity over time, Friedman's Related-Samples Two-Way Analysis of Variance was applied. For correlations, Pearson's (r) correlation coefficients were calculated to explore associations between sitting postural control dynamics (trunk displacement features in the AP and ML directions, along with resultant trunk sway time series) and perceived pain intensity (NPRS Sum of neck, upper back, and lower back pain). As Pearson's r represents both the correlation coefficient and the effect size, it allows for a direct interpretation of the strength of relationships between variables. NPRS scores were summed across spinal regions to create an NPRS index. Summed pain intensity scores were analyzed for each day (Day 1: Monday; Day 3: Wednesday; Day 5: Friday) and period (AM: pre-work; PM: post-work). A significance threshold of $\alpha = 0.05$ was applied.

3. Results

The study sample consisted of 10 participants, 80% of whom identified as female. Physical activity levels, as assessed by the IPAQ-SF, indicated that 30% of participants engaged in low physical activity, 40% in moderate activity, and 30% in high activity levels. The mean age of the participants was 54 years (SD = 6.5). The average BMI was 26.75 kg/m^2 (SD = 6.14), with participants having an average of 18.2 years of work experience (SD = 14.06) and a typical weekly work schedule of approximately 40 h (SD = 4). On average, participants reported spending 9.4 h per day sitting (SD = 3.44), with a reduced average of 4.18 h of sitting on weekends (SD = 1.78). The characteristics of the participants are summarized in Table 1.

Table 1. Sample characterization.

Variable	Outcome
Gender	80% Female (8 Females, 2 Males)
Physical Activity Levels	Low: 30%; Moderate: 40%; High: 30%
Mean Age (years)	54 ± 6.5
Mean BMI (kg/m^2)	26.75 ± 6.14
Work Experience (years)	18.2 ± 14.06
Weekly Work (h)	40 ± 4
Daily Sitting Time (h)	9.4 ± 3.44
Weekend Sitting Time (h)	4.18 ± 1.78

The COPSOQ II results indicated moderate job demands (67.5; SD = 2.7) and neutral perceptions of health and well-being (50.0; SD = 6.1). No offensive behavior was reported (0.0; IQR: 0–10). Social relations and leadership scored moderately (38.1; SD = 3.5), as did values' alignment within the workplace (31.3; SD = 4.8) and the work–individual interface (42.6; SD = 11.8). Work organization and job content (41.7; SD = 4.6) also received moderate ratings.

3.1. Pain Experience

The distribution of reported pain locations among participants revealed that three (30.0%) experienced isolated neck pain, five (50.0%) reported a combination of neck and lower back pain, one (10.0%) had upper back pain, and one (10.0%) experienced pain in both the neck and upper back regions.

The disability levels, assessed using the 11-point NPRS, revealed the following median scores: neck disability, 2.00 (IQR: 0–4); upper back disability, 0.90 (IQR: 0–5); and lower back disability, 0.80 (IQR: 0–5). In terms of classification, 20% of participants reported no disability, 50% reported mild disability, and 30% reported moderate disability for neck pain. For upper back disability, 80% reported no disability, while 20% reported moderate disability. Regarding lower back disability, 70% reported no disability, 10% reported mild disability, and 20% reported moderate disability.

Regarding pain-related distress, also assessed using the NPRS, the median distress scores were as follows: neck distress, 2.50 (IQR: 0–6); upper back distress, 1.10 (IQR: 0–6); and lower back distress, 1.20 (IQR: 0–5). For neck distress, 10% of participants reported no distress, 70% reported mild distress, and 20% reported moderate distress. For upper back distress, 80% reported no distress, and 20% reported moderate distress. For lower back distress, 60% of participants reported no distress, 30% reported mild distress, and 10% reported moderate distress.

Regarding pain intensity, which was assessed both before and after work each day, a detailed description can be found in Table 2. No statistically significant differences were found across days, periods, and pain locations ($p > 0.05$).

Table 2. Pain intensity scores based on the NPRS.

Variable	AM			PM		
	Median	IQR	95% CI	Median	IQR	95% CI
Day 1						
Neck	0.00	4	(−0.26, 3.06)	0.00	2	(−0.61, 3.01)
Upper Back	0.00	1	(−0.47, 2.27)	0.00	1	(−0.55, 2.35)
Lower Back	0.00	5	(0.12, 3.88)	0.00	4	(−0.29, 3.09)
Day 3						
Neck	0.00	3	(−0.27, 2.47)	0.00	3	(−0.22, 2.62)
Upper Back	0.00	0	(−0.63, 1.63)	0.00	1	(−0.55, 2.35)
Lower Back	0.00	0	(0.00, 0.00)	0.00	4	(−0.29, 3.09)
Day 5						
Neck	0.00	3	(−0.23, 2.43)	0.00	3	(−0.30, 2.70)
Upper Back	0.00	1	(−0.37, 1.77)	0.00	5	(−0.02, 3.82)
Lower Back	0.00	3	(−0.17, 2.17)	0.00	4	(−0.09, 3.49)
NPRS Sum						
Day 1	4.0	9	(1.10, 7.50)	2.5	6	(0.54, 6.46)
Day 3	0.0	3	(−0.72, 3.92)	3.5	5	(0.76, 6.24)
Day 5	0.0	6	(−0.32, 5.92)	3.5	8	(0.51, 9.09)

AM: pre-work; PM: post-work; NPRS: Numeric Pain Rating Scale; IQR: interquartile range; CI: Confidence Interval.

3.2. Correlations

Daily pain intensity (NPRS Sum) analysis across six assessment points (Day 1 AM/PM, Day 3 AM/PM, Day 5 AM/PM) revealed occasional correlations with postural sway metrics. While most correlations did not reach statistical significance ($p > 0.05$), several moderate-to-strong correlations were observed, indicating potential relationships that merit further investigation. A summary of significant correlations between the NPRS and trunk sway metrics is provided in Table 3, with comprehensive correlation matrices for both linear and nonlinear sway features available in Appendix A.

For linear measurements (Tables A1–A6), significant correlations with the NPRS Sum were observed at different time points. On Day 1 in the morning, the NPRS Sum had a significant negative correlation with overall sway range ($r = -0.688; p < 0.05$). In contrast, on Day 1 in the afternoon, the NPRS Sum exhibited a positive correlation with overall sway range ($r = 0.750; p < 0.05$) and with range in the AP direction ($r = 0.855; p < 0.01$). Additionally, on Day 5 in the morning, a strong negative correlation between the NPRS Sum and the standard deviation in the AP direction (SD AP) was noted ($r = -0.719; p < 0.05$).

Nonlinear sway parameters showed varied correlations with the NPRS Sum across time points (Tables A7–A12). On Day 3 in the AM, several strong correlations were observed. The Hurst exponents at the scale $H(0)$ in both the AP ($r = -0.812; p < 0.01$) and ML ($r = -0.860; p < 0.01$) directions, as well as at the scale $H(4.5)$ in the AP ($r = -0.786; p < 0.01$) and ML ($r = -0.780; p < 0.01$) directions, were significantly negatively correlated with the NPRS Sum. SaEn in the ML direction also exhibited a significant negative correlation with the NPRS Sum ($r = -0.703; p < 0.05$). On Day 3 in the PM, no significant correlations were found between the NPRS Sum and the nonlinear sway parameters. However, on Day 5 in the PM, the NPRS Sum showed a negative correlation with the Hurst exponent at the scale $H(2)$ in the AP direction ($r = -0.722; p < 0.05$).

Table 3. Significant correlations between NPRS Sum and linear/nonlinear metrics.

	Day	Period	Metric	Direction	Correlation
NPRS vs.	1	AM	Overall range	Negative	−0.688 *
	1	PM	AP range	Positive	0.855 **
	1	PM	Overall range	Positive	0.750 *
	3	AM	H(0) AP	Negative	−0.812 **
	3	AM	H(0) ML	Negative	−0.860 **
	3	AM	H(4.5) AP	Negative	−0.786 **
	3	AM	H(4.5) ML	Negative	−0.780 **
	3	AM	SaEn ML	Negative	−0.703 *
	5	AM	SD AP	Negative	−0.719 *
	5	PM	H(2)	Negative	−0.722 *

Abbreviations: NPRS: Numeric Pain Rating Scale; SD: standard deviation; AP: anteroposterior; ML: mediolateral; H: Hurst exponent. Significance levels: * $p < 0.05$; ** $p < 0.01$.

Furthermore, moderate to strong positive intercorrelations were found among both linear and nonlinear postural sway parameters (Appendix A).

4. Discussion

This study investigated the relationship between pain intensity, measured using the NPRS Sum for neck, upper, and lower back pain, and postural sway characteristics in office workers with chronic spinal pain. IMUs were employed for real-time, field-based posture assessment. Both linear and nonlinear sway metrics were analyzed during pre- and post-work periods on Days 1 (Monday), 3 (Wednesday), and 5 (Friday) to assess their potential as objective indicators of pain intensity within occupational settings.

The findings revealed limited and variable correlations between pain intensity and postural sway metrics across different time points, illustrating the intrinsic intricacy of postural control systems in the context of chronic pain.

4.1. Interpretation of Results

Linear metrics, including range (in mm), mean acceleration (in m/s^2), SD (in m/s^2), velocity (in mm/s), sway path length (in mm), and sway path area (in mm^2), were used to assess postural control. Nonlinear techniques, MF-DFA and SaEn, were applied to capture the postural control complexity, reflecting subtle changes that linear metrics might have missed.

Variations in correlations among linear metrics highlighted the nuances of seated postural dynamics. On Day 1, reduced morning sway variability (negative correlation with overall sway range) indicated more rigid postural control, while increased afternoon fluctuations (positive correlations with overall sway range and AP range) suggested compensatory adjustments. By Day 5, greater AP sway variability (negative correlation with SD) was linked to higher pain intensity. These findings are consistent with previous studies. For instance, Søndergaard et al. [54], reported positive correlations between discomfort and the standard deviations of COP displacement in both the AP and ML directions, alongside negative correlations with SaEn. This suggests that increased sway variability and reduced postural control complexity during seated tasks can be associated with greater perceived discomfort. Similarly, Madeleine et al. [63] observed that prolonged sitting led to a greater SD and lower SaEn in COP signals, reflecting decreased postural complexity and increased discomfort. Overall, these findings highlight the link between postural variability degradation and increased discomfort, reflecting the interplay between adaptive posture control and pain perception.

Correlations between nonlinear metrics and pain intensity varied notably across time points. No significant correlations were observed on Day 1 (AM and PM), Day 3 in the PM, or Day 5 in the AM. However, on Day 3 in the AM, strong negative correlations were observed for $H(0)$ (AP and ML), $H(4.5)$ (AP and ML), and SaEn (ML), suggesting a decline in postural sway complexity. On Day 5 in the PM, a significant negative correlation was also found for $H(2)$ in the AP direction, indicating reduced postural adaptability. This reduction in variability aligns with the concept of a more periodic, less adaptive postural strategy, characterized by the loss of multiscale fractal complexity under pathological conditions [12,64]. These findings suggest that higher pain intensity is correlated with diminished variability at both micro-scale fluctuations ($H(0)$) and larger sway deviations ($H(4.5)$), as well as reduced entropy (SaEn), which reflect a shift toward more rigid, less flexible postural control [12]. The absence of consistent correlations across other periods underscores the dynamic and context-dependent nature of postural regulation in response to pain, consistent with theories of adaptive control in motor behavior [27].

Although most postural sway parameters showed weak correlations with the NPRS Sum, specific linear and nonlinear metrics demonstrated moderate to strong correlations at particular time points, indicating pain-related changes in postural stability. Hypothesis 2, predicting stronger evening (PM) correlations, was not supported. Overall, our results suggest a weak link between pain intensity and postural sway dynamics, likely due to the multifactorial nature of chronic pain, influenced by biopsychosocial factors [26,65,66]. Furthermore, variability in sitting habits and postural adjustments also contributes to inconsistent sway patterns (e.g., "breakers" vs. "prolongers") [56].

Our findings highlight the potential for the development of personalized ergonomic interventions aimed at protecting office workers from prolonged exposure to postural stress and pain. By understanding trunk posture dynamics, tailored strategies can help reduce MSDs and improve comfort, as optimal postures vary between individuals [32].

4.2. Limitations and Future Research

Several limitations should be considered. Data were collected from an adult population with an average age of 54 years (SD = 6.5), while previous studies emphasize age-related differences in variability [49,67], particularly in office workers [55]. Thus, the kinematic measurements in this study may not reflect those of other age groups or occupations. The use of smartphone IMUs, while practical, introduced limitations, as placement variability and daily reapplication increased the risk of random errors in postural sway measurements due to inconsistent placement [68], despite the use of standardized straps and consistent researcher handling.

As this study was conducted in a field setting, variations in cognitive load (e.g., focused computer work) may have influenced postural sway. Prior research suggests that cognitive dual-tasking can reduce postural sway in chronic low back pain, though effects are more pronounced in complex balance tasks [69]. Similar effects were observed in healthy adults, where cognitive demands altered postural complexity without significantly affecting displacement measures [70]. Cognitive task difficulty has also been linked to changes in postural variability, particularly in children and older adults, who demonstrate increased sway area and complexity under more challenging conditions [71]. Future studies should integrate controlled cognitive-load assessments to better isolate the effects of attentional demands on postural control, such as using EEG [72].

Customer service roles in public administration and finance face substantial psychosocial risks. For example, 31% of EU workers report suppressing emotions due to customer anger and abuse [73]. In tax offices, depression has been linked to high trait anxiety, workplace conflicts, and low job satisfaction, making tax workers particularly vulnerable to MSDs [74–77]. These psychosocial hazards limit the applicability of the findings to other office roles, such as programmers and call center staff. However, the non-alarming COPSOQ II results in this study suggest a lower psychosocial risk in the analyzed sample.

While our findings suggest a weak correlation between pain intensity and postural sway metrics, they underscore the complexity of chronic pain management. This highlights the need for individualized, multidimensional approaches to postural assessment and ergonomic interventions, where pain intensity is considered alongside other psychosocial and physical factors. Future interventions may benefit from a combination of sensor data and self-reported measures to provide more accurate assessments of pain and postural dynamics, guiding more effective ergonomic strategies in the workplace.

Although a one-week observation period was chosen to align with this study's primary objectives, future research could benefit from longer observation durations to capture greater variability in postural dynamics and explore potential long-term trends. Additionally, while the small sample size limits the generalizability of the findings, future studies with larger, more diverse samples will offer more robust and conclusive insights. Given the multiple comparisons conducted in this study, the potential for Type I errors must be considered. Future research should apply corrections to account for multiple tests, thereby enhancing the robustness of the findings.

5. Conclusions

Although postural sway parameters showed weak correlations with pain intensity, specific metrics revealed stronger correlations, suggesting potential links between pain and postural stability. These findings highlight the need for more research on motor variability and pain intensity to inform ergonomic interventions. While our findings were not strongly significant, they contribute to assessing postural sway in real-world settings and provide exploratory insights into how movement-based metrics may inform pain assessment, ergonomic interventions, and future rehabilitation strategies for individuals with chronic spinal pain.

Hypothesis 1 was partially supported, with pain intensity correlated with the reduced complexity of postural sway at specific points, although the effects were inconsistent. Hypothesis 2 was not supported, as work activities did not consistently increase post-work pain or reduce variability, suggesting that other factors may influence postural control and pain intensity. Future research should involve larger sample sizes, longitudinal designs, randomized controlled trials, and consider pain location to better explore these relationships. Furthermore, utilizing a full range of digital health resources, including wearable sensors, could provide valuable information on postural dynamics and pain management.

Author Contributions: E.O.: Conceptualization, Writing—original draft, Investigation, Formal analysis. A.C.J.: Formal analysis, Writing—review and editing. L.S.: Formal analysis, Writing—review and editing. P.P.: Investigation, Writing—review and editing. J.P.V.-B.: Supervision, Writing—review and editing. A.R.P.: Supervision, Writing—review and editing. H.G.: Funding acquisition, Resources, Project administration, Supervision, Writing—review and editing. All authors have read and agreed to the published version of the manuscript.

Funding: This study was partially funded by the Portuguese Foundation for Science and Technology (FCT) through the project PREVOCUPAI (DSAIPA/AI/0105/2019). This work also received support provided by the FCT, I.P., and the European Union under the project UIDB/05913/2020—Centre for Research, Education, Innovation, and Intervention in Sport (https://doi.org/10.54499/UIDB/05913/2020). P. Probst was supported by the doctoral grant PRT/BD/152843/2021, financed by the FCT and with funds from the State Budget, under the MIT Portugal Program.

Institutional Review Board Statement: This study was conducted in accordance with the Declaration of Helsinki and approved by the Ethics Committee of NOVA University Lisbon (protocol code: CE/FCT/005/2022).

Informed Consent Statement: Informed consent was obtained from all subjects involved in this study.

Data Availability Statement: The data presented in this study are available upon reasonable request from the corresponding author.

Acknowledgments: The authors wish to extend their thanks to the workers who participated in this study.

Conflicts of Interest: The authors declare no conflicts of interest.

Appendix A

The following tables present the correlation matrices for various sway metrics and pain intensity. Tables A1–A6 summarize the linear correlations between sway metrics and pain intensity across different days and time periods. Tables A7–A12 provide the nonlinear correlation matrices for the same metrics and conditions.

Table A1. Correlation Matrix of Linear Measurements on Day 1 During the AM Period and NPRS Sum (Day 1 AM).

	Mean		SD		Range			Area	Path	Velocity
	AP	ML	AP	ML	AP	ML	Overall			
NPRS Sum	−0.064	−0.348	0.351	0.041	−0.592	−0.461	−0.688 *	−0.552	−0.594	−0.593
Mean AP		0.449	−0.174	−0.013	−0.119	−0.424	−0.253	−0.226	−0.070	−0.073
Mean ML			−0.662 *	−0.099	0.339	−0.112	0.221	0.071	0.057	0.033
SD AP				0.662 *	−0.457	0.257	−0.241	−0.529	−0.383	−0.371
SD ML					−0.328	0.241	−0.168	−0.651 *	−0.580	−0.582
Range AP						0.173	0.904 **	0.612	0.547	0.547
Range ML							0.571	0.475	0.552	0.545
Range Overall								0.706 *	0.700 *	0.698 *
Area									0.956 **	0.954 **
Path										0.999 **

AM: Pre-work; NPRS: Numeric Pain Rating Scale; SD: Standard Deviation; AP: Anteroposterior; ML: Mediolateral; *: $p < 0.05$; **: $p < 0.01$.

Table A2. Correlation Matrix of Linear Measurements on Day 1 During the PM Period and NPRS Sum (Day 1 PM).

	Mean		SD		Range			Area	Path	Velocity
	AP	ML	AP	ML	AP	ML	Overall			
NPRS Sum	0.007	0.199	−0.196	−0.600	0.855 **	0.143	0.750 *	0.345	0.378	0.393
Mean AP		−0.245	0.152	−0.040	−0.061	−0.138	−0.108	−0.318	−0.304	−0.306
Mean ML			0.322	−0.387	−0.026	−0.688 *	−0.234	0.014	−0.106	−0.053
SD AP				0.247	0.032	−0.220	−0.055	−0.118	−0.212	−0.196
SD ML					−0.341	0.377	−0.174	0.150	0.169	0.171
Range AP						0.467	0.965 **	0.582	0.596	0.594
Range ML							0.678 *	0.628	0.718 *	0.678 *
Range Overall								0.660 *	0.698 *	0.685 *
Area									0.984 **	0.987 **
Path										0.997 **

PM: Post-work; NPRS: Numeric Pain Rating Scale; SD: Standard Deviation; AP: Anteroposterior; ML: Mediolateral; *: $p < 0.05$; **: $p < 0.01$.

Table A3. Correlation Matrix of Linear Measurements on Day 3 During the AM Period and NPRS Sum (Day 3 AM).

	Mean		SD		Range			Area	Path	Velocity
	AP	ML	AP	ML	AP	ML	Overall			
NPRS Sum	0.148	0.456	0.095	−0.127	−0.006	−0.368	−0.163	−0.047	0.085	0.059
Mean AP		−0.278	−0.447	−0.449	0.039	−0.068	−0.008	−0.306	−0.074	−0.077
Mean ML			0.375	−0.066	−0.072	−0.497	−0.256	0.211	0.009	−0.017
SD AP				0.765 **	−0.377	−0.382	−0.403	−0.136	−0.305	−0.310
SD ML					−0.333	−0.082	−0.240	−0.170	−0.323	−0.313
Range AP						0.695 *	0.947 **	0.743 *	0.914 **	0.915 **
Range ML							0.888 **	0.550	0.720 *	0.732 *
Range Overall								0.721*	0.905 **	0.911 **
Area									0.887 **	0.889 **
Path										0.999 **

AM: Pre-work; NPRS: Numeric Pain Rating Scale; SD: Standard Deviation; AP: Anteroposterior; ML: Mediolateral; *: $p < 0.05$; **: $p < 0.01$.

Table A4. Correlation Matrix of Linear Measurements on Day 3 During the PM Period and NPRS Sum (Day 3 PM).

	Mean		SD		Range			Area	Path	Velocity
	AP	ML	AP	ML	AP	ML	Overall			
NPRS Sum	0.505	−0.366	−0.011	−0.370	0.573	0.210	0.478	0.214	0.297	0.269
Mean AP		−0.504	0.049	0.031	−0.194	−0.193	−0.236	−0.180	−0.291	−0.279
Mean ML			0.316	0.164	0.067	0.200	0.164	−0.199	−0.088	−0.101
SD AP				0.495	−0.223	0.298	0.026	−0.417	−0.362	−0.373
SD ML					−0.282	0.491	0.024	−0.128	−0.188	−0.139
Range AP						0.588	0.926 **	0.674 *	0.842 **	0.829 **
Range ML							0.843 **	0.433	0.556	0.580
Range Overall								0.591	0.777 **	0.734 **
Area									0.969 **	0.974 **
Path										0.996 **

PM: Post-work; NPRS: Numeric Pain Rating Scale; SD: Standard Deviation; AP: Anteroposterior; ML: Mediolateral; *: $p < 0.05$; **: $p < 0.01$.

Table A5. Correlation Matrix of Linear Measurements on Day 5 During the AM Period and NPRS Sum (Day 5 AM).

	Mean		SD		Range			Area	Path	Velocity
	AP	ML	AP	ML	AP	ML	Overall			
NPRS Sum	0.288	−0.085	−0.719 *	−0.054	−0.134	−0.082	−0.112	−0.247	−0.165	−0.173
Mean AP		−0.286	−0.467	−0.115	0.096	−0.218	0.025	0.086	−0.190	−0.191
Mean ML			0.217	−0.449	−0.295	−0.367	−0.351	−0.291	−0.230	−0.219
SD AP				0.506	0.457	0.363	0.435	0.378	0.393	0.410
SD ML					0.546	0.687 *	0.642 *	0.507	0.568	0.579
Range AP						0.637 *	0.957 **	0.855 **	0.743 *	0.748 *
Range ML							0.826 **	0.730 *	0.907 **	0.908 **
Range Overall								0.912 **	0.878 **	0.883 **
Area									0.879 **	0.885 **
Path										0.999 **

AM: Pre-work; NPRS: Numeric Pain Rating Scale; SD: Standard Deviation; AP: Anteroposterior; ML: Mediolateral; *: $p < 0.05$; **: $p < 0.01$.

Table A6. Correlation Matrix of Linear Measurements on Day 5 During the PM Period and NPRS Sum (Day 5 PM).

	Mean		SD		Range			Area	Path	Velocity
	AP	ML	AP	ML	AP	ML	Overall			
NPRS Sum	−0.229	−0.501	−0.379	−0.391	0.367	0.493	0.429	0.211	0.201	0.182
Mean AP		0.416	0.233	−0.090	−0.254	0.067	−0.162	−0.060	−0.180	−0.197
Mean ML			0.327	0.405	−0.691 *	−0.677 *	−0.717 *	−0.489	−0.501	−0.497
SD AP				−0.116	0.250	0.024	0.182	0.417	0.377	0.397
SD ML					−0.669 *	−0.642 *	−0.680 *	−0.664 *	−0.539	−0.532
Range AP						0.842 **	0.983 **	0.951 **	0.944 **	0.943 **
Range ML							0.926 **	0.759 *	0.806 **	0.775 **
Range Overall								0.918 **	0.929 **	0.916 **
Area									0.941 **	0.944 **
Path										0.996 **

PM: Post-work; NPRS: Numeric Pain Rating Scale; H: Hurst Exponent; SaEn: Sample Entropy; AP: Anteroposterior; ML: Mediolateral; *: $p < 0.05$; **: $p < 0.01$.

Table A7. Correlation Matrix of Nonlinear Measurements on Day 1 During the AM Period and NPRS Sum (Day 1 AM).

	H(−5)		H(0)		H(2)		H(4.5)		SaEn	
	AP	ML	AP	ML	AP	ML	AP	ML	AP	ML
NPRS Sum	0.255	−0.100	0.212	−0.107	−0.300	−0.403	0.098	−0.273	0.263	0.378
H(−5) AP		−0.079	0.221	0.116	0.058	−0.218	0.460	−0.120	−0.061	0.057
H(−5) ML			0.462	0.615	0.712 *	0.486	0.220	0.261	0.211	0.016
H(0) AP				0.231	0.625	0.057	0.555	−0.084	−0.388	−0.065
H(0) ML					0.654 *	0.862 **	0.335	0.787 **	−0.029	−0.486
H(2) AP						0.655 *	0.718 *	0.391	−0.487	−0.513
H(2) ML							0.212	0.864 **	−0.260	−0.750 *
H(4.5) AP								0.072	−0.606	−0.397
H(4.5) ML									−0.083	−0.752 *
SaEn AP										0.671 *

AM: Pre-work; NPRS: Numeric Pain Rating Scale; H: Hurst Exponent; SaEn: Sample Entropy; AP: Anteroposterior; ML: Mediolateral; *: $p < 0.05$; **: $p < 0.01$.

Table A8. Correlation Matrix of Nonlinear Measurements on Day 1 During the PM Period and NPRS Sum (Day 1 PM).

	H(−5)		H(0)		H(2)		H(4.5)		SaEn	
	AP	ML	AP	ML	AP	ML	AP	ML	AP	ML
NPRS Sum	−0.075	0.278	−0.257	0.153	−0.112	−0.236	−0.366	−0.100	−0.372	−0.437
H(−5) AP		0.462	0.533	0.524	0.671 *	−0.044	0.648 *	−0.090	0.146	−0.201
H(−5) ML			0.338	0.733 *	0.252	0.204	0.463	0.241	−0.068	−0.462
H(0) AP				0.745 *	0.639 *	0.278	0.568	−0.069	0.100	−0.177
H(0) ML					0.420	0.030	0.329	0.169	−0.272	−0.589
H(2) AP						0.320	0.674 *	0.032	0.480	0.134
H(2) ML							0.599	0.281	0.688 *	0.573
H(4.5) AP								−0.063	0.601	0.321
H(4.5) ML									0.348	0.189
SaEn AP										0.856 **

PM: Post-work; NPRS: Numeric Pain Rating Scale; H: Hurst Exponent; SaEn: Sample Entropy; AP: Anteroposterior; ML: Mediolateral; *: $p < 0.05$; **: $p < 0.01$.

Table A9. Correlation Matrix of Nonlinear Measurements on Day 3 During the AM Period and NPRS Sum (Day 3 AM).

	H(−5)		H(0)		H(2)		H(4.5)		SaEn	
	AP	ML	AP	ML	AP	ML	AP	ML	AP	ML
NPRS Sum	−0.631	−0.587	−0.812 **	−0.860 **	−0.330	−0.455	−0.786 **	−0.780 **	−0.451	−0.703 *
H(−5) AP		0.932 **	0.708 *	0.728 *	0.005	0.255	0.542	0.627	0.542	0.613
H(−5) ML			0.569	0.714 *	−0.060	0.409	0.575	0.661 *	0.513	0.490
H(0) AP				0.893 **	0.384	0.451	0.765 **	0.764 *	0.342	0.557
H(0) ML					0.281	0.553	0.770 **	0.885 **	0.454	0.500
H(2) AP						0.522	0.613	0.271	−0.454	0.137
H(2) ML							0.667 *	0.633 *	0.075	0.170
H(4.5) AP								0.778 **	0.072	0.475
H(4.5) ML									0.565	0.462
SaEn AP										0.608

AM: Pre-work; NPRS: Numeric Pain Rating Scale; H: Hurst Exponent; SaEn: Sample Entropy; AP: Anteroposterior; ML: Mediolateral; *: $p < 0.05$; **: $p < 0.01$.

Table A10. Correlation Matrix of Nonlinear Measurements on Day 3 During the PM Period and NPRS Sum (Day 3 PM).

	H(−5)		H(0)		H(2)		H(4.5)		SaEn	
	AP	ML	AP	ML	AP	ML	AP	ML	AP	ML
NPRS Sum	−0.195	0.008	−0.207	−0.019	−0.404	0.060	−0.190	0.368	0.260	0.103
H(−5) AP		−0.163	0.923 **	−0.002	0.528	−0.579	0.811 **	−0.207	−0.058	0.365
H(−5) ML			0.099	0.793 **	−0.302	0.179	−0.151	0.530	−0.308	−0.038
H(0) AP				0.219	0.593	−0.562	0.860 **	−0.046	−0.127	0.455
H(0) ML					0.078	0.273	−0.006	0.601	−0.712 *	−0.275
H(2) AP						−0.022	0.780 **	0.014	−0.369	0.285
H(2) ML							−0.257	0.478	−0.331	−0.149
H(4.5) AP								−0.074	−0.012	0.674 *
H(4.5) ML									−0.539	0.023
SaEn AP										0.325

PM: Post-work; NPRS: Numeric Pain Rating Scale; H: Hurst Exponent; SaEn: Sample Entropy; AP: Anteroposterior; ML: Mediolateral; *: $p < 0.05$; **: $p < 0.01$.

Table A11. Correlation Matrix of Nonlinear Measurements on Day 5 During the AM Period and NPRS Sum (Day 5 AM).

	H(−5)		H(0)		H(2)		H(4.5)		SaEN	
	AP	**ML**	**AP**	**ML**	**AP**	**ML**	**AP**	**ML**	**AP**	**ML**
NPRS Sum	−0.012	−0.046	0.129	−0.130	0.129	−0.415	−0.064	−0.308	0.240	0.457
H(−5) AP		0.738 *	0.846 **	0.724 *	0.589	−0.448	0.685 *	0.532	0.350	0.623
H(−5) ML			0.878 **	0.969 **	0.504	0.077	0.848 **	0.755 *	0.176	0.632
H(0) AP				0.888 **	0.550	−0.197	0.856 **	0.728 *	0.388	0.753 *
H(0) ML					0.406	0.085	0.810 **	0.819 **	0.223	0.593
H(2) AP						0.042	0.750 *	0.542	−0.021	0.314
H(2) ML							0.229	0.345	−0.418	−0.442
H(4.5) AP								0.801 **	0.071	0.457
H(4.5) ML									0.283	0.436
SaEn AP										0.769 **

AM: Pre-work; NPRS: Numeric Pain Rating Scale; H: Hurst Exponent; SaEn: Sample Entropy; AP: Anteroposterior; ML: Mediolateral; *: $p < 0.05$; **: $p < 0.01$.

Table A12. Correlation Matrix of Nonlinear Measurements on Day 5 During the PM Period and NPRS Sum (Day 5 PM).

	H(−5)		H(0)		H(2)		H(4.5)		SaEN	
	AP	**ML**	**AP**	**ML**	**AP**	**ML**	**AP**	**ML**	**AP**	**ML**
NPRS Sum	−0.276	−0.280	−0.215	−0.349	−0.722 *	−0.562	−0.317	−0.506	−0.071	−0.309
H(−5) AP		0.995 **	0.742 *	0.542	0.034	0.136	−0.507	0.132	−0.587	0.005
H(−5) ML			0.745 *	0.596	0.070	0.173	−0.530	0.144	−0.592	−0.017
H(0) AP				0.696 *	−0.004	0.445	−0.453	−0.027	−0.318	0.303
H(0) ML					0.326	0.663 *	−0.426	0.352	−0.333	0.161
H(2) AP						0.649 *	0.309	0.721 *	0.387	0.096
H(2) ML							−0.025	0.530	0.404	0.500
H(4.5) AP								−0.001	0.392	0.502
H(4.5) ML									0.330	−0.069
SaEn AP										0.245

PM: Post-work; NPRS: Numeric Pain Rating Scale; H: Hurst Exponent; SaEn: Sample Entropy; AP: Anteroposterior; ML: Mediolateral; *: $p < 0.05$; **: $p < 0.01$.

References

1. Ferreira, M.L.; De Luca, K.; Haile, L.M.; Steinmetz, J.D.; Culbreth, G.T.; Cross, M.; Kopec, J.A.; Ferreira, P.H.; Blyth, F.M.; Buchbinder, R.; et al. Global, regional, and national burden of low back pain, 1990–2020, its attributable risk factors, and projections to 2050: A systematic analysis of the Global Burden of Disease Study 2021. *Lancet Rheumatol.* **2023**, *5*, e316–e329. [CrossRef]
2. Wu, A.M.; Cross, M.; Elliott, J.M.; Culbreth, G.T.; Haile, L.M.; Steinmetz, J.D.; Hagins, H.; Kopec, J.A.; Brooks, P.M.; Woolf, A.D.; et al. Global, regional, and national burden of neck pain, 1990–2020, and projections to 2050: A systematic analysis of the Global Burden of Disease Study 2021. *Lancet Rheumatol.* **2024**, *6*, e142–e155. [CrossRef]
3. Zhang, C.; Zi, S.; Chen, Q.; Zhang, S. The burden, trends, and projections of low back pain attributable to high body mass index globally: An analysis of the global burden of disease study from 1990 to 2021 and projections to 2050. *Front. Med.* **2024**, *11*, 1469298. [CrossRef] [PubMed]
4. GBD 2019 Ageing Collaborators. Global, regional, and national burden of diseases and injuries for adults 70 years and older: Systematic analysis for the Global Burden of Disease 2019 Study. *BMJ* **2022**, *376*, e068208. [CrossRef]
5. Peereboom, K.; Langen, N.; Copsey, S. *Prolonged Static Sitting at Work: Health Effects and Good Practice Advice*; European Agency for Safety and Health at Work: Bilbao, Spain, 2021. [CrossRef]
6. Nunes, A.; Espanha, M.; Teles, J.; Petersen, K.; Arendt-Nielsen, L.; Carnide, F. Neck pain prevalence and associated occupational factors in Portuguese office workers. *Int. J. Ind. Ergon.* **2021**, *85*, 103172. [CrossRef]
7. Mathiassen, S.E. Diversity and variation in biomechanical exposure: What is it, and why would we like to know? *Appl. Ergon.* **2006**, *37*, 419–427. [CrossRef] [PubMed]

8. Wang, Z.; Sato, K.; Nawrin, S.S.; Widatalla, N.S.; Kimura, Y.; Nagatomi, R. Low back pain exacerbation is predictable through motif identification in center of pressure time series recorded during dynamic sitting. *Front. Physiol.* **2021**, *12*, 696077. [CrossRef]
9. Bakator, M.; Ćoćkalo, D.; Makitan, V.; Stanisavljev, S.; Nikolić, M. The three pillars of tomorrow: How Marketing 5.0 builds on Industry 5.0 and impacts Society 5.0? *Heliyon* **2024**, *10*, e36543. [CrossRef]
10. Duggal, A.S.; Malik, P.K.; Gehlot, A.; Singh, R.; Gaba, G.S.; Masud, M.; Al-Amri, J.F. A sequential roadmap to Industry 6.0: Exploring future manufacturing trends. *Iet Commun.* **2022**, *16*, 521–531. [CrossRef]
11. Kadir, B.A.; Broberg, O.; da Conceição, C.S. Current research and future perspectives on human factors and ergonomics in Industry 4.0. *Comput. Ind. Eng.* **2019**, *137*, 106004. [CrossRef]
12. Stergiou, N.; Decker, L.M. Human movement variability, nonlinear dynamics, and pathology: is there a connection? *Hum. Mov. Sci.* **2011**, *30*, 869–888. [CrossRef] [PubMed]
13. Stergiou, N.; Harbourne, R.T.; Cavanaugh, J.T. Optimal movement variability: a new theoretical perspective for neurologic physical therapy. *J. Neurol. Phys. Ther.* **2006**, *30*, 120–129. [CrossRef]
14. Heredia-Rizo, A.M.; Madeleine, P.; Szeto, G.P. Pain mechanisms in computer and smartphone users. In *Features and Assessments of Pain, Anaesthesia, and Analgesia*; Academic Press: Cambridge, MA, USA, 2022; pp. 291–301. [CrossRef]
15. Toomingas, A.; Forsman, M.; Mathiassen, S.E.; Heiden, M.; Nilsson, T. Variation between seated and standing/walking postures among male and female call centre operators. *BMC Public Health* **2012**, *12*, 154. [CrossRef]
16. Wang, H.; Yu, D.; Zeng, Y.; Zhou, T.; Wang, W.; Liu, X.; Pei, Z.; Yu, Y.; Wang, C.; Deng, Y.; et al. Quantifying the impacts of posture changes on office worker productivity: An exploratory study using effective computer interactions as a real-time indicator. *BMC Public Health* **2023**, *23*, 2198. [CrossRef] [PubMed]
17. Sui, W.; Smith, S.T.; Fagan, M.J.; Rollo, S.; Prapavessis, H. The effects of sedentary behaviour interventions on work-related productivity and performance outcomes in real and simulated office work: A systematic review. *Appl. Ergon.* **2019**, *75*, 27–73. [CrossRef]
18. Waongenngarm, P.; Areerak, K.; Janwantanakul, P. The effects of breaks on low back pain, discomfort, and work productivity in office workers: A systematic review of randomized and non-randomized controlled trials. *Appl. Ergon.* **2018**, *68*, 230–239. [CrossRef] [PubMed]
19. Antonaci, F.G.; Olivetti, E.C.; Marcolin, F.; Castiblanco Jimenez, I.A.; Eynard, B.; Vezzetti, E.; Moos, S. Workplace Well-Being in Industry 5.0: A Worker-Centered Systematic Review. *Sensors* **2024**, *24*, 5473. [CrossRef]
20. Lim, S.; D'Souza, C. A narrative review on contemporary and emerging uses of inertial sensing in occupational ergonomics. *Int. J. Ind. Ergon.* **2020**, *76*, 102937. [CrossRef]
21. Jun, D.; Johnston, V.; McPhail, S.M.; O'Leary, S. Are measures of postural behavior using motion sensors in seated office workers reliable? *Hum. Factors* **2019**, *61*, 1141–1161. [CrossRef]
22. Patel, V.; Chesmore, A.; Legner, C.M.; Pandey, S. Trends in workplace wearable technologies and connected-worker solutions for next-generation occupational safety, health, and productivity. *Adv. Intell. Syst.* **2022**, *4*, 2100099. [CrossRef]
23. Lind, C.M.; Abtahi, F.; Forsman, M. Wearable motion capture devices for the prevention of work-related musculoskeletal disorders in ergonomics—An overview of current applications, challenges, and future opportunities. *Sensors* **2023**, *23*, 4259. [CrossRef] [PubMed]
24. Knox, M.F.; Chipchase, L.S.; Schabrun, S.M.; Romero, R.J.; Marshall, P.W. Anticipatory and compensatory postural adjustments in people with low back pain: A systematic review and meta-analysis. *Spine J.* **2018**, *18*, 1934–1949. [CrossRef] [PubMed]
25. Alsubaie, A.M.; Mazaheri, M.; Martinez-Valdes, E.; Falla, D. Is movement variability altered in people with chronic non-specific low back pain? A systematic review. *PloS ONE* **2023**, *18*, e0287029. [CrossRef] [PubMed]
26. Bontrup, C.; Taylor, W.R.; Fliesser, M.; Visscher, R.; Green, T.; Wippert, P.M.; Zemp, R. Low back pain and its relationship with sitting behaviour among sedentary office workers. *Appl. Ergon.* **2019**, *81*, 102894. [CrossRef]
27. Hodges, P.W.; Tucker, K. Moving differently in pain: a new theory to explain the adaptation to pain. *Pain* **2011**, *152*, S90–S98. [CrossRef]
28. Zemp, R.; Fliesser, M.; Wippert, P.M.; Taylor, W.R.; Lorenzetti, S. Occupational sitting behaviour and its relationship with back pain—A pilot study. *Appl. Ergon.* **2016**, *56*, 84–91. [CrossRef]
29. Asgari, M.; Sanjari, M.A.; Mokhtarinia, H.R.; Sedeh, S.M.; Khalaf, K.; Parnianpour, M. The effects of movement speed on kinematic variability and dynamic stability of the trunk in healthy individuals and low back pain patients. *Clin. Biomech.* **2015**, *30*, 682–688. [CrossRef]
30. Mingels, S.; Dankaerts, W.; van Etten, L.; Bruckers, L.; Granitzer, M. Lower spinal postural variability during laptop-work in subjects with cervicogenic headache compared to healthy controls. *Sci. Rep.* **2021**, *11*, 5159. [CrossRef]
31. International Labour Office. *Stress Prevention at Work Checkpoints: Practical Improvements for Stress Prevention in the Workplace, 13.04.5*; International Labour Office: Geneva, Switzerland, 2012; Volume 1.

32. Slater, D.; Korakakis, V.; O'Sullivan, P.; Nolan, D.; O'Sullivan, K. "Sit up straight": Time to Re-evaluate. *J. Orthop. Sport. Phys. Ther.* **2019**, *49*, 562–564. [CrossRef]
33. Treede, R.D.; Rief, W.; Barke, A.; Aziz, Q.; Bennett, M.I.; Benoliel, R.; Cohen, M.; Evers, S.; Finnerup, N.B.; First, M.B.; et al. Chronic pain as a symptom or a disease: the IASP Classification of Chronic Pain for the International Classification of Diseases (ICD-11). *Pain* **2019**, *160*, 19–27. [CrossRef]
34. Oliosi, E.; Probst, P.; Rodrigues, J.; Silva, L.; Zagalo, D.; Cepeda, C.; Gamboa, H. Week-long Multimodal Data Acquisition of Occupational Risk Factors in Public Administration Workers. In Proceedings of the 2023 19th International Conference on Intelligent Environments (IE), Uniciti, Mauritius, 29–30 June 2023; pp. 1–8. [CrossRef]
35. International Association for the Study of Pain (IASP). IASP Announces Revised Definition of Pain. 2020. Available online: https://www.iasp-pain.org/resources/terminology/#pain (accessed on 11 November 2024).
36. Craig, C.L.; Marshall, A.L.; Sjöström, M.; Bauman, A.E.; Booth, M.L.; Ainsworth, B.E.; Pratt, M.; Ekelund, U.; Yngve, A.; Sallis, J.F.; et al. International physical activity questionnaire: 12-country reliability and validity. *Med. Sci. Sports Exerc.* **2003**, *35*, 1381–1395. [CrossRef] [PubMed]
37. Rosário, S.; Azevedo, L.F.; Fonseca, J.A.; Nienhaus, A.; Nübling, M.; da Costa, J.T. The Portuguese long version of the Copenhagen Psychosocial Questionnaire II (COPSOQ II)—A validation study. *J. Occup. Med. Toxicol.* **2017**, *12*, 24. [CrossRef]
38. Pejtersen, J.H.; Kristensen, T.S.; Borg, V.; Bjorner, J.B. The second version of the Copenhagen Psychosocial Questionnaire. *Scand. J. Public Health* **2010**, *38*, 8–24. [CrossRef] [PubMed]
39. Barbado, D.; Irles-Vidal, B.; Prat-Luri, A.; García-Vaquero, M.P.; Vera-Garcia, F.J. Training intensity quantification of core stability exercises based on a smartphone accelerometer. *PLoS ONE* **2018**, *13*, e0208262. [CrossRef] [PubMed]
40. Chung, C.C.; Soangra, R.; Lockhart, T.E. Recurrence quantitative analysis of postural sway using force plate and smartphone. In Proceedings of the Human Factors and Ergonomics Society Annual Meeting, Lisbon, Portugal, 1 September 2014; SAGE Publications Sage CA: Los Angeles, CA, USA, 2014; Volume 58, pp. 1271–1275. [CrossRef]
41. Karlinsky, K.T.; Netz, Y.; Jacobs, J.M.; Ayalon, M.; Yekutieli, Z. Static balance digital endpoints with Mon4t: Smartphone sensors vs. Force plate. *Sensors* **2022**, *22*, 4139. [CrossRef]
42. Zhou, J.; Yu, W.; Zhu, H.; Lo, O.Y.; Gouskova, N.; Travison, T.; Lipsitz, L.A.; Pascual-Leone, A.; Manor, B. A novel smartphone App-based assessment of standing postural control: Demonstration of reliability and sensitivity to aging and task constraints. In Proceedings of the 2020 IEEE International Conference on E-health Networking, Application & Services (HEALTHCOM), Shenzhen, China, 1–2 March 2021; pp. 1–6. [CrossRef]
43. Huang, R.; Kaminishi, K.; Hasegawa, T.; Yozu, A.; Chiba, R.; Ota, J. Estimation of center of pressure information by smartphone sensors for postural control training. In Proceedings of the 2023 45th Annual International Conference of the IEEE Engineering in Medicine & Biology Society (EMBC), Sydney, Australia, 24–27 July 2023; pp. 1–4. [CrossRef]
44. Onuma, R.; Hoshi, F.; Tozawa, R.; Soutome, Y.; Sakai, T.; Jinno, T. Reliability and validity of quantitative evaluation of anticipatory postural adjustments using smartphones. *J. Phys. Ther. Sci.* **2023**, *35*, 553–558. [CrossRef]
45. Prieto, T.E.; Myklebust, J.B.; Hoffmann, R.G.; Lovett, E.G.; Myklebust, B.M. Measures of postural steadiness: differences between healthy young and elderly adults. *IEEE Trans. Biomed. Eng.* **1996**, *43*, 956–966. [CrossRef]
46. Saito, H.; Watanabe, Y.; Kutsuna, T.; Futohashi, T.; Kusumoto, Y.; Chiba, H.; Kubo, M.; Takasaki, H. Spinal movement variability associated with low back pain: A scoping review. *PLoS ONE* **2021**, *16*, e0252141. [CrossRef]
47. Harbourne, R.T.; Stergiou, N. Movement variability and the use of nonlinear tools: principles to guide physical therapist practice. *Phys. Ther.* **2009**, *89*, 267–282. [CrossRef]
48. Deffeyes, J.E.; Harbourne, R.T.; Kyvelidou, A.; Stuberg, W.A.; Stergiou, N. Nonlinear analysis of sitting postural sway indicates developmental delay in infants. *Clin. Biomech.* **2009**, *24*, 564–570. [CrossRef]
49. Stergiou, N.; Kent, J.A.; McGrath, D. Human movement variability and aging. *Kinesiol. Rev.* **2016**, *5*, 15–22. [CrossRef]
50. Carpena, P.; Gómez-Extremera, M.; Bernaola-Galván, P.A. On the validity of detrended fluctuation analysis at short scales. *Entropy* **2021**, *24*, 61. [CrossRef] [PubMed]
51. Kantelhardt, J.W.; Zschiegner, S.A.; Koscielny-Bunde, E.; Havlin, S.; Bunde, A.; Stanley, H.E. Multifractal detrended fluctuation analysis of nonstationary time series. *Phys. Stat. Mech. Its Appl.* **2002**, *316*, 87–114. [CrossRef]
52. Richman, J.S.; Moorman, J.R. Physiological time-series analysis using approximate entropy and sample entropy. *Am. J. Physiol. Heart Circ. Physiol.* **2000**, *278*, H2039–H2049. [CrossRef]
53. van Dieën, J.H.; Koppes, L.L.; Twisk, J.W. Postural sway parameters in seated balancing; their reliability and relationship with balancing performance. *Gait Posture* **2010**, *31*, 42–46. [CrossRef]
54. Søndergaard, K.H.; Olesen, C.G.; Søndergaard, E.K.; De Zee, M.; Madeleine, P. The variability and complexity of sitting postural control are associated with discomfort. *J. Biomech.* **2010**, *43*, 1997–2001. [CrossRef]

55. Madeleine, P.; Marandi, R.Z.; Norheim, K.L.; Andersen, J.B.; Samani, A. Sitting dynamics during computer work are age-dependent. *Appl. Ergon.* **2021**, *93*, 103391. [CrossRef]
56. Arippa, F.; Nguyen, A.; Pau, M.; Harris-Adamson, C. Postural strategies among office workers during a prolonged sitting bout. *Appl. Ergon.* **2022**, *102*, 103723. [CrossRef]
57. Hermann, S. Exploring sitting posture and discomfort using nonlinear analysis methods. *IEEE Trans. Inf. Technol. Biomed.* **2005**, *9*, 392–401. [CrossRef]
58. Oliosi, E.; Júlio, A.; Probst, P.; Silva, L.; Vilas-Boas, J.P.; Pinheiro, A.R.; Gamboa, H. Exploring the Real-Time Variability and Complexity of Sitting Patterns in Office Workers with Non-Specific Chronic Spinal Pain and Pain-Free Individuals. *Sensors* **2024**, *24*, 4750. [CrossRef]
59. Ainsworth, B.E.; Haskell, W.L.; Whitt, M.C.; Irwin, M.L.; Swartz, A.M.; Strath, S.J.; O Brien, W.L.; Bassett, D.R.; Schmitz, K.H.; Emplaincourt, P.O.; et al. Compendium of physical activities: An update of activity codes and MET intensities. *Med. Sci. Sports Exerc.* **2000**, *32*, S498–S504. [CrossRef]
60. Mortazavi, B.; Alsharufa, N.; Lee, S.I.; Lan, M.; Sarrafzadeh, M.; Chronley, M.; Roberts, C.K. MET calculations from on-body accelerometers for exergaming movements. In Proceedings of the 2013 IEEE International Conference on Body Sensor Networks, Cambridge, MA, USA, 6–9 May 2013; pp. 1–6. [CrossRef]
61. Ohlendorf, D.; Pflaum, J.; Wischnewski, C.; Schamberger, S.; Erbe, C.; Wanke, E.M.; Holzgreve, F.; Groneberg, D.A. Standard reference values of the postural control in healthy female adults aged between 31 and 40 years in Germany: an observational study. *J. Physiol. Anthropol.* **2020**, *39*, 27. [CrossRef] [PubMed]
62. Mendes, F.; Probst, P.; Oliosi, E.; Silva, L.; Cepeda, C.; Gamboa, H. Analysis of Postural Variability of Office Workers Using Inertial Sensors. In Proceedings of the BIOSIGNALS, Lisbon, Portugal, 16–18 February 2023; pp. 273–280. [CrossRef]
63. Madeleine, P. Dynamics of seated computer work before and after prolonged constrained sitting. *J. Appl. Biomech.* **2012**, *28*, 297–303. [CrossRef] [PubMed]
64. Goldberger, A.L. Fractal variability versus pathologic periodicity: complexity loss and stereotypy in disease. *Perspect. Biol. Med.* **1997**, *40*, 543–561. [CrossRef] [PubMed]
65. Gatchel, R.J.; Peng, Y.B.; Peters, M.L.; Fuchs, P.N.; Turk, D.C. The biopsychosocial approach to chronic pain: scientific advances and future directions. *Psychol. Bull.* **2007**, *133*, 581. [CrossRef]
66. O'Sullivan, K.; O'Sullivan, P.; O'Keeffe, M.; O'Sullivan, L.; Dankaerts, W. The effect of dynamic sitting on trunk muscle activation: A systematic review. *Appl. Ergon.* **2013**, *44*, 628–635. [CrossRef]
67. van Emmerik, R.E.; van Wegen, E.E. On variability and stability in human movement. *J. Appl. Biomech.* **2000**, *16*, 394–406. [CrossRef]
68. Davidson, J.M.; Callaghan, J.P. A week-long field study of seated pelvis and lumbar spine kinematics during office work. *Appl. Ergon.* **2025**, *122*, 104374. [CrossRef]
69. Van Daele, U.; Hagman, F.; Truijen, S.; Vorlat, P.; Van Gheluwe, B.; Vaes, P. Decrease in postural sway and trunk stiffness during cognitive dual-task in nonspecific chronic low back pain patients, performance compared to healthy control subjects. *Spine* **2010**, *35*, 583–589. [CrossRef]
70. Cavanaugh, J.T.; Mercer, V.S.; Stergiou, N. Approximate entropy detects the effect of a secondary cognitive task on postural control in healthy young adults: A methodological report. *J. Neuroeng. Rehabil.* **2007**, *4*, 42. [CrossRef]
71. Shafizadeh, M.; Parvinpour, S.; Balali, M.; Shabani, M. Effects of age and task difficulty on postural sway, variability and complexity. *Adapt. Behav.* **2021**, *29*, 617–625. [CrossRef]
72. Bibbo, D.; Conforto, S.; Schmid, M.; Battisti, F. The Influence of Different Levels of Cognitive Engagement on the Seated Postural Sway. *Electronics* **2020**, *9*, 601. [CrossRef]
73. Mockałło, Z. Stress-Inducing Customer Behaviors and Wellbeing in Tax Administration Workers: What Is the Role of Emotional Labor? In *Emotional Labor in Work with Patients and Clients*; CRC Press: Boca Raton, FL, USA, 2020; pp. 7–28.
74. Issever, H.; Ozdilli, K.; Altunkaynak, O.; Onen, L.; Disci, R. Depression in tax office workers in Istanbul and its affecting factors. *Indoor Built Environ.* **2008**, *17*, 414–420. [CrossRef]
75. Nieminen, L.K.; Pyysalo, L.M.; Kankaanpää, M.J. Prognostic factors for pain chronicity in low back pain: A systematic review. *Pain Rep.* **2021**, *6*, e919. [CrossRef]
76. Timmers, I.; Quaedflieg, C.W.; Hsu, C.; Heathcote, L.C.; Rovnaghi, C.R.; Simons, L.E. The interaction between stress and chronic pain through the lens of threat learning. *Neurosci. Biobehav. Rev.* **2019**, *107*, 641–655. [CrossRef]
77. Wainwright, E.; Bevan, S.; Blyth, F.M.; Khalatbari-Soltani, S.; Sullivan, M.J.; Walker-Bone, K.; Eccleston, C. Pain, work, and the workplace: A topical review. *Pain* **2022**, *163*, 408–414. [CrossRef]

sensors

MDPI

Article

Electrodermal Activity Analysis at Different Body Locations

Patricia Gamboa [1,2,*], Rui Varandas [1,2], Katrin Mrotzeck [2], Hugo Plácido da Silva [2,3] and Cláudia Quaresma [1,*]

1 LIBPhys (Laboratory for Instrumentation, Biomedical Engineering and Radiation Physics), NOVA School of Science and Technology, 2829-516 Caparica, Portugal; r.varandas@campus.fct.unl.pt
2 PLUX—Wireless Biosignals S.A., 1050-059 Lisboa, Portugal; katrin.mrotzeck@gmail.com (K.M.)
3 IT—Instituto de Telecomunicações, 1049-001 Lisboa, Portugal
* Correspondence: pg.neves@campus.fct.unl.pt (P.G.); q.claudia@fct.unl.pt (C.Q.)

Abstract: Electrodermal activity (EDA) reflects the variation in the electrical conductance of the skin in response to sweat secretion, constituting a non-invasive measure of the sympathetic nervous system. This system intervenes in reactions to stress and is strongly activated in emotional states. In most cases, EDA signals are collected from the hand (fingers or palms), which is not an ideal location for a sensor when the participant has to use their hands during tasks or activities. This study aims to explore alternative locations for retrieving EDA signals (e.g., the chest, back, and forehead). EDA signals from 25 healthy participants were collected using a protocol involving different physical stimuli that have been reported to induce an electrodermal response. The features extracted included the Skin Conductance Response (SCR) height, SCR amplitude, and peak prominence. An analysis of these features and the analysis of the correlation between the standard position with the different locations suggested that the chest, while a possible alternative for EDA signal collection, presents some weak results, and further evaluation of this site is needed. Additionally, the forehead should be excluded as an alternative site, at least in short-term measurements.

Keywords: electrodermal activity; alternative site; skin conductance response; skin conductance level

1. Introduction

The Autonomic Nervous System (ANS) controls most of the body's visceral functions [1], innervating the endocrine glands, the exocrine glands (e.g., sweat glands), and the viscera. It is divided into the sympathetic and parasympathetic nervous systems and operates involuntarily through autonomic reflexes and central control [2]. Electrodermal activity (EDA) is a manifestation of the activity of the eccrine sweat glands, which are innervated by the ANS [3]. The EDA is considered to be a peripheral indicator of sympathetic activation [4], and it refers to the variation in the electrical conductance of the skin in response to sweat secretion [5].

The EDA response is categorized by a tonic component and a phasic component. The tonic component refers to gradual and soft changes in the EDA response, which occur in the absence of stimuli [6]. The most common measure of this component is the Skin Conductance Level (SCL). Research suggests its variations seem to reflect the global changes in the autonomic excitation and occur typically in a period of dozens of seconds to minutes [6], in the absence of stimuli [7]. On the other hand, the phasic component, designated by the Skin Conductance Response (SCR), refers to sudden and rapid changes in the EDA response [6]. These phasic responses of conductivity seem to correspond to arousal states, with SCR amplitudes providing information on the intensity of those states [8]. The EDA signal reflects a combination of different processes—attentional, affective, motivational [1]—and it has been used in different studies targeting emotional arousal [9] and stress [10].

The human body contains between 1.6 and 4.0 million eccrine sweat glands in total, with densities per square centimeter of 64 on the back, 181 on the forehead, 600–700 on the palms and soles (Sato et al., 1989, as cited in [11]), and 20 on the chest (Wilke et al., 2004, as cited in [12]). Most researchers use the palms or the volar surfaces of the fingers as active sites for EDA recording, and this is the preferred Standard Position (SP) for EDA collection [11]. However, as the hands are usually used in tasks or activities performed during experimental studies or daily monitoring, research has been conducted to investigate EDA signals retrieved from different body locations.

Several studies have investigated the relationship between the signal retrieved from the fingers (SP) and other body locations, such as the wrist [13,14], feet [15,16], or ankle [13]. However, few studies explore several locations simultaneously.

One study investigated SCR in the context of emotion elicitation through the visualization of emotional film clips, comparing 16 different recording positions in 17 participants [17]. The highest SCL and SCR were observed for the forehead, foot, fingers, and shoulders. Conversely, the lowest SCR was found for the arm, armpit, thigh, buttock, back, and abdomen. The highest correlations between the fingers (SP) and other positions were found for the foot, followed by the forehead, which was among the top three most responsive body locations for SCL and SCRs. Thus, the authors suggest that sensors could be embedded into headbands or headphones to unobtrusively measure EDA. However, in addition to a small sample size, the study also had an imbalanced gender ratio (five females).

Another study compared multiple nonpalmar sites (e.g., the wrist, abductor hallucis of the foot, foot arch, toes, and forehead) with the fingers [18], during the visualization of 19 images from the International Affective Picture System (IAPS; Lang, Bradley & Cuthbert, 2008, as cited in [18]) and an arithmetic stress task. The results revealed that nonpalmar sites are generally less responsive, with the wrist providing the lowest SCL values and the toes the highest, obtaining SCL values closer to the ones obtained from the fingers. Within-participant correlations between the fingers and other sites were higher for the plantar sites and lowest for the forehead, followed by the wrist [18]. In conclusion, toes are the most equivalent alternative in terms of responsiveness to stimuli, followed by the abductor hallucis location (recommended by Boucsein, 2012, as cited by [18]).

In another study, 115 participants performed a breathing exercise (4 min long) and listened to four musical segments (conveying different emotions) and one emotionally neutral computer-generated tone (lasting 7 s each), while EDA was measured from five anatomical sites bilaterally (finger, foot, wrist, shoulder, and calf [19]). The response magnitudes of SCRs to breathing exercises, music segments, and neutral tones were higher at the feet (most likely due to the high density of eccrine sweat glands). Within-subject correlations were also higher for the feet, followed by the wrists (when comparing these locations with the fingers), in all tasks. In summary, among the sites explored in this study, feet are the recommended alternative location for EDA collection. Even though lower SCR amplitudes were found for the wrists (when compared to the fingers), authors recommend this alternative site if the feet are not available. Furthermore, they also highlight that with adequate hydration time (20 min), the calves become comparable to the wrists in terms of response frequency, magnitude and correlation [19]. However, the sample was composed predominantly of females (n = 89). Another limitation identified is related to the hydration time, which might be shorter than the amount of time needed for the alternate sites to become electrodermally active. Also, the wide range of ambient temperature in the experiment may have affected the results [19].

A more recent study compared the SP with three other body locations (forehead, neck and foot) in 23 participants [20]. A high correlation between EDA signals from the SP and the foot was obtained, even when analyzing the phasic and tonic components separately. Again, the authors highlight the foot as the best alternative location for EDA acquisition. Moreover, the forehead was considered to be the most robust against motion artifacts and, with adequate hydration (although this could be an issue for short-time applications), it may become more responsive and provide a more accurate SCR. One limitation of this study is the gender balance of the sample (four females), which makes it difficult to generalize the findings.

The present study focuses on analyzing EDA collected in different body locations (forehead, back, and chest) and comparing these signals to the ones retrieved at the SP for EDA acquisition (fingers on the non-dominant hand). The motivation for this study was set in the context of selecting an alternative EDA site, other than the SP, for the collection of EDA signals from Medical First Responders participating in the H2020 project MED1stMR (Medical First Responder Training using a Mixed-Reality Approach featuring haptic feedback for enhanced realism—is an H2020 project that developed scenarios of mass casualty incidents to train Medical First Responders in several different skills, including first triage. The project involved the collection of participants' biosignals, including EDA and ECG signals (https://www.med1stmr.eu/, accessed on 16 December 2024)), since the participants were required to wear gloves on their hands, which were used to command avatars in a virtual reality scenario (therefore, it was not feasible to have EDA sensors on the hands or fingers as well).

Nonetheless, results can be extended to support studies where the hands are used when performing tasks or activities (using a specific item, writing, etc.). This research includes body locations that are less commonly studied in EDA research, and thus holds relevance for validating the reliability and consistency of EDA signals from non-standard sites. Determining whether EDA can be reliably measured at alternative sites is essential for facilitating unobtrusive biosignal collection. This could significantly improve device usability and enable the deployment of portable devices to be used with various populations and settings.

The novelty of this study lies in its exploration of less commonly studied body locations for EDA measurement, addressing a gap in the literature regarding non-standard EDA collection sites. Furthermore, by examining whether EDA can be reliably measured at alternative sites, the study contributes to the development of more unobtrusive biosignal collection systems, which is particularly valuable for scenarios where hand usage is restricted (e.g., writing, using tools). This work has practical implications for improving wearable device usability, facilitating the deployment of portable technologies across diverse populations and settings.

2. Materials and Methods

2.1. Data Collection

The physiological data were collected using biosignalsplux acquisition devices from PLUX (PLUX—Wireless Biosignals, S.A., Lisbon, Portugal, https://www.pluxbiosignals.com/, accessed on 16 December 2024), at 10 Hz and 16-bit resolution, with pre-gelled Ag/AgCl electrodes. The EDA data were collected using an exosomatic approach, with an external constant current applied between two electrodes.

EDA data were collected from four different body locations: the fingers, forehead, back and chest. The sample comprised 25 healthy participants (aged 18–51 years old, M = 29.3, SD = 8.9; 14 females). The data collection was performed in an area specifically designated for this purpose, namely a room containing two researchers and each participant. This study was approved by the Ethics Committee of the NOVA School of Science and Technology (protocol code CE-FCT-006-2022).

The inclusion criteria were as follows: aged above 18 years old; no pathology associated; alcohol consumption limited to no more than two times per week (as alcohol is a known psychotropic depressant of the central nervous system [21]); no consumption of psychotropic drugs; no medication (except occasionally); no caffeine consumption in the three previous hours (as caffeine intake leads to elevated electrodermal activity [22]).

To all participants that met the inclusion criteria and gave consent for their participation, the following protocol was applied. First, the study was briefly explained and informed consent was collected. Then, participants answered questions related to the sample characterization and to their health and well-being. Afterwards, each pair of EDA electrodes was positioned in the following locations (see Figure 1):

1. On the hand (SP/gold standard): one of the electrodes was placed on the proximal phalange of the index finger and of the middle finger, on the non-dominant hand;
2. On the anterior face of the torso (chest): the two electrodes were placed next to each other, on the *Rectus Abdominis*, at the sternum level;
3. On the posterior face and superior part of the torso (back): the two electrodes were placed next to each other, on the inferior zone of the trapezius muscle;
4. On the forehead: the two electrodes were placed next to each other, on the frontal area, approximately 2 cm above the procerus.

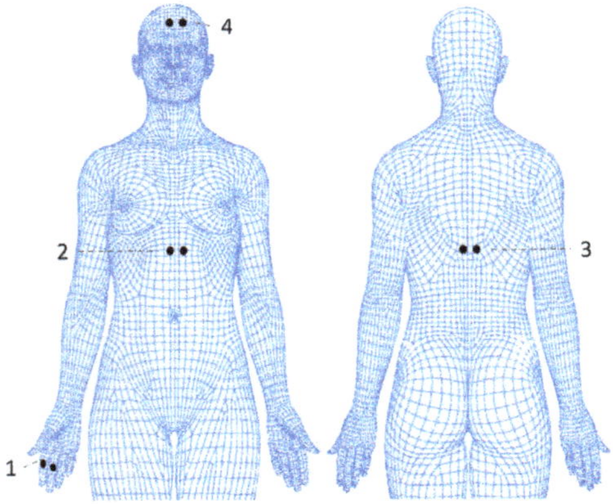

Figure 1. Electrodes positioning (1—fingers of non-dominant hand; 2—chest; 3—back; 4—forehead).

To ensure consistency in electrode placement and facilitate reliable comparisons across participants, we selected a specific location on the forehead—2 cm above the procerus—for all measurements.

After placing the electrodes, a performance test to verify the correct positioning and respective visualization of the EDA signal was performed, followed by a 5 min sample acquisition period to increase the electrodermal contact with the sweat glands ducts [23].

The experiment itself included a 3 min EDA signal acquisition to characterize each individual baseline and the EDA signal acquisition during the performance of tasks that induced an electrodermal response. These tasks were performed by one of the researchers, who very carefully applied the materials/items to the skin surface of the subject to allow them to feel the physical sensation of touching different materials, so that the subject did not need to move. The items/materials used for touch sensation included a mug with hot water inside; a cooling pad; sandpaper; cotton; and a needle (stimuli that generate an electrodermal response according to [24]). An additional task—holding breath—was added [23].

The acquisition of the EDA signal from the four different locations was not performed simultaneously. Each signal was acquired using a different device to avoid any potential mutual interference between the signals, using a customized sync cable to enable the acquisition of signals (using two devices) while ensuring precise temporal synchronization of the recorded data.

The experience consisted of three rounds: SP was compared with the chest; then SP was compared with the back; and lastly, SP was compared with the forehead. There was a baseline period of 3 min before each round and tasks were applied in a randomized sequence for each round. Each of the tasks was interpolated by a 30 s period of rest.

After the data collection, electrodes were removed, and the areas where they were placed were cleaned.

The diagram presented in Figure 2 summarizes the protocol described above.

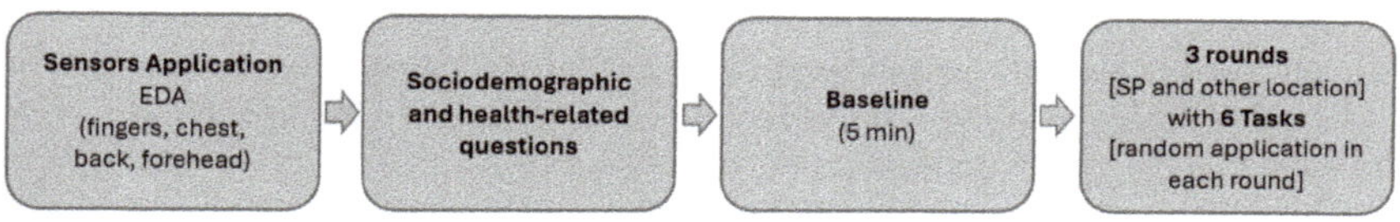

Figure 2. Diagram of the experimental procedure: from sensor attachment to task performance.

2.2. Data Processing

The acquired EDA signal was filtered using a low-pass filter with a bandwidth of 0–3 Hz, as specified in the sensor datasheet (https://support.pluxbiosignals.com/wp-content/uploads/2021/11/Electrodermal_Activity_EDA_Datasheet.pdf, accessed on 16 December 2024). We have also applied a bandpass filter with a bandwidth of 0.045–0.25 Hz.

The tools used for EDA analysis included Python 3.10.9 (Anaconda, Inc., Location Austin, TX, USA) programming language using the NeuroKit2 [25] and SciPy (https://scipy.org/citing-scipy/, accessed on 16 December 2024) packages. Extracted features included the SCR onset, SCR latency or rise time, SCR peak amplitude, and SCR peak prominence (see Figure 3).

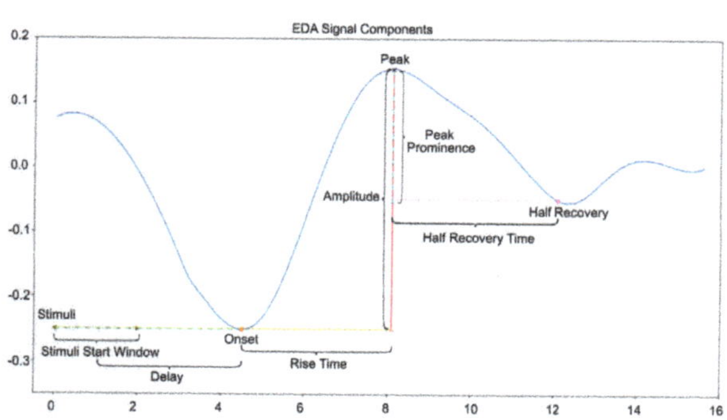

Figure 3. Typical EDA signal response pattern and relevant features.

SCR height includes the tonic and phasic components, while SCR amplitude excludes the tonic component. SCR peak prominence was also calculated, and it measures how much a peak rises above the surrounding baseline of the signal. It represents the vertical distance between the peak and its lowest contour line. The threshold 0.02 µS was chosen to be the same as in [17], so that the results could be compared more directly, and also to consider the literature that suggests thresholds between 0.015 µS and 0.3 µS [26]. This threshold was considered as the minimum value for each response. Everything below this threshold was ignored to avoid detection of features that were caused by non-task-related artifacts such as movements. Specific time windows in which stimuli were applied were analyzed. For the correlation analysis, we considered the complete time window, whereas for the SCR analysis, we only considered the first peak appearing after applying the stimuli.

3. Results

3.1. SCR Results by Location

After applying the NeuroKit2 EDA tool [25] to the time windows of the events, we extracted the features for all peaks that appeared within the time windows that were above the mentioned threshold. Afterwards, we only considered the first peak of each time window, averaging the results across all participants with the same sensor position and task. The primary rationale for considering only the first peak was our interest in examining the EDA feedback immediately following the initial stimulus, as this event's time point could be precisely defined, unlike subsequent stimuli/events within the same time window. Furthermore, this approach was chosen to enhance comparability across different tasks and sensor positions, recognizing that each stimulus might elicit distinct responses over time and a different number of detectable responses. By isolating the first peak, we aimed to ensure consistency and reliability in our analysis across conditions.

Table 1 displays the SCR results by position, presenting the mean value (in µS) and standard deviation in brackets, for the following features: height, amplitude and prominence.

Table 1. SCR results by location (in µS).

Location	SCR Height	SCR Amplitude	SCR Prominence
SP	0.19 (0.31)	0.34 (0.48)	0.26 (0.43)
Chest	0.05 (0.10)	0.17 (0.18)	0.07 (0.13)
SP	0.33 (0.44)	0.75 (0.99)	0.40 (0.52)
Back	0.03 (0.09)	0.21 (0.24)	0.04 (0.13)
SP	0.06 (0.06)	0.10 (0.09)	0.07 (0.08)
Forehead	0.01 (0.03)	0.02 (0.00)	0.01 (0.01)

As shown in Table 1, the chest was the location for which the values obtained were closer to the SP in the three features (even though the results were lower than the ones obtained for the SP) . The forehead was the position that resulted in the lowest values of all the positions in all features. Figure 4 depicts a boxplot comparing the positions, regarding SCR Height, SCR Amplitude, and SCR Prominence.

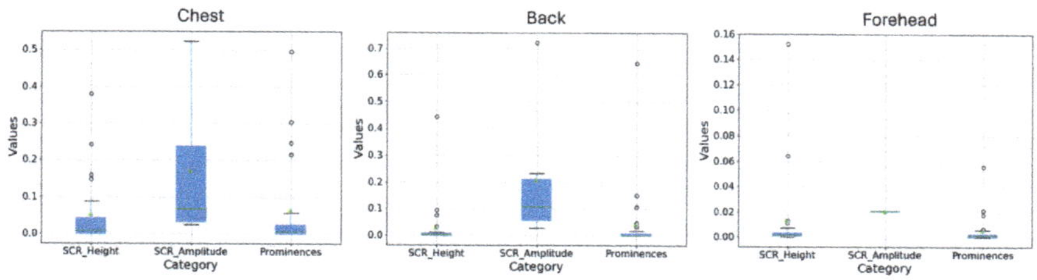

Figure 4. SCR Height, SCR Amplitude, and SCR Prominence per location.

Regarding the amplitude, the peak amplitude of the SCR appears to be the feature that reflects values closer to the SP value (0.17 µS on the chest and 0.21 µS on the back). This suggests that peak amplitude may be a reliable feature for comparing physiological responses across different sensor placements and stimulus conditions.

3.2. Correlations with the Standard Position

The correlations between the EDA signals collected at the SP (fingers) and the alternative locations (chest, back, and forehead) were calculated using Pearson's correlation coefficient [27] for both the tonic and phasic components of the EDA, as presented in Table 2.

As indicated in the table, the EDA signals recorded from the chest exhibit a higher correlation with those collected at the SP, for both the phasic and tonic components, in comparison to other locations, for all tasks except the breathing task.

On the other hand, with the exception of the hot water task, the forehead displayed lower and, in some cases, negative correlations with the EDA from the SP, for both the phasic and tonic components of the EDA.

Table 2. Correlation coefficients between EDA signals from the SP and other locations.

Location	Task	Tonic	Phasic
Chest	Hot	0.526	0.357
	Sandpaper	0.401	0.285
	Pin	0.551	0.244
	Cold	0.069	0.192
	Cotton	0.359	0.234
	Breath	0.041	0.253
Back	Hot	0.462	0.143
	Sandpaper	0.190	0.114
	Pin	0.054	0.084
	Cold	0.105	0.243
	Cotton	0.026	0.068
	Breath	0.219	0.167
Forehead	Hot	0.501	0.110
	Sandpaper	0.105	0.116
	Pin	−0.316	0.211
	Cold	−0.175	−0.057
	Cotton	−0.222	0.087
	Breath	0.080	0.122

When computing the mean value for all tasks for each position, the chest yielded the highest values for both the tonic (0.325) and phasic (0.261) components of the EDA. In contrast, the back produced notably lower values (0.176 for tonic and 0.137 for phasic) and the forehead presented the lowest values (−0.005 for tonic and 0.098 for phasic).

These results suggest that, among the alternative measurement sites analyzed, the chest demonstrates relatively stronger signal responsiveness, while the back indicates weaker EDA responsiveness, and the forehead, with a near-zero tonic value and the lowest phasic value, appears to be the least effective site for EDA measurement.

Figure 5 presents the phasic component around the first peak of the hot water task, for the different locations (SP1—SP round 1—and chest; SP2—SP round 2—and back; SP3—SP round 3—and forehead, respectively), for one of the participants.

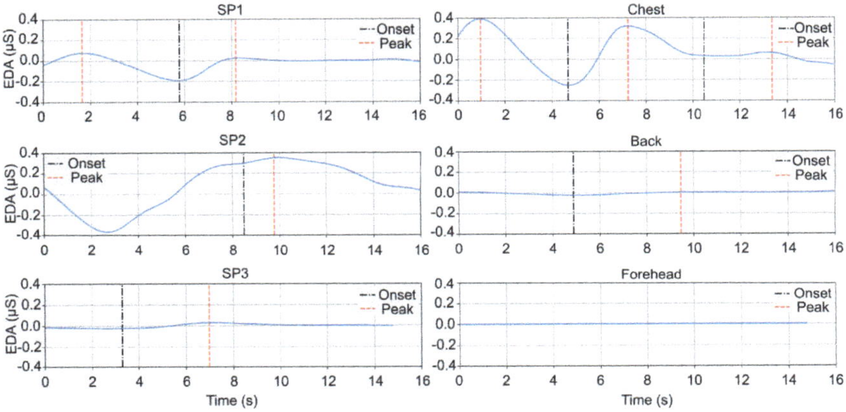

Figure 5. Phasic component of hot water task, for the different locations, for one of the participants.

The EDA response for the chest follows a similar trend to SP1, showing a clear onset and peak. On the other hand, the back shows a much weaker EDA response compared to SP2, with the signal remaining nearly flat. The forehead EDA signal is flat, with no clear onset or peak. These findings seem to support the exclusion of the back and forehead as viable sites for EDA measurement.

4. Discussion

This study explored EDA signal collection from multiple locations on the body, specifically the chest, back, and forehead, comparing them to the standard position (fingers). The objective was to determine viable alternative locations for EDA measurement, particularly when the hands are unavailable due to task performance. Our findings provide meaningful insights into the suitability of alternative EDA collection sites, contributing to advancements in wearable sensor technology and real-world biosignal monitoring applications.

The chest showed relatively better suitability for EDA collection compared to the back and forehead, based on several key indicators. First, it consistently demonstrated signal features that approximated those of the SP across the analyzed parameters, including SCR height, amplitude, and prominence. Secondly, the chest also presented the highest correlation values with the SP for both tonic and phasic components (Table 2), suggesting that it may capture autonomic nervous system responses with acceptable reliability.

Conversely, the forehead consistently produced low and sometimes negative correlations, indicating that this site may not be reliable for EDA collection in short-term applications. Factors such as lower sweat gland density likely contributed to this reduced performance. These findings align with previous research suggesting that forehead EDA signals require specific conditions, such as extended hydration periods, to produce reliable measurements [20]. However, unlike our findings, previous research reported a moderate correlation between EDA measured at the forehead and finger EDA, with the correlation being notably lower for the phasic component [20]. In [17], this site also recorded the highest SCL and the second-highest SCRs value among the 16 locations explored. Regarding correlation with the SP, amongst the 15 alternative sites explored, the forehead ranked fifth highest, while the chest placed ninth, still showing a moderate positive correlation. The back ranked 14th, displaying a low–moderate positive correlation.

In our study, the back also showed poor performance, with correlations lower than those of the chest but still higher than those observed for the forehead. Its performance was task-dependent, particularly in response to thermal stimuli such as the hot water task. This variability suggests that the back may be conditionally useful, depending on the specific monitoring context. Further investigation into task-dependent variability and its influence on sensor reliability at different body locations should be developed.

Considering the results presented in Tables 1 and 2, we suggest that, while the chest may serve as an alternative site for EDA data collection, its reliability remains limited. Additionally, the forehead should be excluded as a suitable alternative location, particularly for short-term biosignal acquisitions.

A comparison of experimental methodologies reveals differences between our protocol and the one followed by [20], where participants had to relax in a supine position, perform the Stroop Task (a neuropsychological test used to assess the ability to inhibit cognitive interference [28]), walk at 3mph, and lift a dumbbell (each task lasting 120 s). We focused on collecting EDA data while participants experienced the sensation of different materials/items coming into contact with the skin. While these had been reported as stimuli that generate electrodermal response [24], our findings suggest that certain tasks were more effective at inducing noticeable responses than others. Notably, the hot water task consistently generated strong responses across all sensor positions, while the sandpaper and pin tasks were particularly effective when sensors were positioned on the chest. These results highlight the variability in response intensity depending on the nature of the stimuli and sensor placement. Future studies should explore alternative, non-harmful stimuli that may generate more robust and consistent electrodermal responses, contributing to the refining of methodologies for studying EDA.

Ensuring gender diversity in research samples is another fundamental aspect to ensure that we reach conclusions that can be generalized and that are inclusive. In our study, particular attention was given to achieving a balanced sample to ensure adequate female representation. Indeed, 56% of our sample was composed of women, addressing a common limitation found in similar studies (e.g., [20]) and strengthening the relevance and applicability of our results across genders.

Finally, our study was not conducted without some limitations. The sample size was relatively small and derived from a convenience sample, which may limit the generalizability of the findings. Furthermore, EDA acquisitions were conducted sequentially rather than simultaneously, leading to variability in SP values across different rounds of data collection, conditioning the comparison of results between location sites.

Future research should focus on collecting data from larger sample sizes using randomized sampling techniques and standardizing acquisition protocols to improve the reliability and comparability of results. Increasing the sample size would also enable more detailed analyses of demographic variables such as gender and age, thereby expanding the understanding of EDA signals and their variability. This is particularly relevant for enhancing the accuracy and robustness of applications in relation to stress monitoring and emotion recognition. By accounting for demographic factors, these applications could be refined to deliver more personalized and context-sensitive assessments, thereby improving their effectiveness in real-world contexts, including mental health monitoring, workplace productivity, and adaptive human-computer interaction systems.

Several practical and methodological aspects emerged during this study. The decision to analyze only the first SCR peak following each stimulus minimized signal contamination from overlapping responses, ensuring that the results primarily reflected initial autonomic responses rather than cumulative effects. However, future studies should consider multi-peak analysis to capture more complex response patterns. The sequential rather than simultaneous data acquisition may have constrained the generalizability of the findings; thus, future studies implementing simultaneous multi-site recordings would improve data reliability. Additionally, incorporating a wider range of tasks and environmental conditions would provide a more comprehensive evaluation of alternative EDA measurement sites. Future studies could also aim to explore EDA measurement in more naturalistic settings to complement our findings. Finally, future research could incorporate simultaneous respiratory monitoring (using inductive respiration or accelerometer signals) to quantify and account for signal influences due to breathing frequencies.

In summary, the chest shows some potential as an alternative site but still presents a weaker response than the standard finger placement. More research is needed to further characterize the chest as a feasible alternative site for EDA measurement. This alternative placement would be important, especially in scenarios where hand-based monitoring is impractical. The back may serve as a complementary site, particularly when task-specific responses are considered. The forehead, however, appears unsuitable for short-term EDA monitoring due to its inconsistent signal quality. These findings can contribute to the development of more versatile wearable biosensors and expand the possibilities for real-world EDA monitoring in contexts such as stress detection, human–computer interaction, and rehabilitation therapies.

5. Conclusions

This study collected EDA signals from three different body locations (chest, back, and forehead) and compared them to the finger EDA, which is considered the standard position for EDA collection. To the best of our knowledge, this is the first study to explore EDA from different sites using physical stimuli that induce electrodermal activity, with a gender-balanced sample. Based on the results, we conclude that although the chest may serve as an alternative site for EDA collection, it is not an ideal replacement for the standard finger placement. Additionally, the forehead should be ruled out as a viable site, particularly for short-term measurements.

Author Contributions: Conceptualization, P.G. and K.M.; methodology, P.G., K.M. and C.Q.; software, R.V. and K.M.; formal analysis, P.G., K.M. and R.V.; investigation, P.G. and K.M.; data curation, K.M.; writing—original draft preparation, P.G.; writing—review and editing, P.G., H.P.d.S. and C.Q.; supervision, H.P.d.S. and C.Q.; project administration, P.G.; funding acquisition, P.G., R.V., H.P.d.S. and C.Q. All authors have read and agreed to the published version of the manuscript.

Funding: This work was partly supported by Fundação para a Ciência e Tecnologia, under PhD grant PD/BDE/150672/2020 and the European Union's Horizon 2020 Research and Innovation Program MED1stMR under grant agreement No 101021775. This work was also supported by national funds from Fundação para a Ciência e Tecnologia, through the DOI 10.54499/UIDB/04559/2020 (LIBPhys-UNL) andUID/50008 (Instituto de Telecomunicações).

Institutional Review Board Statement: The study was conducted in accordance with the Declaration of Helsinki and approved by the Ethics Committee of NOVA University of Lisbon, Faculty of Sciences and Technology (protocol code CE-FCT-006-2022, approved on the 7 November 2022).

Informed Consent Statement: Informed consent was obtained from all participants involved in the study.

Data Availability Statement: The data are being prepared for publication. At this moment, data are only available from the corresponding author upon request.

Conflicts of Interest: The study used material from the company PLUX, where some of the authors worked at the time and are affiliated with.

Abbreviations

The following abbreviations are used in this manuscript:

ANS	Autonomic Nervous System
EDA	Electrodermal Activity
SCL	Skin Conductance Level
SCR	Skin Conductance Response
SP	Standard Position

References

1. Critchley, H.; Nagai, Y. Electrodermal Activity (EDA). In *Encyclopedia of Behavioral Medicine*; Gellman, M.D., Turner, J.R., Eds.; Springer: New York, NY, USA, 2013; pp. 666–669.
2. Berne, R.; Levy, M. *Fisiologia [Physiology]*; Guanabara Koogan: Rio de Janeiro, Brazil, 1996.
3. Bari, D.; Yacoob, H. *Electrodermal Activity: Simultaneous Recordings*; IntechOpen: London, UK, 2019.
4. Posada-Quintero, H.F.; Florian, J.P.; Orjuela-Cañón, A.D.; Chon, K.H. Electrodermal Activity Is Sensitive to Cognitive Stress under Water. *Front. Physiol.* **2018**, *8*, 1128. .. [CrossRef] [PubMed]
5. Ali, M.; Mosa, A.H.; Machot, F.A.; Kyamakya, K. Emotion Recognition Involving Physiological and Speech Signals: A Comprehensive Review. In *Recent Advances in Nonlinear Dynamics and Synchronization: With Selected Applications in Electrical Engineering, Neurocomputing, and Transportation*; Kyamakya, K., Mathis, W., Stoop, R., Chedjou, J.C., Li, Z., Eds.; Studies in Systems, Decision and Control; Springer International Publishing: Cham, Switzerland, 2018; pp. 287–302.
6. Braithwaite, J.; Watson, D.; Jones, R.; Rowe, M. A Guide for Analysing Electrodermal Activity (EDA) & Skin Conductance Responses (SCRs) for Psychological Experiments. In *Technical Report Technical Report*, 2nd ed.; University of Birmingham, UK, Selective Attention & Awareness Laboratory (SAAL) Behavioural Brain Sciences Centre: Birmingham, UK, 2015.
7. Vavrinsky, E.; Stopjakova, V.; Kopani, M.; Kosnacova, H. The Concept of Advanced Multi-Sensor Monitoring of Human Stress. *Sensors* **2021**, *21*, 3499. [CrossRef] [PubMed]
8. Benedek, M.; Kaernbach, C. Decomposition of skin conductance data by means of nonnegative deconvolution. *Psychophysiology* **2010**, *47*, 647–658. [CrossRef] [PubMed]
9. Bradley, M.M.; Lang, P.J. Emotion and motivation. In *Handbook of Psychophysiology*, 3rd ed.; Cambridge University Press: New York, NY, USA, 2007; pp. 581–607.
10. Reinhardt, T.; Schmahl, C.; Wüst, S.; Bohus, M. Salivary cortisol, heart rate, electrodermal activity and subjective stress responses to the Mannheim Multicomponent Stress Test (MMST). *Psychiatry Res.* **2012**, *198*, 106–111. [CrossRef] [PubMed]
11. Boucsein, W. *Electrodermal Activity*; Springer: Boston, MA, USA, 2012.
12. Wilke, K.; Martin, A.; Terstegen, L.; Biel, S.S. A short history of sweat gland biology. *Int. J. Cosmet. Sci.* **2007**, *29*, 169–179. [CrossRef] [PubMed]
13. Ferguson, B.J.; Hamlin, T.; Lantz, J.F.; Villavicencio, T.; Coles, J.; Beversdorf, D.Q. Examining the Association Between Electrodermal Activity and Problem Behavior in Severe Autism Spectrum Disorder: A Feasibility Study. *Front. Psychiatry* **2019**, *10*, 654. [CrossRef] [PubMed]
14. Klimek, A.; Mannheim, I.; Schouten, G.; Wouters, E.J.M.; Peeters, M.W.H. Wearables measuring electrodermal activity to assess perceived stress in care: A scoping review. *Acta Neuropsychiatr.* **2023**, *24*, 1–11.
15. Kappeler-Setz, C.; Gravenhorst, F.; Schumm, J.; Arnrich, B.; Tröster, G. Towards long term monitoring of electrodermal activity in daily life. *Pers. Ubiquitous Comput.* **2013**, *17*, 261–271. [CrossRef]
16. Ferreira, A.F.; da Silva, H.P.; Alves, H.; Marques, N.; Fred, A. Feasibility of Electrodermal Activity and Photoplethysmography Data Acquisition at the Foot Using a Sock Form Factor. *Sensors* **2023**, *23*, 620. [CrossRef] [PubMed]
17. van Dooren, M.; de Vries, J.J.G.G.J.; Janssen, J.H. Emotional sweating across the body: Comparing 16 different skin conductance measurement locations. *Physiol. Behav.* **2012**, *106*, 298–304. [CrossRef] [PubMed]

18. Payne, A.F.H.; Schell, A.M.; Dawson, M.E. Lapses in skin conductance responding across anatomical sites: Comparison of fingers, feet, forehead, and wrist. *Psychophysiology* **2016**, *53*, 1084–1092. [CrossRef] [PubMed]
19. Kasos, K.; Kekecs, Z.; Csirmaz, L.; Zimonyi, S.; Vikor, F.; Kasos, E.; Veres, A.; Kotyuk, E.; Szekely, A. Bilateral comparison of traditional and alternate electrodermal measurement sites. *Psychophysiology* **2020**, *57*, e13645. [CrossRef] [PubMed]
20. Hossain, M.B.; Kong, Y.; Posada-Quintero, H.F.; Chon, K.H. Comparison of Electrodermal Activity from Multiple Body Locations Based on Standard EDA Indices' Quality and Robustness against Motion Artifact. *Sensors* **2022**, *22*, 3177. [CrossRef] [PubMed]
21. Costardi, J.V.V.; Nampo, R.A.T.; Silva, G.L.; Ribeiro, M.A.F.; Stella, H.J.; Stella, M.B.; Malheiros, S.V.P. A review on alcohol: From the central action mechanism to chemical dependency. *Rev. Assoc. Médica Bras.* **2015**, *61*, 381–387. .. [CrossRef] [PubMed]
22. Davidson, R.A.; Smith, B.D. Caffeine and novelty: Effects on electrodermal activity and performance. *Physiol. Behav.* **1991**, *49*, 1169–1175. [CrossRef] [PubMed]
23. Boucsein, W.; Fowles, D.C.; Grimnes, S.; Ben-Shakhar, G.; Roth, W.T.; Dawson, M.E.; Filion, D.L. Society for Psychophysiological Research Ad Hoc Committee on Electrodermal Measures. Publication recommendations for electrodermal measurements. *Psychophysiology* **2012**, *49*, 1017–1034. [CrossRef] [PubMed]
24. Quaresma, C.; Gomes, M.; Cardoso, H.; Ferreira, N.; Vigário, R.; Quintão, C.; Fonseca, M. An Integrated System Combining Virtual Reality with a Glove with Biosensors for Neuropathic Pain: A Concept Validation. In *Advances in Human Factors and Systems Interaction. AHFE 2018. Advances in Intelligent Systems and Computing*; Nunes, I.L., Ed.; Springer: Cham, Switzerland, 2019; pp. 274–284. [CrossRef]
25. Makowski, D.; Pham, T.; Lau, Z.J.; Brammer, J.C.; Lespinasse, F.; Pham, H.; Schölzel, C.; Chen, S.H.A. NeuroKit2: A Python toolbox for neurophysiological signal processing. *Behav. Res. Methods* **2021**, *53*, 1689–1696. [CrossRef] [PubMed]
26. Schmidt, S.; Walach, H. Electrodermal activity (EDA): State-of-the-art measurement and techniques for parapsychological purposes. *J. Parapsychol.* **2000**, *64*, 139–163.
27. Chao, C.C.J. Correlation, Pearson. In *The SAGE Encyclopedia of Communication Research Methods*; SAGE Publications, Inc.: Thousand Oaks, CA, USA, 2017; pp. 267–270.
28. Scarpina, F.; Tagini, S. The Stroop Color and Word Test. *Front. Psychol.* **2017**, *8*, 557. [CrossRef] [PubMed]

sensors

MDPI

Article

Assessing Physiological Stress Responses in Student Nurses Using Mixed Reality Training

Kamelia Sepanloo [1], Daniel Shevelev [2], Young-Jun Son [1], Shravan Aras [3] and Janine E. Hinton [4,*]

1 Edwardson School of Industrial Engineering, Purdue University, West Lafayette, IN 47907, USA; ksepanlo@purdue.edu (K.S.); yjson@purdue.edu (Y.-J.S.)
2 School of Information Science, University of Arizona, Tucson, AZ 85721, USA; dshevelev@arizona.edu
3 Center for Biomedical Informatics and Biostatistics, University of Arizona, Tucson, AZ 85721, USA; shravanaras@arizona.edu
4 College of Nursing, University of Arizona, Tucson, AZ 85721, USA
* Correspondence: hintonje@arizona.edu; Tel.: +1-(520)-626-6154

Abstract: This study explores nursing students' stress responses while they are being trained in a mixed reality (MR) setting that replicates highly stressful clinical scenarios. Using measurements of physiological indices such as heart rate, electrodermal activity, and skin temperature, the study assesses the level of stress when the students interact with digital patients whose vital signs and symptoms interact dynamically to respond to student inputs. The simulation consists of six segments, during which critical events like hypotension and hypoxia occur, and the patient's condition changes based on the nurse's clinical decisions. Machine learning algorithms were then used to analyze the nurse's physiological data and to classify different levels of stress. Among the models tested, the Stacking Classifier demonstrated the highest classification accuracy of 96.4%, outperforming both Random Forest (96.18%) and Gradient Boosting (95.35%). The results showed clear patterns of stress during the simulation segments. Statistical analysis also found significant differences in stress responses and identified key physiological markers linked to each stress level. This pioneering study demonstrates the effectiveness of MR as a training tool for healthcare professionals in high-pressured scenarios and lays the groundwork for further studies on stress management, adaptive training procedures, and real-time detection and intervention in MR-based nursing training.

Keywords: physiological measures analysis; wearable sensors; mixed reality; nursing

1. Introduction

Stress is a dominant concern in the nursing field, and it greatly impacts the general well-being of nurses and patient care quality. Various studies emphasized reducing the stress level among medical professionals. A study conducted by [1] focused on the psychological effect of stress experienced by medical personnel serving at the frontline amidst the COVID-19 pandemic. Loss of control, personal illness, and susceptibility to infection were among the variables the study recognized as significant sources of stress. Similarly, ref. [2] emphasized the need to examine the level of stress among nurses in acute care to be able to establish the stressors that can compromise the provision of quality patient care.

Stress levels were shown through research to impact the competency and work performance of nurses, specifically in ICU settings. The environment of the ICU and the emotional impact of working in areas with high levels of stress are contributing factors to the stress of nurses [3]. Workload was shown to be associated with physiological stress responses in nurses; hence, it is essential to eliminate work overload and have sufficient rest to prevent stress elevation [4]. Moreover, studies focusing on specific nursing departments reveal that stress levels can vary significantly between different specializations. Research shows that nurses working in internal medicine departments report higher stress levels than their surgical counterparts, suggesting that the work environment and patient characteristics play critical roles in stress experiences [5].

There is evidence that high levels of stress in nursing students are related to low academic performance and satisfaction. For instance, ref. [6] confirmed that increased levels of stress while learning online, particularly during the COVID-19 pandemic, led to decreased satisfaction and poorer academic performance in nursing students. Similarly, ref. [7] confirmed that common stressors included academic workload and clinical environment problems, which cumulatively impacted students' learning experiences. This is also emphasized by [8], who confirmed that stressors in clinical education greatly influence students' learning abilities and overall educational performance. In support of this, ref. [9] explored the perspectives of nursing educators and undergraduate nursing students engaging in mixed reality-based remote simulations. Their study highlighted that integrating mixed reality into nursing education not only enhanced students' engagement but also exposed them to realistic clinical stressors, providing opportunities to develop stress management strategies in a safe learning environment.

Several recent studies emphasized the importance of utilizing physiological measures in occupational stress quantification among nurses. Some of the key physiological correlations such as heart rate, electrodermal activity, and skin temperature are crucial in ascertaining stress in nurses [10]. For instance, ref. [11] utilized wearable ECG devices to assess heart rate and HRV among nurses, establishing a correlation between these physiological metrics and subjective stress responses, thus reinforcing HRV's applicability in occupational health assessments. Similarly, ref. [12] demonstrated the effectiveness of various wearable sensors, including EDA, in monitoring stress in intensive care unit (ICU) nurses in real-time. However, further studies are needed in taking advantage of physiological measures in continuous stress and fatigue monitoring in nursing due to the existence of research gaps [13].

Additionally, immersive virtual scenarios with real-time feedback have been applied in psychological stress management, with encouraging results in enhancing coping skills and self-efficacy among nurses [14]. Virtual reality (VR) training was found to elicit similar stress responses to realistic face-to-face scenarios, demonstrating the effectiveness of VR in simulating high-stress environments for stress monitoring [15]. Furthermore, ref. [16] conducted a systematic review of virtual reality simulation effectiveness in nursing and midwifery education with a focus on its superiority in enhancing students' procedural knowledge. Similarly, ref. [17] reviewed the role of digitally assisted mindfulness interventions in improving self-regulation and sustaining mental health. Their systematic review emphasized that incorporating digital tools into mindfulness practices significantly improved individuals' ability to manage stress, suggesting potential applications of such technologies in nursing education to enhance mental resilience.

The continuous monitoring of physiological parameters during immersive training sessions can give valuable feedback on the levels of stress in nurses and allow the tailoring of interventions to reduce occupational stress more effectively [18]. The findings from [19] indicate that while various technology-delivered interventions exist, the integration of MR into stress management programs tailored for nursing is still limited. Therefore, further research is needed to explore the potential of mixed reality environment in nursing education, particularly regarding stress management [20,21].

Therefore, this study conducted a novel experiment to assess the stress levels of nurse learners in a mixed reality environment that was designed to simulate actual healthcare scenarios. The learners were equipped with an Empatica E4 wristband (manufactured by Empatica Inc. based in Cambridge, Massachusetts) to capture the key indicators of heart rate, electrodermal activity, and skin temperature. These markers were continuously recorded as the learners interacted with digital patients through the segments of the simulation. In recording real-time physiological data, the goal was to determine the change in stress level throughout the simulation and how it impacted clinical performance.

2. Experiment Design

The experiment was facilitated using a Microsoft HoloLens 2 MR headset (manufactured by Microsoft Inc., Redmond, WA, USA). All the digital patients and medical equipment were developed using the Unity 3D game engine (version 2022.3.19). Figure 1 shows a learner using the system, and Figure 2 shows what they viewed inside the headset.

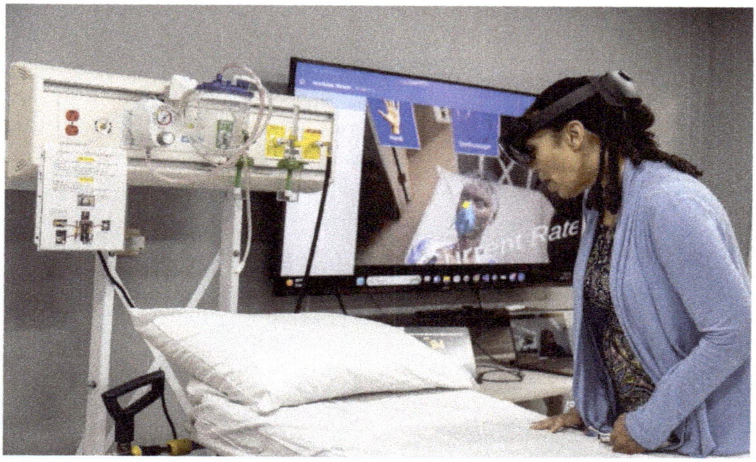

Figure 1. Learner engaged in the experiment, interacting with the digital patient and equipment within a physical environment.

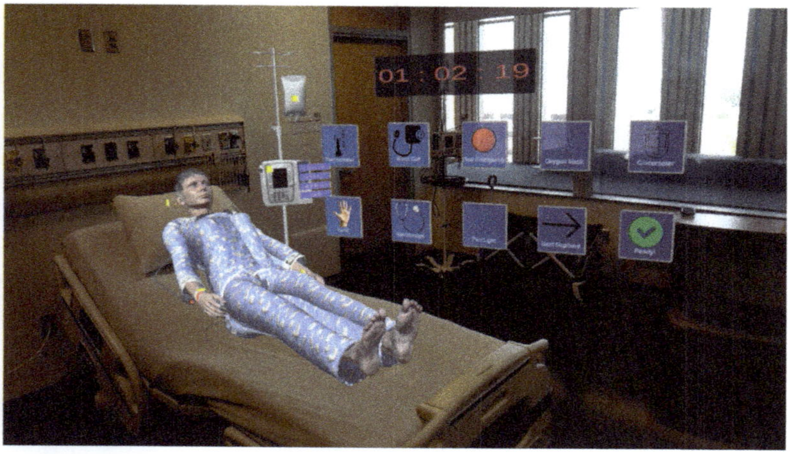

Figure 2. View inside of the HoloLens Headset.

Through the headset, the learner experienced a blend of digital and real elements, with digital patients and medical equipment overlaid onto the real-world objects. The digital patients were also equipped with an advanced conversational artificial intelligence (AI) model that allowed them to communicate naturally with the learner during the simulation. This model was developed using MindMeld conversational AI platform in Python 3.11.7, and could respond to the learner's questions, actions, and remarks, simulating the interaction in a more realist way as a natural conversation with a patient. This contributed to realism, mimicking what nurses normally encounter in real life. The patient's facial expressions also changed based on the health condition, responding to what learner has intervened and therefore made the whole experience more realistic [22].

Each training session took a duration of approximately 2 h per learner. At the beginning, the learners were given a tutorial to become familiar with the system and learn to use the digital equipment. Upon its completion, they were then introduced to an overview of the patient's situation, medical history, physical findings, nursing recommendations, and orders from the physician. After preparing, the learners started the session and worked with the digital patient. They controlled the pace of simulation by pressing a "Next Segment" button, moving the scenario 2 h ahead, for a total of six segments. Depending on the learners' actions and decisions, the status of the patient may improve or degrade. However, the patient would encounter hypotension and hypoxia at some point, simulating a medical emergency. At the end of the experiment, the learners were given a set of debriefing questions where they stated their objectives, patients' needs, risks, and interventions during the simulation.

The main goal of the experiment was to measure the learner's stress and perform analysis of features with respect to it while using the MR system. To that end, the physiological signals of the learners were captured with the Empatica E4 wearable sensor, which tracks heart rate, electrodermal activity, and skin temperature. As an initial step for the training, the physiological data of learners were recorded for 10 min to identify each learner's pre-simulation initial stress level. This baseline measurement was taken as a reference basis for measuring any changes in stress during the simulation.

3. Methodology

3.1. Pre-Processing and Feature Extraction

Pre-processing is a crucial step in working with physiological data as it enables us to denoise the data, deal with missing values and prepare the data for proper analysis and modeling. For this purpose, a Python script was developed to preprocess the data, select significant features and prepare it for machine learning. Some of the key libraries utilized in the script are "pandas" for data manipulation and data arrangement, "numpy" for calculation operations, and "scipy" for statistical functionality. Figure 3 demonstrates all the steps followed in this pre-processing.

The process began with using each learner's Heart Rate (HR), Skin Temperature (TEMP), and Electrodermal Activity (EDA) data. Since these signals have different sampling rates, they were first resampled to a unified rate of 4 Hz to ensure consistent data alignment and reduce information loss. Next, the data were cleaned to ensure that high-quality data were used in the model. A small percentage (1.02%) of missing values were present in the dataset. Therefore, missing values in each signal (EDA, HR, and TEMP) were replaced with the median of the respective feature, ensuring that data imputation did not distort the overall signal characteristics.

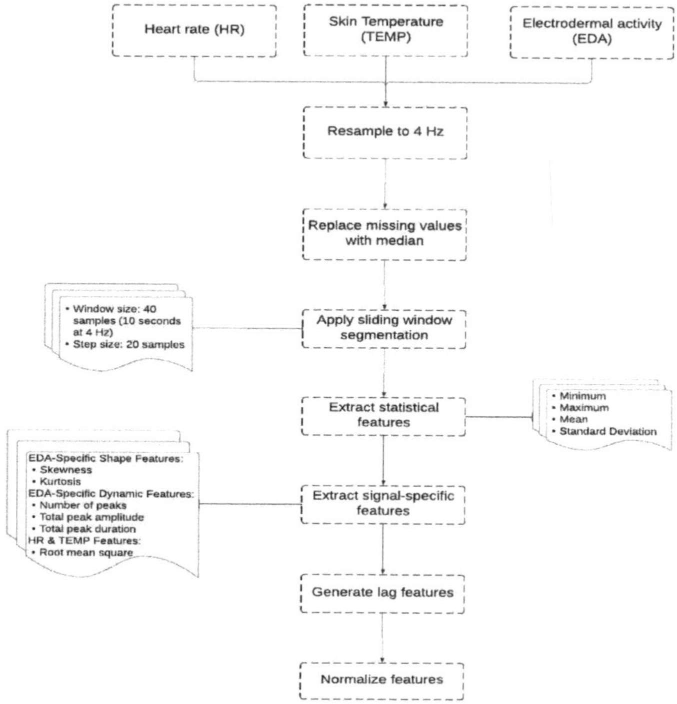

Figure 3. Steps of the data preprocessing.

To extract relevant features, a sliding window technique was employed with a window size of 40 samples and a step size of 20 samples (50% overlap). Within each window, we computed statistical descriptors (minimum, maximum, mean, and standard deviation) for EDA, HR, and TEMP. For the EDA signal, additional shape-related features (skewness and kurtosis) were calculated to capture asymmetry and tailedness. Furthermore, EDA-specific dynamic features were derived using peak analysis, including the number of peaks (indicative of phasic responses), total peak amplitude, and total peak duration (both representing the intensity and temporal extent of EDA fluctuations).

The HR and TEMP signals had their root mean square (RMS) of first differences computed to quantify variability and short-term fluctuations within the window. In total, this resulted in 18 features describing the windowed physiological activity.

To account for temporal dependencies and trends in physiological responses, lagged features were generated. Specifically, the mean values of EDA, HR, and TEMP over the previous 1 to 10 windows were concatenated to the current feature vector. This yielded 30 additional lag-based features, which, combined with the 18 current-window features, formed a comprehensive feature set of 48 dimensions.

Prior to training the machine learning models, all features were normalized using min-max scaling to rescale their values into the [0, 1] range. Although min-max scaling can be sensitive to outliers, it was appropriate in this context because the windowed features exhibited stable ranges, and no extreme outliers were present after preprocessing.

3.2. Stress Detection Models

The models in this study were trained using the AffectiveROAD dataset [23], which was specifically designed to collect a broad set of physiological and environmental measurements in actual driving conditions. Drivers wore Empatica E4 wristbands and Zephyr

BioHarness 3 chest straps (manufactured by Zephyr Technology Corporation, Annapolis, MD, USA) which recorded physiological signals including electrodermal activity from both wrists, heart rate, breathing rate, and skin temperature. In addition to these physiological signals, the dataset includes contextual data such as GPS location, in-car temperature, humidity, sound level, and synchronized video recordings of both the vehicle interior and the external driving environment. A continuous, real-time stress metric was also recorded during each drive. This metric was annotated by an observer seated in the rear seat of the vehicle, who used a slider to indicate the perceived overall stress level on a scale from low (0) to high (1). After each driving session, the driver reviewed the video footage and validated or corrected the stress annotations to ensure their accuracy. This rich dataset is particularly beneficial for the investigation of levels of stress and attention in the participants. The class labels in our models were assigned according to the mean stress levels throughout the session: 'no stress' for class 0, 'medium stress' for class 1, and 'high stress' for class 2. These thresholds were initially established using the AffectiveROAD dataset and further validated by participant survey response [24].

We used the Random Forest Classifier and Gradient Boosting Classifier as two base models. For each base classifier, a randomized search strategy was applied over a predefined hyperparameter space, with 100 iterations. The Random Forest classifier was tuned across the following hyperparameters: number of estimators (n_estimators, range 50–300), maximum tree depth (max_depth, range 10–30), number of features considered at each split (max_features, either 'sqrt' or 'log2'), minimum samples required to split an internal node (min_samples_split, range 2–20), minimum samples required at a leaf node (min_samples_leaf, range 1–10), and bootstrap sampling (bootstrap, either True or False). For the Gradient Boosting classifier, the tuned hyperparameters included n_estimators (range 50–300), max_depth (range 3–10), and learning_rate (continuous uniform distribution between 0.01 and 0.31). We then employed nested cross-validation using two levels of Stratified 5-Fold cross-validation. In inner cross-validation, the training dataset was split into 5 folds to optimize the hyperparameters. In outer cross-validation, the entire dataset was split into 5 folds to evaluate the model with best-performing inner cross-validation hyperparameters.

The reason why the Stratified K-Folds method was employed in this study is because the dataset was imbalanced, and this ensured that class distribution was the same in each fold. After hyperparameter tuning, the best hyperparameters were selected, and the models were trained on the training set. Their performance was then measured on the test set, using precision, recall, and F1 score metrics. The performance statistics of each base model are presented in Table 1 (for Random Forest) and Table 2 (for Gradient Boosting).

Table 1. Random Forest test set performance.

Metric	Class 0	Class 1	Class 2
Precision	0.99	0.95	0.98
Recall	0.99	0.94	0.98
F1 Score	0.99	0.94	0.98
Support	1082	450	957
Accuracy	0.98	0.98	0.98
Macro Avg Precision	0.97	0.97	0.97
Macro Avg Recall	0.97	0.97	0.97
Macro Avg F1 Score	0.97	0.97	0.97
Macro Avg Precision	0.98	0.98	0.98
Weighted Avg Recall	0.98	0.98	0.98
Weighted Avg F1 Score	0.98	0.98	0.98

Table 2. Gradient Boosting test set performance.

Metric	Class 0	Class 1	Class 2
Precision	0.99	0.96	0.96
Recall	0.99	0.91	0.98
F1 Score	0.99	0.93	0.97
Support	1082	450	957
Accuracy	0.97	0.97	0.97
Macro Avg Precision	0.97	0.97	0.97
Macro Avg Recall	0.96	0.96	0.98
Macro Avg F1 Score	0.96	0.96	0.97
Macro Avg Precision	0.97	0.97	0.97
Weighted Avg Recall	0.97	0.97	0.97
Weighted Avg F1 Score	0.97	0.97	0.97

The Random Forest model performed well in nested cross-validation and testing. It averaged 96.18% accuracy in cross-validation, indicating that the model is capable of generalizing to new data. The best hyperparameters had a high number of trees (178 estimators), a deep tree structure (maximum depth of 29), and log2 for feature selection. On the test data, the model achieved 98% accuracy with high precision and recall in all classes. The precision and recall values in class 0 and class 2 were close to 1, whereas in class 1, where the lowest result was obtained, the corresponding precision and recall values were at 0.95 and 0.94.

The Gradient Boosting model also performed well, although slightly lower than the Random Forest. Its nested cross-validation scores averaged 95.35%, which reflected good performance but with greater sensitivity to parameter variation. The optimized parameters were a learning rate of 0.228 and depth of 9. In the test set, it had an overall accuracy of 97%. The performance metrics were high for all classes, particularly for classes 0 and 2. Class 1 had a lower recall of 0.91 in comparison to Random Forest but possessed high precision at 0.96.

The results of inner and outer cross-validation scores showed no overfitting. Overfitting would generally occur when a model has high performance on training data but low performance on unseen data, and this would reflect in a large gap between training and validation scores. However, the model results show consistent performance in inner and outer loops with no significant differences in scores.

In addition, a Stacking Classifier was employed to combine the Random Forest and Gradient Boosting models' classification outcomes. Stacking is designed to take advantage of each model's strengths, with the potential to enhance overall predictive accuracy. The stacked model also underwent an identical process of testing, and performance metrics were generated to verify its capacity to generalize to unseen data. The model achieved the best performance with cross-validation accuracy at 96.4%.

This indicated that the merging of the power of both models gave improved performance. The Stacking model also achieved an accuracy of 98% in the test set, the same as the Random Forest (as seen in Table 3). Recall, accuracy, and F1 scores across all the classes were high with high performance in class 2 and competitive scores in classes 0 and 1. This confirmed that the stacking approach worked in combining the strengths of the individual models as they complemented one another, resulting in overall better classification performance.

Table 3. Stacking classifier test set performance.

Metric	Class 0	Class 1	Class 2
Precision	0.99	0.93	0.98
Recall	0.99	0.94	0.97
F1 Score	0.99	0.94	0.98
Support	1082	450	957
Accuracy	0.98	0.98	0.98
Macro Avg Precision	0.97	0.97	0.97
Macro Avg Recall	0.97	0.97	0.97
Macro Avg F1 Score	0.97	0.97	0.97
Macro Avg Precision	0.98	0.98	0.98
Weighted Avg Recall	0.98	0.98	0.98
Weighted Avg F1 Score	0.98	0.98	0.98

The selection of physiological features, such as heart rate, skin temperature, and electrodermal activity was guided by prior literature indicating their strong association with sympathetic nervous system activation and stress responses. Electrodermal activity, in particular, has been widely validated as a sensitive marker of acute stress and arousal in both laboratory and applied settings, which justified its prioritization. The machine learning models (Random Forest, Gradient Boosting, and Stacking Classifier) were selected due to their robustness, capacity to handle complex, non-linear relationships, and proven high performance in prior stress classification studies. Random Forest offers interpretability and resistance to overfitting; Gradient Boosting enhances predictive power through iterative refinement; and the Stacking Classifier capitalizes on model complementarity to improve generalization. These models align with our research objective of developing a reliable and accurate classification framework to assess stress levels from physiological data within the MR simulation.

We also evaluated several other machine learning models to ensure thorough analysis of the data. These included Logistic Regression, Support Vector Machine (SVM), K-Neighbors, and Adaptive Boosting. Tables 4–7 display the optimal hyperparameters and classification reports for each model. Despite the capabilities of these individual algorithms, the Stacking Classifier consistently outperformed them and showed its ability to effectively combine the predictive strengths of both the Random Forest and Gradient Boosting models.

Table 4. Logistic regression.

Metric	Value
Fitting Details	5 folds for each of 45 hyperparameter candidates, totaling 225 fits
Best Parameters	{'C': 0.001, 'max iteration': 100, 'solver': liblinear}
Best Accuracy	0.6105
Test Set Accuracy	0.6102
Test Set Precision	0.6180
Test Set Recall	0.4957
Test Set F1 Score	0.4513

Table 5. Support Vector Machine (SVM).

Metric	Value
Fitting Details	5 folds for each of 24 hyperparameter candidates, totaling 120 fits
Best Parameters	{'C': 100, 'gamma': 'scale', 'kernel': radial basis function}
Best Accuracy	0.7612

Table 5. *Cont.*

Metric	Value
Test Set Accuracy	0.7794
Test Set Precision	0.7473
Test Set Recall	0.7231
Test Set F1 Score	0.7311

Table 6. K-Neighbors.

Metric	Value
Fitting Details	5 folds for each of 16 hyperparameter candidates, totaling 80 fits
Best Parameters	{'metric': Manhattan, 'number of neighbors': 3, 'weights': distance}
Best Accuracy	0.9054
Test Set Accuracy	0.9274
Test Set Precision	0.9118
Test Set Recall	0.9113
Test Set F1 Score	0.9115

Table 7. Adaptive Boosting.

Metric	Value
Fitting Details	5 folds for each of 125 hyperparameter candidates, totaling 625 fits
Best Parameters	{'base estimator max depth': 5, 'learning rate': 0.1, 'number of estimators': 300}
Best Accuracy	0.9035
Test Set Accuracy	0.9206
Test Set Precision	0.9197
Test Set Recall	0.8954
Test Set F1 Score	0.9049

3.3. Features Analysis

To illustrate the impact of each feature in prediction results, feature importance scores were calculated using the Mean Decrease in Impurity (MDI) method, as implemented in the scikit-learn library. This approach quantifies the contribution of each feature to the predictive performance of the ensemble model by measuring the extent to which the feature reduces node impurity across all trees.

Specifically, the importance of a feature f was calculated as the total reduction in the criterion (Gini impurity) brought by all splits on f across all trees, averaged and normalized. Formally, the feature importance I(f) for feature f can be represented as:

$$\mathrm{I}() = \frac{1}{T}\sum\nolimits_{t=1}^{T} \sum\nolimits_{n \in N_f^t} \Delta i(n)$$

where T is the total number of trees in the ensemble, N_f^t denotes the set of nodes where feature f was used to split in tree t, and $\Delta i(n)$ represents the impurity decrease at node n. To ensure comparability between models, raw feature importance values were then normalized such that the sum of all importances for each model equaled one. Normalization was achieved by dividing each importance score by the total sum of importances.

Figure 4 indicates the most significant features that were identified through each model. As illustrated in the figure, in the Random Forest model, the highest feature score was the mean value of EDA (EDA_Mean), which suggested that changes in EDA_Mean hold significant information about stress. Following EDA_Mean, EDA minimum value (EDA_Min) and skin temperature maximum value (TEMP_Max) were ranked second. Such features contribute to understanding the extremes and ranges of the values of EDA and temperature, which are important in assessing stress.

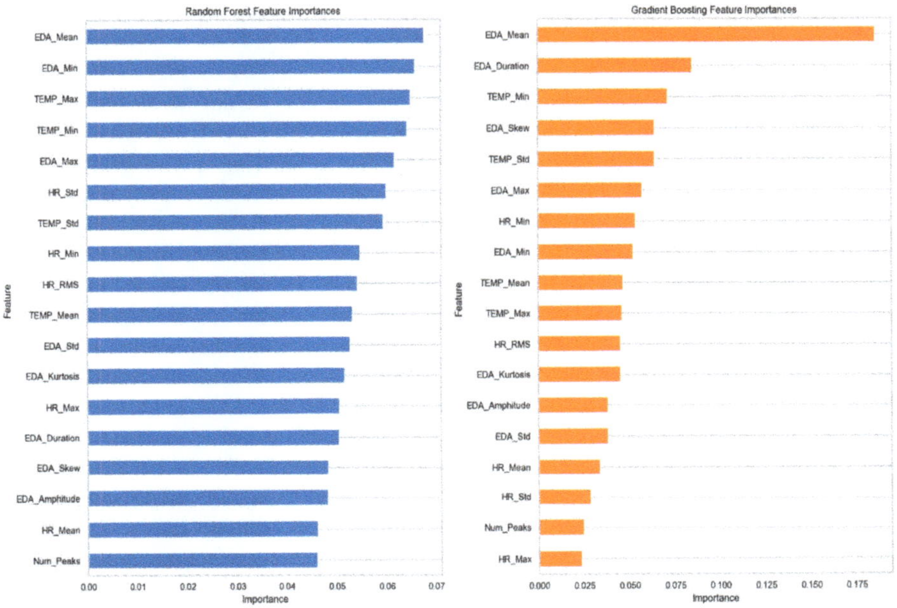

Figure 4. Normalized feature importance from Random Forest and Gradient Boosting models.

Skin temperature minimum value (TEMP_Min) and EDA maximum value (EDA_Max) also improved the model's predictive ability by providing more information about temperature extremes and peak EDA values, respectively. Factors like heart rate standard deviation (HR_Std), temperature standard deviation (TEMP_Std), and heart rate minimum value (HR_Min) were of lesser importance but still played a role in capturing fluctuations related to stress intensity.

On the other hand, the Gradient Boosting model attributed more weight to EDA_Mean. EDA_Duration was also an important feature in this model, and it represents the total time that the EDA signal stayed elevated within the time window. Minimum temperature (TEMP_Min) was another important feature for Gradient Boosting; however, EDA skewness value (EDA_Skew) and EDA amplitude value (EDA_Amplitude) were features but to a lesser degree than EDA_Mean and EDA_Duration, meaning that while they were significant, their influence was slight.

In comparing both models, EDA_Mean is a significant feature in both Gradient Boosting and Random Forest but is more significant in Gradient Boosting. This discrepancy is what indicates that Gradient Boosting's modeling approach is more capable of identifying the mean EDA value in the case of stress. The different level of significance of features like EDA_Min and TEMP_Min across the models indicated that both models utilize different data parameters. Random Forest may be more attuned to changes in these features, while Gradient Boosting may be able to detect more subtle patterns of stress.

Secondly, we examined the correlation between these features presented in Figure 5. The correlation matrix indicates that all three metrics correlate which confirm that changes in one metric are related to changes in the others.

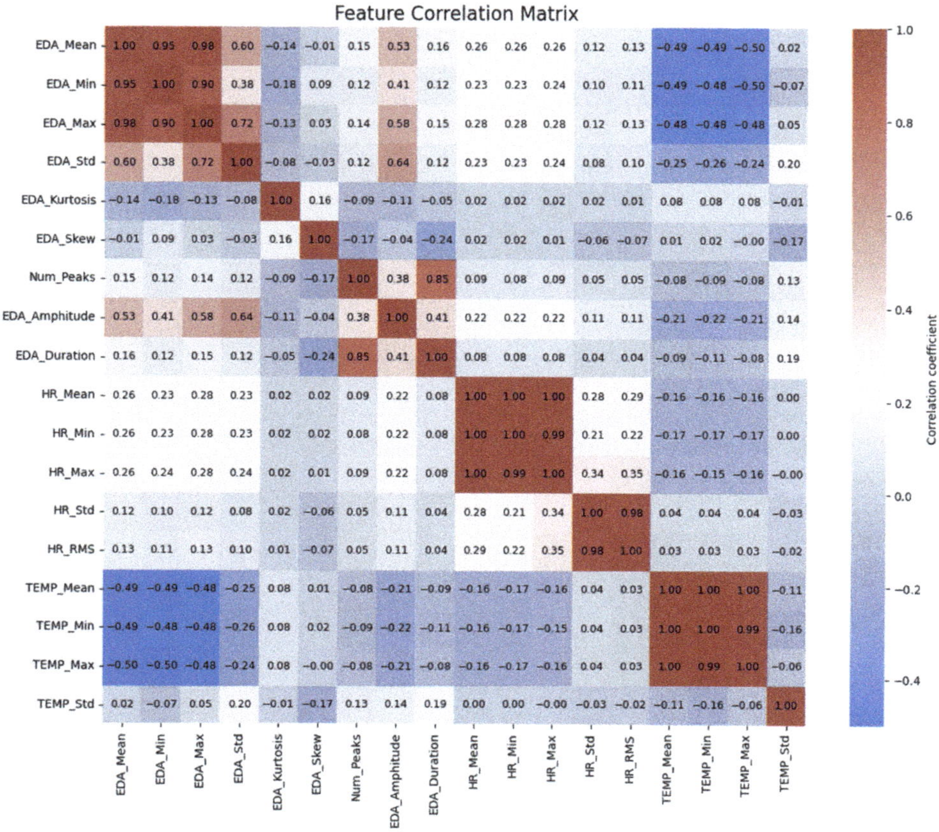

Figure 5. Correlation matrix of the features.

The correlation matrix further reveals interrelationships among the physiological measurements. Firstly, it shows an inverse relationship between body temperature and EDA. In other words, EDA_Mean is inversely related to TEMP_Mean (−0.49), TEMP_Min (−0.49), and TEMP_Max (−0.50). This relationship persists across the measurements of EDA, because EDA_Max is also inversely related to TEMP_Mean (−0.50). This suggests that with increases in stress levels, as indicated by EDA increases, there is an accompanying decrease in skin temperature. This inverse effect suggests a physiological phenomenon in which increased stress or arousal is accompanied by a decrease in surface temperature as vasoconstriction redirects blood to the core of the body [25].

In addition, EDA is positively correlated with heart rate. EDA_Mean is correlated with HR_Mean (0.26) and HR_Max (0.26), indicating that higher levels of EDA are associated with increased heart rates. This confirms that as individuals experience more stress, their heart rate increases. The same goes for EDA_Min, but with a poorer though still significant correlation with HR_Mean (0.23), indicating that even the lowest values of EDA are in some way associated with heart rate means.

EDA amplitude and duration also yield useful information. EDA_Amplitude is positively related to both EDA_Mean (0.53) and EDA_Max (0.58) at a moderate level, suggesting that larger fluctuation in skin conductance is associated with larger overall levels of EDA. Moreover, EDA_Duration is positively related to HR_Min (0.29), which means that longer durations of high electrodermal activity are associated with lower minimum heart rates. This could imply that long-lasting stress responses are associated with a decrease in the baseline heart rate.

Finally, relations are seen between the distribution measures of EDA, i.e., kurtosis and skewness. EDA_Kurtosis is positively correlated with EDA_Std (0.72) at high significance levels, such that increased deviation from the mean is associated with more variability in EDA. EDA_Skew, on the other hand, is not highly correlated with other variables, and this suggests that asymmetry in EDA distributions is unlikely to have a significant in-fluence on other physiological variables. These findings offer a glimpse into the intricate relationship between EDA, heart rate, and temperature and how they all react as a coordinated system to stress in the body.

4. Pilot Study Results

A total of nine pre-licensure nursing students and three nurse faculty members of the University of Arizona College of Nursing, aged between 20 and 49 years (mean = 29.6, SD = 10.1), volunteered to participate in our pilot study approved by the IRB. Each participant spent approximately 2 h on the experiment, yielding a total of 86,400 s of data collected. The participant demographic information is indicated in Table 8, offering a mix of levels of education and experience that reflect a diverse group of participants in the study.

Table 8. Demographics of study participants.

Demographics	Percentage of Participants
Nursing Education	
Less than one semester of nursing courses	25%
One to two semesters of nursing courses	42%
Bachelor's degree	8%
Master's degree	25%
Experience Level	
No experience	33%
Less than 2 years	8%
2 to 5 years	17%
6 to 10 years	25%
21 to 25 years	17%
Types of healthcare simulations participated in	
Standardized patient	33%
Manikin	50%
Virtual screen-based	17%
Virtual with headset	17%
Mixed reality with headset	8%
Experience with Virtual Reality headset	8%
Very little	58%
None	50%
Experience with Mixed Reality headset	
Very little	67%
None	58%

A representation of the distribution of time over different stress levels for all the subjects in our experiment is given in Figure 6. This result gives a clear view of stress level distributions across subjects by showing how much time each subject spent in each of the different stress states. Additionally, the participants' answers to the debriefing questions at the end of the simulation are summarized in Table 9.

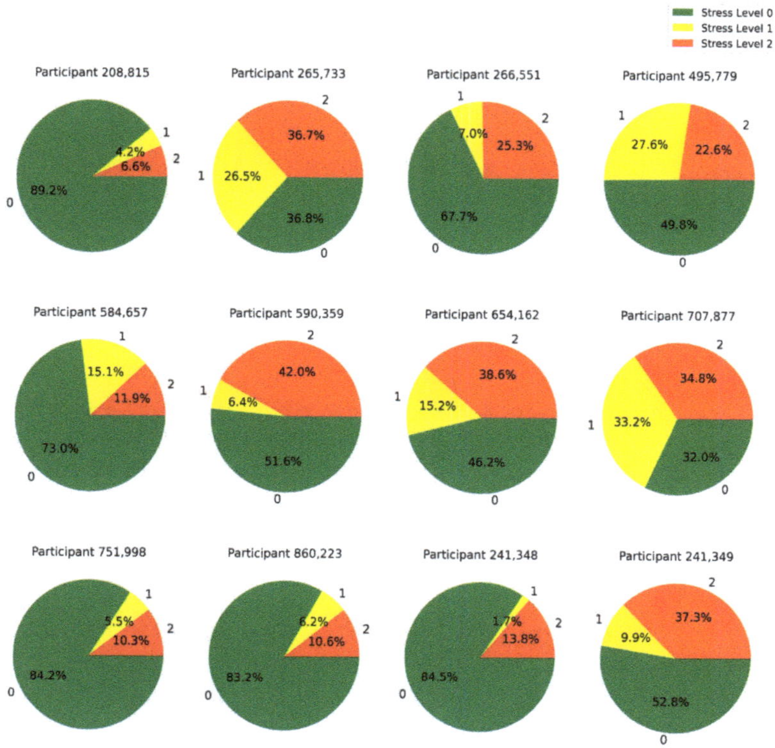

Figure 6. Distribution of time spent by each learner across different stress levels: 0 (low), 1 (medium), and 2 (high).

Table 9. Summary of participants' simulation goals, patient priorities, risks, required equipment, actions taken, and success.

Participant Number	Goal During Simulation	Patient's Priority Needs	Patient's Risks	Essential Items	Actions Taken	Succesfull?
208,815	Keeping my patient alive	Watching for hypovolemia and sepsis	Sepsis, hypovolemic shock, hemorrhage	Oxygen, Blood pressure, IV pump/suction	Recognized low blood pressure, patient unresponsive, called rapid response, initiated protocols	Yes
265,733	Contribute to education and patient survival	Blood pressure, perfusion to major organs	Loss of oxygenation, internal bleeding	IV fluids, Oxygen, electrolytes	Adjusted IV rate, monitored vitals, called rapid response, bolus of Lactated Ringer's, 4L O_2	No
266,551	Becoming oriented with virtual tools	Assessing the patient	Impaired gastric motility, altered bowel habits, pressure injury	Oxygen, call light, Blood pressure machine	Thorough assessment, evaluated chart before engaging	No
495,779	Improve patient assessment skills	Follow doctors' orders, monitor vitals	Pulmonary embolism, low O_2, hypertension	Ambu bag, supplemental O_2, code cart	Assessed patient, applied oxygen	Yes

Table 9. *Cont.*

Participant Number	Goal During Simulation	Patient's Priority Needs	Patient's Risks	Essential Items	Actions Taken	Succesfull?
584,657	Learn AR benefits for nursing education	Pain and infection control	Sepsis, severe pain, malnutrition	Ambu bag, IV, monitors	Monitored vitals, IV fluids, assessment, used call light, reviewed orders	Yes
590,359	Checking vitals, administering IV, oxygen	Oxygen, IV	Blood infection, sepsis, hypotension	Oxygen, IVs, blood glucose	Used oxygen mask, administered IV	No
654,162	Implement interventions, monitor vitals	Oxygen, NG suction, IV bolus, vital sign observation	Hypotension, hypoxia, pain	Oxygen, suction, IV bolus	Adjusted IV rate, turned on O_2/suction, administered bolus, notified MD, monitored vitals	No
707,877	Provide competent care in a safe environment	Addressing safety errors, pain management, responding to sepsis	Cardiac arrhythmias, organ failure, death	Ambu bag, oxygen source, code cart	Verified call light, placed patient on suction, changed IVF rate, called rapid response, followed protocol	No
751,998	Learn MR, use HoloLens, navigate space	Fluid resuscitation, oxygen, antibiotics	Septic shock, severe hypotension, hypoxemia	Pressure bag, surgical team, vasopressors	Locked bed, raised side rails, administered fluids, called rapid response, updated provider, assessed for deterioration	Yes
860,223	Maintain patient's O_2, ensure breathing, contact provider	Oxygen, chest pain, circulation	Heart attack, low O_2, circulation loss	EKG, heart shock kit, CPR equipment	Increased oxygen, positioned patient upright, monitored BP	No
241,348	Practice nursing and critical thinking	Oxygenation, monitoring chest pain, breathing pattern, BP	Myocardial infarction, pulmonary embolism, stroke	Oxygen, IV site, AED	Administered oxygen, constant monitoring, called rapid response and provider	Yes
241,349	Follow hypotension protocol, manage NG tube suction	Stabilizing vitals	Infection, low O_2, hypotension	Oxygen, suction, code cart	Lowered bed, monitored vitals, called rapid response and doctor, applied oxygen, allowed family access	No

Based on Figure 6 and Table 9, we identified that all participants who experienced stress levels of 2 for more than 25% of the simulation time, reported that they were not successful in fully treating the patient. This highlights the point that stress level 2 during the training had an impact on the participants' performance outcomes. This insight can be used to further personalize the training by decreasing the complexity of the simulation or offering supportive cues in the mixed reality environment when the stress reaches level 2.

4.1. Scenario-Based Validation

To ensure the applicability of the stress classification model to actual settings, we employed scenario-based validation within the context of the pilot study. This validation involved a critical segment of the simulation (segment 4) in which participants had to react to an emergency medicine scenario where the patient was on the verge of developing hypotension and hypoxia; situations that need prompt and effective decision-making.

The result of this validation showed that the model correctly classified all participants as being under a higher level of stress (Stress Level 1 or Stress level 2) during the emergency scenario. This consistent classification across all test populations suggests that the model is sensitive and accurate in detecting heightened stress reactions to critical, high-stakes situations.

This scenario-based validation supports both the accuracy of the model's classifications and its practical value in real clinical settings. The model holds significant potential for use in training environments focused on understanding and managing stress, as it accurately reflects the stress responses typically seen in such situations. This can help improve clinical performance and patient outcomes.

4.2. Variation in Physiological Markers Across Stress Levels

To further analyze the stress levels, Figures 7–9 illustrate the way mean heart rates, skin temperature, and electrodermal activity vary amongst learners across the different stress levels.

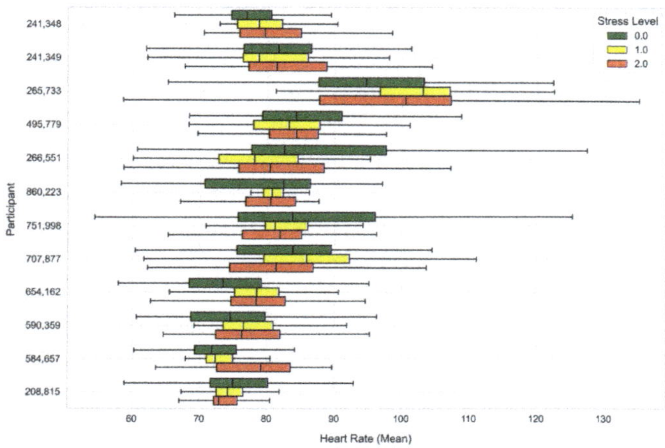

Figure 7. Average heart rate across stress levels for each learner.

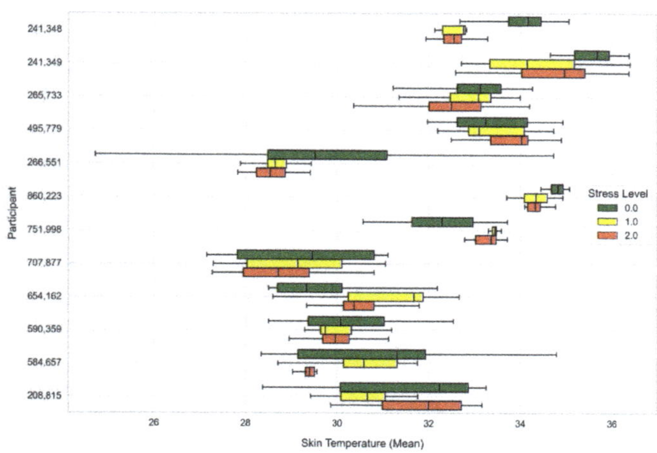

Figure 8. Average skin temperature across stress levels for each learner.

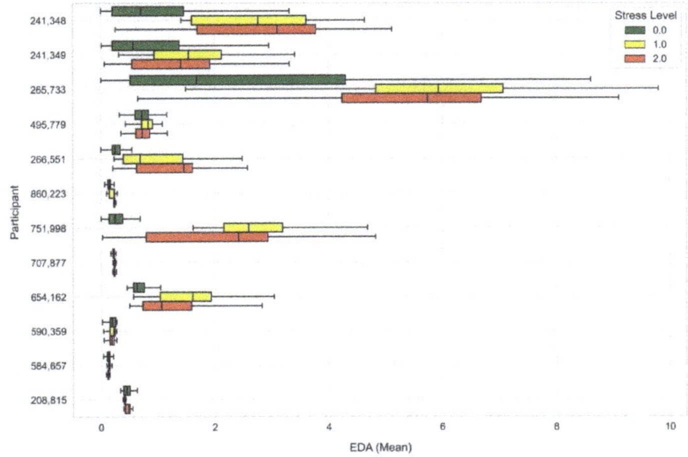

Figure 9. Average electrodermal activity across stress levels for each learner.

We then used paired *t*-tests to determine differences in physiological measurements across the three levels of stress (Stress Level 0, 1, and 2). The analysis was performed over 86,400 s of data and the summaries of the results are presented in Tables 10 and 11.

Table 10. Mean comparison results.

Metric	Stress Level 0	Stress Level 1	Stress Level 2
Heart Rate Mean	82.23	86.30	84.79
Skin Tempreture Mean	31.81	31.49	31.23
Electrodermal Activity Mean	0.68	2.09	1.87

Table 11. T-test results.

Comparison	T-Statistics	*p*-Value	Significance
Stress Level 1 vs. Stress Level 0 (HR_Mean)	13.7554	$p < 0.001$	Statistically significant
Stress Level 2 vs. Stress Level 0 (HR_Mean)	11.0204	$p < 0.001$	Statistically significant
Stress Level 1 vs. Stress Level 0 (TEMP_Mean)	−6.8260	$p < 0.001$	Statistically significant
Stress Level 2 vs. Stress Level 0 (TEMP_Mean)	−14.7139	$p < 0.001$	Statistically significant
Stress Level 1 vs. Stress Level 0 (EDA_Mean)	28.2458	$p < 0.001$	Statistically significant
Stress Level 2 vs. Stress Level 0 (EDA_Mean)	36.7045	$p < 0.001$	Statistically significant

There were considerable differences in heart rate in both analyses. Under Stress Level 1, the heart rate was significantly higher compared to Stress Level 0 (t-statistic = 13.7554, *p*-value $\approx$ 0.0), indicating a substantial increase in heart rate with elevated stress. Similarly, the comparison of Stress Level 2 versus Stress Level 0 also showed an increase in heart rate at significance level (t-statistic = 11.0204, *p*-value $\approx$ 0.0).

Mean skin temperature showed significant decrease through levels of stress. Stress Level 1 recorded a lower skin temperature than Stress Level 0 (t-statistic = −6.8260, *p*-value $\approx$ 0.0), and the difference was even larger at Stress Level 2 (t-statistic = −14.7139, *p*-value $\approx$ 0.0).

EDA also recorded significant differences by levels of stress, where under Stress Level 1 was significantly higher than Stress Level 0 (t-statistic = 28.2458, *p*-value $\approx$ 0.0), and the same significant rise was achieved under Stress Level 2 compared to Stress Level 0 (t-statistic = 36.7045, *p*-value $\approx$ 0.0). The rise in EDA is reflective of heightened sympathetic nervous system activity, leading to heightened sweating and greater skin conductance due to stress.

In conclusion, the outcome of the *t*-test indicated that heart rate, skin temperature, and electrodermal activity varied significantly with the variation in stress level. In other words, such physiological measures could be reliable indicators for the assessment of stress and may aid in the design of effective stress management interventions within the mixed reality settings.

4.3. Participants Feedback

Participants reported that the MR simulations presented realistic and engaging clinical scenarios that elicited cognitive and emotional demands similar to real-world patient care. Many noted feeling mentally challenged when prioritizing patient needs such as fluid resuscitation, oxygen administration, and infection management. The integration of digital patients who could communicate and respond added an additional layer of realism that increased situational awareness and heightened stress, particularly when monitoring for critical risks like hypotension.

While several participants acknowledged moments of increased stress due to managing complex tasks and interpreting patient responses, they also highlighted that the simulation environment provided a safe space to practice under pressure without risking patient safety. One participant emphasized, "Keeping my patient alive was my primary focus, which made the experience intense but rewarding". Another shared, "I was constantly watching for signs of deterioration, which kept me engaged and aware of time pressures".

Participants consistently expressed that the MR simulations enhanced their clinical competence and decision-making skills. They appreciated the opportunity to interact with digital patients using both verbal communication and physical actions, such as administering oxygen or preparing vasopressors. Several participants stated that the experience improved their understanding of prioritizing care under dynamic clinical conditions.

Most participants rated the MR system as superior or comparable to traditional manikin-based training. They found that the interactive and immersive nature of the simulation helped solidify nursing procedures and improve communication skills with patients. One participant noted, "Compared to a manikin, this felt more realistic, and it helped me better prepare for actual patient interactions".

5. Conclusions

Stress is a significant concern in the nursing field that impacts both the nurses' health and the quality of patient care. To address the issue, we conducted an experiment aimed at measuring levels of stress in nursing students in a mixed reality training system. In the experiment, subjects were exposed to digital patients and clinical equipment, replicating real-life health environments.

The research included 2 h training per learner, divided into six segments. Learners were exposed to clinical scenarios developed to replicate high-pressure healthcare environments, and they directly interacted with the digital patients. The virtual patients had been integrated with a conversational AI model that allowed for natural-sounding voice interactions. In addition, the patient's facial expressions were scripted to react based on their medical condition and emotional state, adding to the realism of the simulation.

Physiological signals such as heart rate, electrodermal activity, and skin temperature were continuously recorded using the Empatica E4 wristband. These measurements were employed as objective indices to assess the nurses' stress levels during the simulation. Physiological signals were pre-processed to achieve accuracy and consistency for all measurements. Afterwards, statistical measures such as mean, standard deviation, skewness, and kurtosis were extracted for each physiological signal. Additionally, dynamic changes in the signals such as peak detection in electrodermal activity and root mean square values in heart rate and temperature were examined.

A Stacking Classifier of Gradient Boosting and Random Forest was then used to classify the participant's level of stress. Nested cross-validation was implemented for hyperparameter tuning and model selection. The Stacking Classifier performed the best among all, which had a 98% accuracy on the test set. The model combined well the strengths of Random Forest and Gradient Boosting and achieved superior predictive power in classifying stress levels.

Our findings highlight that the high-pressured mixed reality training environment significantly impacts the physiological level of stress in nursing students. Participants displayed measurable responses to stress, with elevations in heart rates and electrodermal activity on high-stress sections of the simulation.

The findings of this study can inform the integration of MR simulations into nursing education to enhance both technical competencies and stress management skills. For example, MR scenarios replicating high-acuity patient care situations could be embedded into simulation-based courses to allow students to practice managing stress while making clinical decisions in a safe environment. Additionally, MR modules could be used as refresher training for practicing nurses in critical care or emergency settings to maintain readiness and resilience. These applications support a more experiential, self-regulated approach to developing both clinical and emotional competencies essential for high-stakes healthcare delivery.

6. Discussion and Future Work

Although this study identified nursing students' stress levels in MR settings, there are certain avenues for future research that can assist in improving the understanding and application of MR in nursing education.

An important avenue for future research involves investigating the long-term impact of MR-based training on stress management and clinical performance. Although the present study focused on immediate stress responses during simulation sessions, it remains unknown whether repeated exposure to MR scenarios can enhance nurses' resilience and stress-coping skills in real clinical environments. Longitudinal studies assessing retention of stress-management strategies and transferability to practice (potentially through follow-up assessments weeks or months post-training) would provide valuable insights into the sustained benefits of this approach. Such research could also explore whether MR-based training reduces stress-induced decision errors or improves patient outcomes in high-pressure clinical scenarios.

Another course for future work will be real-time stress detection with adaptive interventions during training. Since this study was aimed at recording physiological data, for example, heart rate, skin temperature, and electrodermal activity in order to measure the level of stress, future research could involve real-time analysis of these data with mechanisms for automated feedback. For example, adaptive systems can be programmed to offer relaxation techniques, such as guided breathing, when heightened levels of stress are detected. This real-time feedback would enhance the learning experience by enabling nursing students to manage their levels of stress more effectively, so they are buffered during stressful training exercises but still reap the benefits of the pressure that comes with realistic environments.

This would also give a more profound understanding of the stress level by varying the physiological data that is recorded. Whereas the experiment made use of heart rate, electrodermal activity, and skin temperature, future experiments may consider using other biomarkers, such as respiratory rate or brain-wave activity (EEG), thereby adding more proof of the multi-responses of the physiological systems occurring under stress in XR environments. In addition, the inclusion of these markers could increase the accuracy of stress detection, allowing for a more comprehensive view of the nurse's physiological state during training.

Additionally, the relatively small sample size of our study limits the generalizability of the results. The participants were drawn from a specific population of nursing students within a single institution, which may not fully represent the broader diversity of practicing nurses or students from different educational backgrounds. Future research should aim to replicate and extend these findings using larger and more diverse participant groups to enhance external validity and deepen the understanding of individual differences in stress responses within extended reality environments.

Furthermore, monitoring physiological data in educational settings raises important ethical considerations that warrant careful attention. Participants' privacy must be safeguarded through secure storage of sensor data, anonymization protocols, and clear communication about data usage. Consent procedures explicitly outlined the nature of data collection, how data would be used, and participants' right to withdraw at any time without penalty. Additionally, continuous monitoring during simulations may introduce psychological discomfort or heightened self-awareness, potentially influencing behavior. To mitigate this, participants were thoroughly briefed and given opportunities to express concerns. Future applications of such technologies in education should prioritize transparency, minimize intrusiveness, and ensure that physiological monitoring is framed as a tool to enhance learning, not as an evaluative measure that could induce anxiety or judgment.

By addressing these areas in future research, MR-based training for nurses can be an even more powerful, more specific, and more effective way of preparing healthcare professionals to manage high-stress environments with greater resilience and effectiveness.

Author Contributions: Conceptualization, K.S., Y.-J.S., S.A. and J.E.H.; methodology, K.S., Y.-J.S., S.A. and J.H; software, K.S., D.S.; validation, K.S., Y.-J.S., S.A. and J.H; formal analysis, K.S., Y.-J.S., S.A. and J.E.H.; investigation, K.S., Y.-J.S., S.A. and J.E.H.; resources, K.S., Y.-J.S., S.A. and J.E.H.; data curation, K.S., Y.-J.S., S.A. and J.H; writing—original draft preparation, K.S., Y.-J.S., S.A. and J.H; writing—review and editing, K.S., Y.-J.S., S.A. and J.H; visualization, K.S., Y.-J.S., S.A. and J.E.H.; supervision, Y.-J.S., S.A. and J.E.H.; funding acquisition, Y.-J.S., S.A. and J.E.H. All authors have read and agreed to the published version of the manuscript.

Funding: This study was funded in part by the Center for University Education Scholarship (CUES) at University of Arizona, Sensor Lab Seed Grants to Advance Innovative Research at University of Arizona, and Edwardson School of Industrial Engineering at Purdue University. Any views, findings, or recommendations hereby expressed are those of the authors only.

Institutional Review Board Statement: This study was approved by the Human Research Ethics committee (IRB) of the University of Arizona, STUDY00001862. All participants in this experiment were provided with information regarding its objectives. Furthermore, all data have been anonymized to ensure participant privacy.

Informed Consent Statement: Informed consent was obtained from all subjects involved in the study.

Data Availability Statement: The data supporting the findings of the study is not publicly available but can be accessed by contacting the corresponding author directly.

Conflicts of Interest: The authors declare no conflicts of interest.

References

1. Cai, H.; Tu, B.; Ma, J.; Chen, L.; Fu, L.; Jiang, Y.; Zhuang, Q. Psychological impacts and coping strategies of front-line medical staff during COVID-19 outbreak in Hunan, China. *Med. Sci. Monit.* **2020**, *26*, e924171-1–e924171-16. [CrossRef] [PubMed]
2. Almazan, J.U.; Albougami, A.S.; Alamri, M.S. Exploring nurses' work-related stress in an acute care hospital in KSA. *J. Taibah. Univ. Med. Sci.* **2019**, *14*, 376–382. [CrossRef] [PubMed]
3. Kibria, M.G. Prevalence of Stress and Coping Mechanism Among Staff Nurses of Intensive Care Unit in a Selected Hospital. *Int. J. Neurosurg.* **2018**, *2*, 8. [CrossRef]
4. de Cássia de Marchi Barcellos Dalri, R.; da Silva, L.A.; Mendes, A.M.O.C.; do Carmo Cruz Robazzi, M.L. Nurses' workload and its relation with physiological stress reactions. *Rev. Lat. Am. Enferm.* **2014**, *22*, 959–965. [CrossRef]
5. Kundrata, D.; Pukljak, Z.; Repustić, M.; Rotim, C.; Friganović, A.; Kurtović, B. Coping with stress of nurses employed in the internal medicine and surgical departments. *Croat. Nurs. J.* **2022**, *6*, 33–43. [CrossRef]
6. Oducado, R.M.F.; Estoque, H. Online Learning in Nursing Education During the COVID-19 Pandemic: Stress, Satisfaction, and Academic Performance. *J. Nurs. Pract.* **2021**, *4*, 143–153. [CrossRef]
7. Pulido-Martos, M.; Augusto-Landa, J.M.; Lopez-Zafra, E. Sources of stress in nursing students: A systematic review of quantitative studies. *Int. Nurs. Rev.* **2012**, *59*, 15–25. [CrossRef]
8. Ghorbanzadeh, K.; Ilka, N.; Pishkhani, M.K.; Jafari, M.; Sadeghi, H. Explaining the Clinical Education Stressors in Nursing Students: A Qualitative Study. *J. Qual. Res. Health Sci.* **2023**, *12*, 152–158. [CrossRef]
9. Jas Deol, M.N. Remote Simulation-Based Learning Using a Mixed Reality Device: Perspectives of Nursing Educators and Undergraduate Nursing Students. *Nurs. Prax. New Zealand* **2024**, *40*, 1–10.
10. Ahmadi, N.; Sasangohar, F.; Nisar, T.; Danesh, V.; Larsen, E.; Sultana, I.; Bosetti, R. Quantifying Occupational Stress in Intensive Care Unit Nurses: An Applied Naturalistic Study of Correlations Among Stress, Heart Rate, Electrodermal Activity, and Skin Temperature. *Hum. Factors J. Hum. Factors Ergon. Soc.* **2022**, *64*, 159–172. [CrossRef]
11. Li, X.; Zhu, W.; Sui, X.; Zhang, A.; Chi, L.; Lv, L. Assessing workplace stress among nurses using heart rate variability analysis with wearable ecg device–a pilot study. *Front. Public Health* **2022**, *9*, 810577. [CrossRef] [PubMed]
12. Zhang, Q.; Sasangohar, F.; Saravanan, P.; Ahmadi, N.; Nisar, T.; Danesh, V.; Masud, F. Real-time stress monitoring for intensive care unit (icu) nurses. *Proc. Hum. Factors Ergon. Soc. Annu. Meet.* **2022**, *66*, 779–782. [CrossRef]
13. Alkhawaldeh, J.M.A.; Soh, K.L.; Mukhtar, F.B.M.; Ooi, C.P. Effectiveness of stress management interventional programme on occupational stress for nurses: A systematic review. *J. Nurs. Manag.* **2020**, *28*, 209–220. [CrossRef]
14. Gaggioli, A.; Pallavicini, F.; Morganti, L.; Serino, S.; Scaratti, C.; Briguglio, M.; Crifaci, G.; Vetrano, N.; Giulintano, A.; Bernava, G.; et al. Experiential Virtual Scenarios With Real-Time Monitoring (Interreality) for the Management of Psychological Stress: A Block Randomized Controlled Trial. *J. Med. Internet Res.* **2014**, *16*, e167. [CrossRef]
15. Martaindale, M.H.; Sandel, W.L.; Duron, A.; McAllister, M.J. Can a Virtual Reality Training Scenario Elicit Similar Stress Response as a Realistic Scenario-Based Training Scenario? *Police Q.* **2024**, *27*, 109–129. [CrossRef]
16. Saab, M.M.P.; McCarthy, M.; O'Mahony, B.M.; Cooke, E.M.; Hegarty, J.P.; Murphy, D.P.; Walshe, N.M.; Noonan, B.D. Virtual Reality Simulation in Nursing and Midwifery Education. *CIN Comput. Inform. Nurs.* **2023**, *41*, 815–824. [CrossRef]
17. Mitsea, E.; Drigas, A.; Skianis, C. Digitally assisted mindfulness in training self-regulation skills for sustainable mental health: A systematic review. *Behav. Sci.* **2023**, *13*, 1008. [CrossRef]
18. Gutiérrez-Fernández, A.; Fernández-Llamas, C.; Vázquez-Casares, A.M.; Mauriz, E.; Riego-del-Castillo, V.; John, N.W. Immersive haptic simulation for training nurses in emergency medical procedures. *Vis. Comput.* **2024**, *40*, 7527–7537. [CrossRef]
19. Velana, M.; Rinkenauer, G. Individual-level interventions for decreasing job-related stress and enhancing coping strategies among nurses: A systematic review. *Front. Psychol.* **2021**, *12*, 708696. [CrossRef]
20. Aguinaga-Ontoso, I.; Guillen-Aguinaga, L.; Guillen-Aguinaga, S. Evaluation of Mixed reality in undergraduate nursing education. A systematic review. *Eur. J. Public Health* **2021**, *31* (Suppl. S3), ckab165–ckab312. [CrossRef]
21. Kim, K.J.; Choi, M.J.; Kim, K.J. Effects of nursing simulation using mixed reality: A scoping review. *Healthcare* **2021**, *9*, 947. [CrossRef] [PubMed]
22. Sepanloo, K.; Shevelev, D.; Islam, M.T.; Son, Y.-J.; Aras, S.; Hinton, J.E. Improving nursing education through an AI-enhanced mixed reality training platform: Development and pilot evaluation. In *Educational Technology Research and Development*; Springer: Berlin/Heidelberg, Germany, 2025. [CrossRef]
23. El Haouij, N.; Poggi, J.-M.; Sevestre-Ghalila, S.; Ghozi, R.; Jaïdane, M. AffectiveROAD system and database to assess driver's attention. In Proceedings of the 33rd Annual ACM Symposium on Applied Computing, New York, NY, USA, 9–13 April 2018; pp. 800–803. [CrossRef]

24. Hosseini, S.; Gottumukkala, R.; Katragadda, S.; Bhupatiraju, R.T.; Ashkar, Z.; Borst, C.W.; Cochran, K. A multimodal sensor dataset for continuous stress detection of nurses in a hospital. *Sci. Data* **2022**, *9*, 255. [CrossRef] [PubMed]
25. Jerem, P.; Romero, L.M. It's cool to be stressed: Body surface temperatures track sympathetic nervous system activation during acute stress. *J. Exp. Biol.* **2023**, *226*, jeb246552. [CrossRef]

sensors

MDPI

Article

Attention-Enhanced CNN-LSTM Model for Exercise Oxygen Consumption Prediction with Multi-Source Temporal Features

Zhen Wang, Yingzhe Song, Lei Pang *, Shanjun Li * and Gang Sun

Institute of Artificial Intelligence in Sports, Capital University of Physical Education and Sports, Beijing 100191, China; wangzhen23@cupes.edu.cn (Z.W.); songyingzhe2022@cupes.edu.cn (Y.S.); sungang@cupes.edu.cn (G.S.)
* Correspondence: panglei@cupes.edu.cn (L.P.); lishanjun@cupes.edu.cn (S.L.)

Abstract

Dynamic oxygen uptake (VO_2) reflects moment-to-moment changes in oxygen consumption during exercise and underpins training design, performance enhancement, and clinical decision-making. We tackled two key obstacles—the limited fusion of heterogeneous sensor data and inadequate modeling of long-range temporal patterns—by integrating wearable accelerometer and heart-rate streams with a convolutional neural network–LSTM (CNN-LSTM) architecture and optional attention modules. Physiological signals and VO_2 were recorded from 21 adults through resting assessment and cardiopulmonary exercise testing. The results showed that pairing accelerometer with heart-rate inputs improves prediction compared with considering the heart rate alone. The baseline CNN-LSTM reached $R^2 = 0.946$, outperforming a plain LSTM ($R^2 = 0.926$) thanks to stronger local spatio-temporal feature extraction. Introducing a spatial attention mechanism raised accuracy further ($R^2 = 0.962$), whereas temporal attention reduced it ($R^2 = 0.930$), indicating that attention success depends on how well the attended features align with exercise dynamics. Stacking both attentions (spatio-temporal) yielded $R^2 = 0.960$, slightly below the value for spatial attention alone, implying that added complexity does not guarantee better performance. Across all models, prediction errors grew during high-intensity bouts, highlighting a bottleneck in capturing non-linear physiological responses under heavy load. These findings inform architecture selection for wearable metabolic monitoring and clarify when attention mechanisms add value.

Keywords: oxygen uptake; deep learning; neural network; attention mechanism

1. Introduction

Cardiorespiratory fitness is an important indicator of all-cause mortality risk [1] and also plays a key role in endurance performance [2]. Oxygen consumption (VO_2) and its dynamic response during exercise are widely used in the assessment of cardiorespiratory fitness. The analysis of VO_2 during exercise provides important physiological information about the components of the aerobic metabolism system, including the cardiopulmonary and muscular systems [3]. Furthermore, abnormal oxygen consumption responses during exercise may precede clinical manifestations of disease, thereby demonstrating significant practical value in disease warning and exercise risk screening [4].

Traditional oxygen consumption monitoring relies on laboratory metabolic chambers (such as the TrueOne 2400, ParvoMedic Inc., Salt Lake City, UT, USA), which can obtain energy metabolism data at rest and during exercise through high-precision gas analysis systems. However, their operation is strictly limited to laboratory environments, and the

 https://doi.org/10.3390/s25134062

equipment is bulky and expensive, making it difficult to meet the dynamic monitoring requirements of sports venues [5]. Portable oxygen consumption monitoring devices currently available on the market (such as K5, Cosmed S.r.l., Rome, Italy and VO_2 Master, VO_2 Master Health Sensors Inc., Vernon, BC, Canada) have broken through the limitations of laboratory environments and enabled the on-site detection of respiratory data during exercise. However, during testing, factors such as wearing respiratory masks that alter the natural breathing pattern of participants, frequent gas calibration procedures, and the high cost of equipment purchase resulted in a certain degree of error between the actual measured oxygen uptake data of exercisers and their true physiological values [6].

The development of wearable sensor technology has provided new ideas for non-invasive oxygen consumption monitoring. Early studies primarily used the heart rate (HR) as an assessment indicator and employed traditional statistical models such as linear regression [7] to estimate oxygen uptake at each moment during exercise [8]. However, the above studies did not fully explore the dynamic information contained in the evolution of heart rate sequences over time. In recent years, artificial intelligence technologies represented by deep learning have opened up more development opportunities for real-time, dynamic oxygen consumption calculations. Deep learning algorithms can more deeply explore the relationship between other physiological signals and oxygen consumption, making oxygen consumption monitoring during exercise more convenient and accurate. Therefore, recent studies have begun to focus on utilizing the time-dependent nature of oxygen uptake during exercise and its correlation with multiple physiological indicators, combined with more complex deep learning prediction models to predict real-time oxygen uptake responses during exercise [9].

A multi-indicator model refers to an oxygen consumption prediction model that uses multiple relevant factors from different data sources as inputs. Typical input indicators include static characteristics (e.g., age, BMI, etc.) and dynamic movement characteristics (e.g., heart rate, acceleration, etc.). They are associated with oxygen consumption by reflecting metabolic basis and exercise intensity. When performing in-depth information mining on the above multi-dimensional features, convolutional neural networks (CNNs) are commonly used because they can extract potential features from adjacent input indicators as spatial features in deep learning models [10]. However, there is no spatial adjacency relationship between the characteristics during the movement process similar to image pixels, and the order of the indicators does not have a clear spatial structure. Therefore, although local convolutions using CNNs can extract some potential features, it is still difficult to comprehensively capture the complex potential relationships between multiple indicators.

A time series refers to the temporal correlation between monitored data sequences. Indicators such as the heart rate, acceleration, and oxygen consumption during exercise tend to change with the duration of exercise, and past data sequences are correlated with future data sequences. Long Short-Term Memory (LSTM) networks are capable of remembering time series information. However, as the time series in the data lengthens, LSTM may not remember early data points well enough [11], requiring further improvement to strengthen temporal modeling.

In summary, existing VO_2 prediction studies still have shortcomings in the deep integration of multi-indicator information, the modeling of long-term dependencies in temporal features, and the dynamic extraction of key features. This paper proposes an oxygen consumption prediction model based on the CNN-LSTM structure and incorporates spatial and temporal attention mechanisms into the model to enhance prediction performance. As shown in Figure 1, the main tasks are as follows: (1) conducting resting experiments and cardiopulmonary exercise tests (CPETs) to collect physiological data, (2) constructing

LSTM and CNN-LSTM dynamic oxygen consumption prediction models based on input features derived from the integration of static and dynamic indicators, and, (3) based on the CNN-LSTM model, adding a time, space, and spatio-temporal attention mechanism to construct an oxygen consumption prediction model and conduct a comparative analysis.

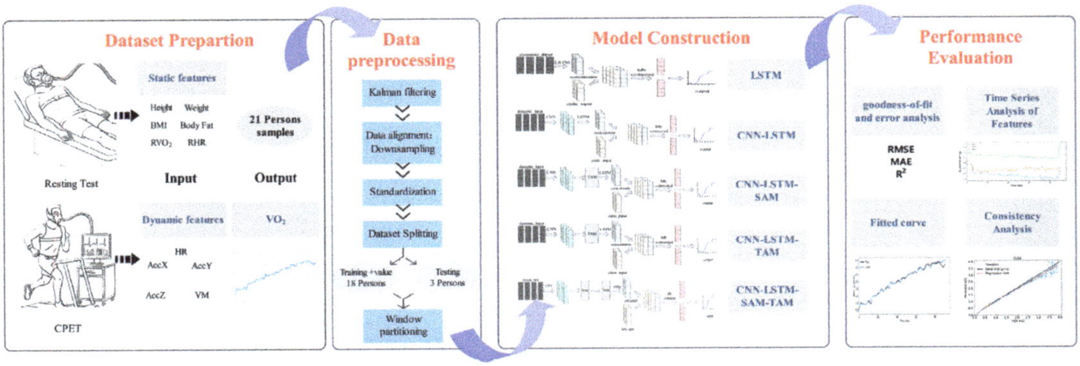

Figure 1. Attention-CNN-LSTM framework for VO_2 prediction using multi-source temporal features.

2. Materials and Methods

2.1. Participants

This study recruited 21 participants, including 14 males and 7 females, aged between 21 and 28 years. Table 1 shows the demographic characteristics of the subjects. This study was approved by the Institutional Review Board, and all participants signed written informed consent forms. Each participant underwent a health assessment screening to assess potential risks, had had no hospitalization records in the past six months, and was able to complete the Physical Activity Readiness Questionnaire (PAR-Q) for the physical activity programmed. We excluded participants with medical implantable electronic devices, those who had sustained running injuries, or those at high risk of injury.

Table 1. Basic information of the subjects.

	Male (n = 14)	Female (n = 7)
Age	24 ± 3	25 ± 3
Height (cm)	176 ± 8	163 ± 5
Weight (kg)	70.6 ± 13.3	52.3 ± 6
BMI	22.8 ± 3	19.8 ± 1.5
Body fat percentage (%)	16.2 ± 5.8	23.7 ± 3.4

2.2. Experimental Design and Data Collection

The data sources included two parts: resting test and CPET. Before the resting test, subjects were asked to fast for at least 4 h and refrain from consuming caffeinated beverages or alcohol for 24 h. They were also asked to avoid strenuous exercise for 48 h before the test to ensure that they were in a resting state before the test. Each subject was asked to close their eyes and lie still for 15 min before the test began to ensure that they were completely relaxed. After the resting testing began, the subjects continued to lie quietly with their eyes closed and wore a heart rate belt (H10, Polar Electro Oy, Kempele, Finland) with a sampling frequency of 1 Hz. At the same time, a gas metabolism analyzer (Powercube-Ergo, Ganshorn, Niederlauer, Germany) was used to conduct a 10-min resting oxygen uptake test, with a sampling frequency of 0.1 Hz. The device recorded their breathing data and heart rates.

Before the CPET, the subjects first did a 10-min slow jog to warm up. After entering the formal testing phase, participants used a treadmill to perform incremental exercise according to the Ramp protocol [12], with the treadmill speed increasing by 1 km/h per minute and the incline remaining at 0%. During the test, accelerometers (WT901BLECL5.0, Witmotion, Shenzhen, China) were worn on the wrists of the subjects' non-dominant hands to collect acceleration data at a frequency of 10 Hz. Heart rate belts collected heart rate data and gas metabolism analyzers collected and recorded oxygen consumption during exercise. The test was terminated when the subject met any two of the following criteria: heart rate reached 90% of maximum heart rate; Respiratory Quotient > 1.15; Rating of Perceived Exertion > 17; oxygen uptake plateaued. The maximum heart rate was calculated using the following equation: HRmax = 208 − 0.7 × age.

2.3. Data Preprocessing

For multi-source heterogeneous data such as heart rate, acceleration, and gas parameters during exercise, time synchronization was first performed based on the experimental records before preprocessing. To suppress random noise and obtain smooth one-dimensional acceleration estimates, this study applied a Kalman filter to the original acceleration signals. The following example uses the original acceleration sequence (a_x) on the X-axis to illustrate the implementation details of the Kalman filter. The remaining Y- and Z-axis signals use the same model and hyperparameters and are processed independently in parallel. The sampling frequency of the original acceleration data is 10 Hz ($\Delta t = 0.1$ s). The filter uses a one-dimensional random walk assumption, and its state-observation model is $x_k = x_{k-1} + w_{k-1}, z_k = x_k + v_k$. Here, x_k denotes the 'true' X-axis acceleration (in units of g) of frame k, z_k denotes the corresponding raw measurement value, $w_{k-1} \sim N(0, Q)$, and $v_k \sim N(0, R)$. Based on the stationary segment noise calibration and Allan variance analysis, the parameters are set as $A = H = 1$, $Q = 0.01g^2$, and $R = 0.10g^2$. The initial state estimate is set as the first frame measurement $x_0 = a_x(0)$, and the initial covariance $P_0 = 1g^2$. After that, the three directional accelerations are combined into a scalar composite value, *VM*.

$$VM = \sqrt{AccX^2 + AccY^2 + AccZ^2} \tag{1}$$

To address the issue of accelerometer sampling frequency being higher than heart rate belt frequency, a down sampling method was used to align the accelerometer data with the heart rate data. After that, the features were divided into dynamic features and static features (Table 2) and standardized using Z-scores (Equation (2)).

$$X' = \frac{X - \mu}{\sigma} \tag{2}$$

μ represents the mean of all sample data and σ represents the standard deviation of all sample data.

To coordinate the sampling frequency of the gas analyzer with other devices, a 10-s non-overlapping time window was constructed, and the dynamic characteristics within the window were serialized in 1-s increments. The absolute oxygen consumption values collected by the gas analyzer were used as label values for each window of the model. The missing acceleration and heart rate values in the window were filled in using the average values in this window.

Table 2. Classification of dynamic and static characteristics.

Feature Category	Feature
Static Features	Weight (kg) Height (m) BMI (kg/m^2) Body fat percentage (%) Resting oxygen consumption (L/min) Resting heart rate (Beats/min)
Dynamic Features	Exercise heart rate (Beats/min) X-axis acceleration (G) Y-axis acceleration (G) Z-axis acceleration (G) VM (G)

2.4. *Model Construction*

2.4.1. Attention Mechanism

Attention mechanisms (AMs) are often used to solve temporal and spatial problems encountered in modeling. By dynamically allocating weights to different indicators or time steps, AMs can highlight key information based on their correlations, thereby assisting predictive models in more accurately capturing key features [13]. This study adopted three attention mechanisms to optimize the spatio-temporal features of multi-source heterogeneous data for oxygen consumption prediction: Spatial Attention Module (SAM), Temporal Attention Module (TAM), and Spatio-temporal Attention Module (STAM). SAM can extract potential features from multiple input variables and analyze their importance to the predicted target indicator. This solves the limitation of CNNs in feature modeling of adjacent input indicators. TAM focuses on the most critical part of time sequence in accurate time prediction. It assigns corresponding weights, reducing the time information that LSTM needs to remember [14].

(1) Time Attention Mechanism (TAM)

The Squeeze-Excitation (SE) module is a temporal attention mechanism that enhances the representational capacity of convolutional neural networks through dynamic channel feature re-labelling [15]. The actual implementation process is shown in Figure 2. In the figure, X represents the input data, C' and C represent time series, W' and W represent spatial dimensions (multiple indicators), F represents feature maps, F_{tr} represents convolution, F_{sq} represents feature map compression, F_{ex} represents feature map excitation, and $Fscale$ represents feature re-calibration.

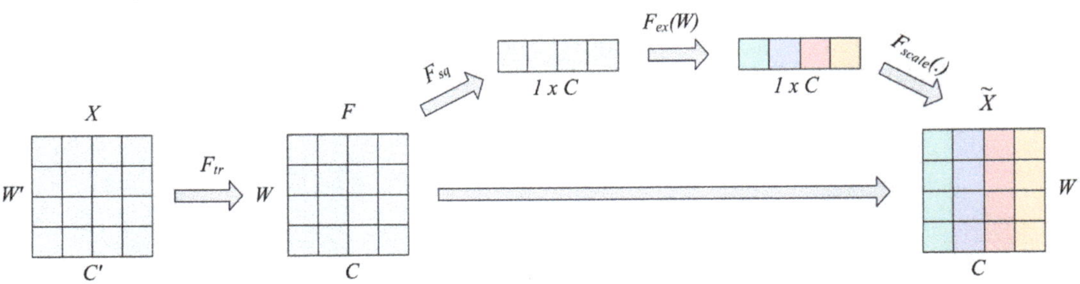

Figure 2. Squeeze-Excitation (SE) module.

The core idea of this mechanism lies in explicitly modeling the non-linear interaction between channel dimensions. Specifically, it consists of two stages:

a. Squeeze: Spatial features (channel number C and two-dimensional spatial dimensions $H \times W$) are compressed along the spatial dimension into channel description vectors through global average pooling. Compared with the $C \times H \times W$ structure of image data, this paper omits the spatial dimension $H \times W$ of the time series and retains only the time channel C and the spatial dimension W composed of multiple indicators. The calculation method is shown in Equation (3). F_C denotes the feature matrix F on the Cth channel and $F_C(i)$ denotes its value at the ith time step.

$$F_C = F[:, C] \in R^W,\ Z_C = \frac{1}{W}\sum_{i=1}^{W} F_C(i) \tag{3}$$

b. Excitation: We introduce a fully connected layer with a bottleneck structure to generate channel attention weights S:

$$S = \sigma(W_2 \cdot \delta(W_1 \cdot Z)) \tag{4}$$

$W_1 \in R^{\frac{C}{r} \times C}$ and $W_2 \in R^{C \times \frac{C}{r}}$ are learnable parameters (r is the dimension reduction ratio), δ is the Relu activation function, and σ is the Sigmoid gate function.

Finally, the original features are re-calibrated using channel-wise weight S_C.

$$F'_C = S_C \cdot F_C \tag{5}$$

(2) Spatial Attention Mechanism (SAM)

According to the spatial attention mechanism mentioned by Woo in their study [16], we define 'spatial attention' as modeling the importance of feature dimensions at different positions in a time series to characterize 'which feature dimensions should be focused on at different time steps'.

The SAM implementation process is shown in Figure 3, where C represents the time series, W represents the spatial dimension (multiple indicators), F represents the feature map, F_{st} represents feature concatenation, F_{tr} represents convolution, and M represents the spatial attention map. First, we perform maximum-pooling and average-pooling operations on the input features F along the time dimension C to obtain two one-dimensional representations: $F^S_{avg}, F^S_{max} \in R^{1 \times W}$. These two representations reflect the average response intensity and strongest response across all time steps for each feature dimension, thereby comprehensively modeling the importance of each dimension. Subsequently, we concatenate the two in the channel dimension to form a $2 \times W$ fusion feature representation, which is then inputted into a one-dimensional convolutional layer to extract local structural information and generate attention weights. Finally, the output is normalized using the Sigmoid function to obtain the spatial attention map $M_S \in R^{1 \times W}$, which is then multiplied element-wise with the original input features (F) to achieve weighted adjustment in feature dimension. The calculation equations are shown in Equations (6) and (7).

$$M_S(F) = \sigma(f([AvgPool(F); MaxPool(F)])) = \sigma(f([F^S_{avg}; F^S_{max}])) \tag{6}$$

$$F\prime = M_S(F) \otimes F \tag{7}$$

(3) Spatio-temporal Attention Mechanism (STAM)

The Spatio-temporal Attention Mechanism consists of a TAM and a SAM (Figure 4), which can jointly model the temporal dynamics of time series and the multi-indicator spatial correlation. This mechanism adopts a cascading structure: input features first pass through TAM, which aggregates information along the indicator dimension to generate temporal step importance weights, highlighting key temporal segments. Subsequently, pooling is performed along the time axis and the dependencies between multiple indicators are learned, and indicator weights are generated through convolution. Finally, the temporal and spatial attention weights are applied to the input features in stages to refine the features in both the temporal and metric dimensions.

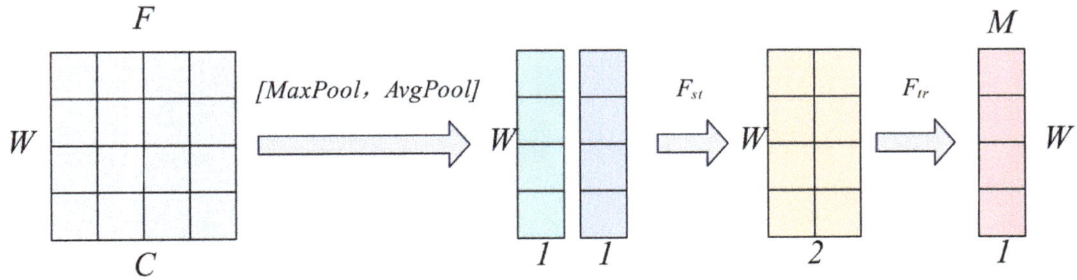

Figure 3. Spatial attention mechanism.

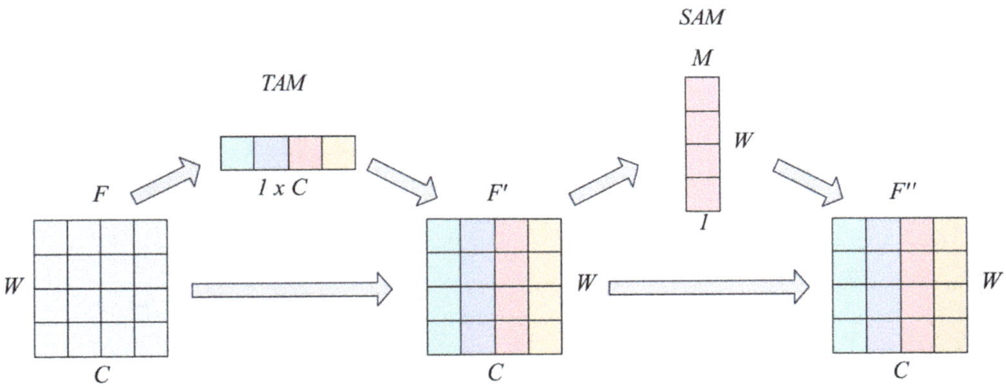

Figure 4. Spatio-temporal Attention Mechanism.

2.4.2. VO_2 Prediction Model

This paper proposes a deep learning model for dynamic oxygen uptake prediction. First, to validate the effectiveness of CNNs for multi-indicator fusion, an independent LSTM model (Figure 5A) was constructed, which directly receives raw time-series inputs and ignores spatial feature extraction across indicators. Second, we constructed a CNN-LSTM model and used it as the baseline model for this study (Figure 5B). It extracts spatial features between multiple indicators through convolution operations and captures time dependency using LSTM.

In order to improve the model's sensitivity to key features, we introduced the three attention mechanisms described in Section 2.4.1 to the baseline model. The CNN-TAM-LSTM (CLTA) model embeds TAM before the LSTM layer (Figure 5C), aggregates the mean and maximum values along the indicator dimension, generates time step weights, and enhances the feature responses of key time periods. The CNN-SAM-LSTM model (CLSA) embeds SAM before the LSTM layer (Figure 5D) to learn indicator importance weights through time dimension pooling. CNN-SAM-TAM-LSTM (CLSTA) cascades SAM and TAM (Figure 5E) achieve joint optimization of temporal sensitivity and indicator correlation.

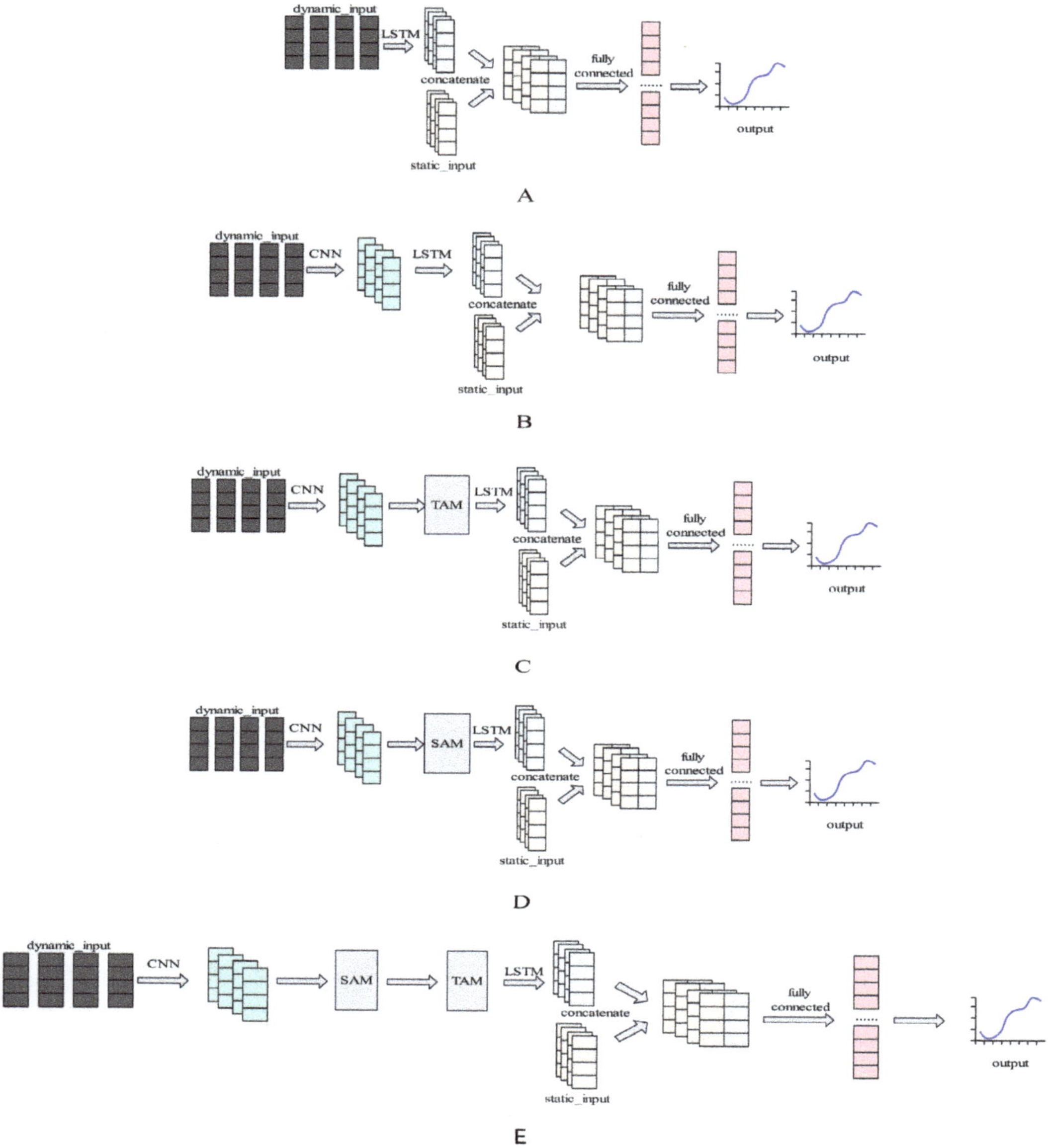

Figure 5. Structure of oxygen uptake prediction models: (**A**)—LSTM; (**B**)—CNN-LSTM; (**C**)—CLTA; (**D**)—CLSA; (**E**)—CLSTA.

The model inputs six static features and five dynamic features (Table 2) separately and predicts the oxygen uptake at the current time step as the output. Using the Adam optimizer, the learning rate is set to 0.001 and the batch size is set to 32. We divide the data of all 21 people into two groups: 3 people as an independent test set and the remaining 18 people for six-fold cross-validation. In each round of division, we divide the 18 people into 6 groups, take 1 group as the validation set in turn, and use the remaining 5 groups as the training set. The specific parameters of each layer of the model are shown in Table 3.

Table 3. Model structure.

	Dynamic Feature Input Layer	Static Feature Input Layer	CNN	SAM	TAM	LSTM	Output Layer
Number of neurons	10 × 5	6	64	64	64	128	1
Activation functions	\	\	ReLU	Sigmoid	Sigmoid	Tanh	Linear

2.5. Model Evaluation Indicators

In order to comprehensively quantify the accuracy, stability, and time alignment capability of the dynamic oxygen uptake prediction model, this study comprehensively selected evaluation indicators.

(1) Root Mean Square Error (RMSE)

$$RMSE = \sqrt{\frac{1}{N}\sum_{i=1}^{N}(y_i - \hat{y}_i)^2} \quad (8)$$

We measure the average deviation between the predicted value and the actual value. N is the total number of samples; y_i and $\hat{y}_i$ are the true value and predicted value of the i-th sample, respectively.

(2) Mean Absolute Error (MAE)

$$MAE = \frac{1}{N}\sum_{i=1}^{N}|y_i - \hat{y}_i| \quad (9)$$

We calculate the absolute average value of the prediction error. The symbols have the same meanings as in the RMSE equation.

(3) Deciding Coefficient (R^2)

$$R^2 = 1 - \frac{\sum_{i=1}^{N}(y_i - \hat{y}_i)^2}{\sum_{i=1}^{N}(y_i - \overline{y}_i)^2}, \overline{y} = \frac{1}{N}\sum_{i=1}^{N} y_i \quad (10)$$

We evaluate the explanatory power of the model for changes in oxygen uptake, ranging from [0, 1], where values closer to 1 indicate a higher degree of model fit. $\overline{y}$ represents the arithmetic mean of the actual oxygen uptake values, and the meanings of the other symbols are the same as in the RMSE equation.

3. Results

3.1. Sequential Dynamic Characteristics

We plotted the time-series changes in the dynamic indicators (including triaxial acceleration, heart rate, VM, and oxygen uptake) of a subject during exercise with increasing load, as shown in Figure 6. The dynamic response patterns of the physiological indicators of this subject were consistent with the group data in this study and can be used as typical examples to intuitively illustrate common patterns. The three-axis acceleration signals (Figure 6A) showed obvious fluctuations at the beginning of the movement due to the insufficient coordination of movements. After entering the stable running phase, the acceleration of each axis showed rhythmic fluctuations around the average value due to the regular alternation of steps. Finally, during the sprinting phase, the violent kicking movements and large trunk swings together led to a significant increase in the intensity of the fluctuations. The heart rate (Figure 6B) increased gradually from the resting value with the increase in random exercise intensity and remained generally upward throughout the exercise, approaching the maximum heart rate at the end. The amplitude of VM (Figure 6C) increased continuously with increasing movement intensity. Due to vector synthesis, single-axis-specific noise was suppressed, and the local variance was significantly lower than that of single-axis data. VO_2 rose slowly in the initial stage and eventually reached a plateau as intensity continued to increase, tending toward the individual's maximum oxygen uptake (Figure 6D).

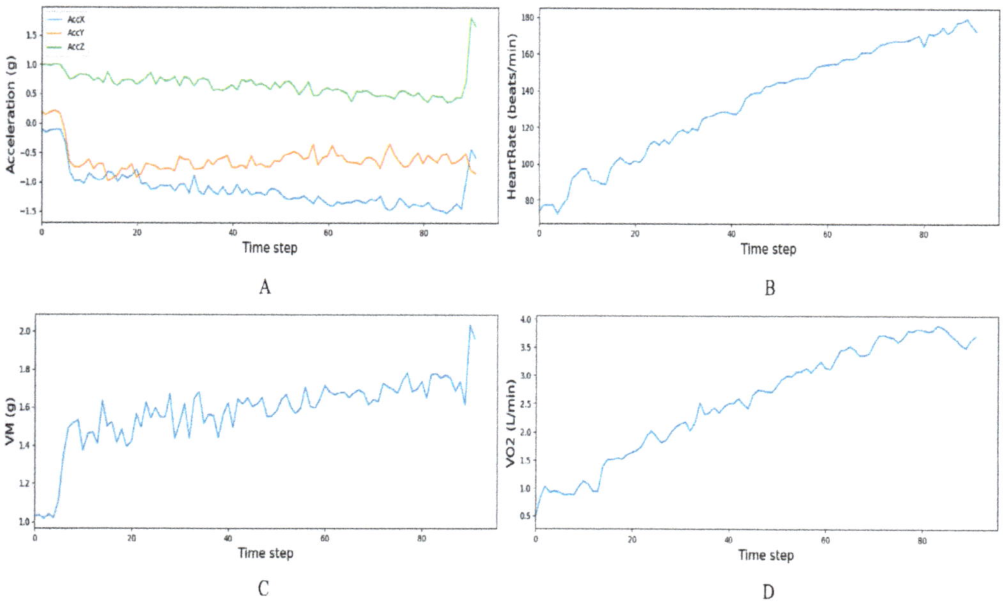

Figure 6. Time dynamics of three-axis acceleration, heart rate, VM, and oxygen uptake during incremental exercise: (**A**)—three-axis acceleration, (**B**)—heart rate, (**C**)—VM, and (**D**)—VO_2.

3.2. *Construction of VO_2 Prediction Model Based on Dynamic-Static Feature Fusion*

In developing the oxygen uptake prediction model, an LSTM network was initially constructed to process time-series data. In order to compare and analyze the impact of integrating different dynamic indicators with static indicators on the performance of the prediction model, static features plus heart rate and static features plus acceleration data and the heart rate were used as model inputs. In Table 4, the RMSE, MAE, and R^2 values for the training set, validation set, and test set after six-fold cross-validation are given. The results indicate that relying solely on heart rate signals to predict VO_2 during exercise is less effective overall than models that combine heart rate and acceleration signals. Among these, after adding the acceleration signal, the RMSE of the LSTM model on the test set decreased from 0.3335 to 0.2317, and R^2 increased from 0.8882 to 0.9460, indicating that the model could more accurately and reliably characterize changes in VO_2. This result was consistent with the dynamic characteristic analysis in Section 3.1. It was precisely because acceleration could capture short-term violent movements and other intensity fluctuations that it compensated for the delay in heart rate response to VO_2 changes, thereby significantly improving the estimation accuracy of energy expenditure and oxygen consumption.

A CNN can extract deep features more effectively, so we further compared the performance of the LSTM and CNN-LSTM models in dynamic VO_2 prediction. The results showed that all models performed better on the training set than on the test set. The models minimized the loss function during the training phase while the test phase measured their generalization ability on unseen data. Therefore, a certain degree of performance degradation was normal. The hybrid model with a CNN layer (CNN-LSTM) outperformed the pure LSTM model in VO_2 prediction accuracy. When using heart rate and static characteristics as input variables, the CNN-LSTM model achieved an RMSE of 0.3232 on the test set, which was better than the corresponding LSTM model's 0.3335; R^2 was improved from 0.8882 for the LSTM model to 0.8950. After adding acceleration data to the input variables, the CNN-LSTM model achieved an RMSE of 0.2317 on the test set, outperforming the corresponding LSTM model's 0.2720; the R^2 value improved from 0.9256 for the LSTM model to 0.9460. This indicates that the introduction of the convolutional structure effectively enhanced the model's ability to capture real VO_2 change trends.

Table 4. Performance comparison of feature combinations and models for VO_2 prediction.

Feature	Model	Train			Validation			Test		
		RMSE	MAE	R^2	RMSE	MAE	R^2	RMSE	MAE	R^2
HR + Static Features	LSTM	0.0851	0.0626	0.9918	0.2006	0.1342	0.9536	0.3335	0.2305	0.8882
	CNN-LSTM	0.0306	0.0224	0.9981	0.2095	0.1477	0.9499	0.3232	0.2950	0.8950
HR + Acc Data + Static Features	LSTM	0.0892	0.0649	0.9908	0.1031	0.0764	0.9871	0.2720	0.2078	0.9256
	CNN-LSTM	0.0044	0.0035	1.0000	0.0504	0.0302	0.9971	0.2317	0.1566	0.9460

3.3. VO_2 Prediction Model with Integrated Attention Mechanism

Attention mechanisms are generally believed to enable models to learn to 'focus on key points' when processing information, like humans do, thereby improving their ability to model complex data and their interpretability. This section proposes a dynamic VO_2 prediction model based on the fusion of time, space, and spatio-temporal attention in the CNN-LSTM model. Since the combination of heart rate and acceleration data with static characteristics is beneficial to model performance, this combination will be used as input in subsequent analyses. The results are shown in Table 5. Compared with the original CNN-LSTM model without the attention mechanism in Section 3.2, the performance of the model was significantly improved after introducing the Spatial Attention Module (CLSA). On both the validation set and the test set, the CLSA model achieved lower RMSE and MAE values and higher R^2 values (the R^2 value on the test set increased from 0.9460 to 0.9621) compared to the best-performing CNN-LSTM model in Section 3.2. In contrast, the CLTA model, which only introduced time attention, did not bring any performance gains. The error on the test set was even slightly higher than that of the original model (RMSE = 0.2648, MAE = 0.1881, R^2 = 0.9295).

Table 5. Comparison of VO_2 prediction performance metrics across models on training, validation, and test sets.

Model	Train			Validation			Test		
	RMSE	MAE	R^2	RMSE	MAE	R^2	RMSE	MAE	R^2
CLSA	0.005	0.0038	1.0000	0.0517	0.0290	0.9968	0.1942	0.1241	0.9621
CLTA	0.0051	0.0040	1.0000	0.0519	0.0285	0.9968	0.2648	0.1881	0.9295
CLSTA	0.0041	0.0031	1.0000	0.0609	0.0304	0.9955	0.2030	0.1279	0.9586

At the same time, the CLSTA model, which combined temporal and spatial attention, achieved extremely high goodness of fit on the training set (training set R^2 = 1.000), but its performance in the validation and testing phases (testing set R^2 = 0.9586) was not optimal (as shown in Figure 6), being slightly inferior to the CLSA model containing only spatial attention (testing set R^2 = 0.9621).

3.4. VO_2 Prediction Performance Across Exercise Intensity Zones

As shown in Figure 7, the model fit well at the initial time steps of the experiment, but its performance declined in the later stages. For an in-depth analysis, this paper presents the scatter plot regression results of the predicted values and actual VO_2 values of the five models on the test dataset (containing data from three individuals) in Figure 8. The intensity grading thresholds were based on the guidelines proposed by the American College of Sports Medicine (ACSM) in the 11th edition of the 'Exercise Testing and Prescription Guidelines': low intensity (<46% VO_2max, <1.80 L·min^{-1}), moderate intensity (46–63% VO_2max, 1.80–2.47 L·min^{-1}), and high intensity (≥64% VO_2max, ≥2.51 L·min^{-1}) [17]. At low intensities, all five models showed a tendency to overestimate, with LSTM showing the largest deviation. As the intensity reached moderate levels, the model prediction shifted to a slight underestimation. Convolutional feature extraction effectively converged the error, with the CNN-LSTM slope approaching 1 and the CLSA points being the most concentrated. During high-intensity exercise, all models showed underestimated prediction errors that were significantly larger than those in the moderate-to-low intensity stages, indicating that the models had difficulty accurately capturing VO_2 changes in this intensity range. Among them, LSTM performed the worst, while CLSA and CLSTA, which fused channel attention, were closest to the ideal line. The performance of the five models was consistent with the R^2 ranking in Tables 4 and 5, indicating that 'convolutional feature extraction + spatial attention' is an effective means of suppressing errors and improving R^2.

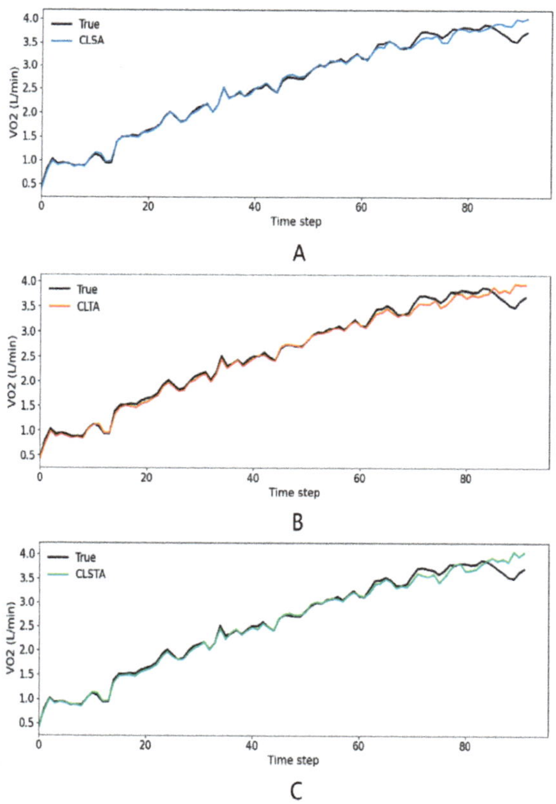

Figure 7. Predicted vs. actual VO_2 curves during exercise from different models: (**A**) CLSA, (**B**) CLTA, and (**C**) CLSTA.

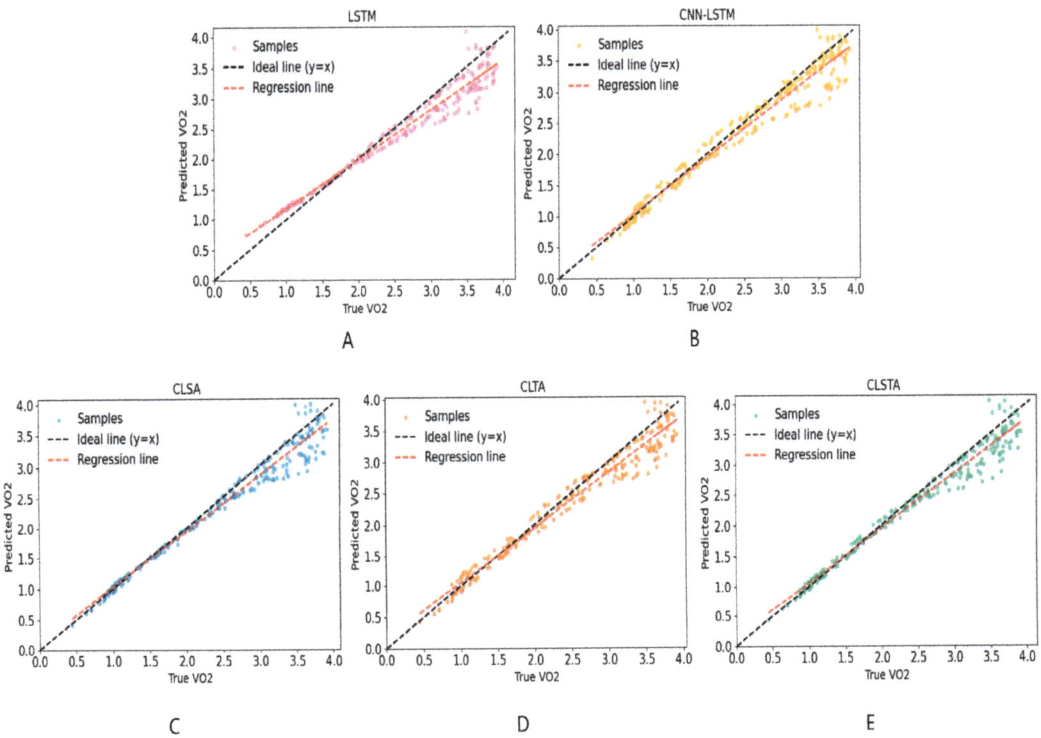

Figure 8. Predicted vs. true VO_2 scatter-regression plots on the test set for five models: (**A**)—LSTM, (**B**)—CNN-LSTM, (**C**)—CLSA, (**D**)—CLTA, and (**E**)—CLSTA.

4. Discussion

Previous studies predicting VO_2 during exercise were limited in terms of both 'input dimensions' and 'model depth.' Most studies only used heart rate, or simply added breathing parameters on top of that; on the other hand, algorithms mainly relied on simple regression or RNN models without the systematic exploration of feature extraction. Lu et al. (2024) used a backpropagation neural network with chest strap ECG/PPG-HR combined with respiratory rate and minute ventilation as input variables to obtain an MAE of 165 $mL \cdot min^{-1}$ [18]. Bangaru et al. (2025) used forearm IMU + electromyography signals and a Bi-LSTM to achieve a lower error of 1.26 $mL \cdot kg^{-1} \cdot min^{-1}$, but this required additional sensor deployment [19]. To address the above limitations, this study constructed and compared five models—LSTM, CNN-LSTM, CLSA, CLTA, and CLSTA—within the same dataset. These models combined spatial, temporal, and spatio-temporal attention mechanisms and were evaluated for their performance in predicting oxygen consumption during exercise. Compared with previous studies, we attempted to use commonly available and easily collected three-axis accelerometers and heart rate as dynamic input variables. At the algorithm level, we not only introduced a convolution module to extract local motion patterns but also systematically examined the benefits and limitations of the attention mechanism. The CLSA model with the best performance in the model constructed in this study achieved an R^2 of 0.96, which was an improvement over previous studies. The results showed the following. (1) Combining accelerometer and heart rate data improved the accuracy of oxygen uptake prediction compared to using the heart rate alone. (2) The introduction of the CNN module improved model performance compared to using the LSTM model alone. (3) The introduction of attention mechanisms led to performance fluctuations. Among them, the SAM could improve model performance while the TAM alone did not improve model performance compared to the baseline CNN-LSTM, indicating that attention mechanisms do not always bring gains. At the same time, the CLSTA model, which simply stacked spatial and temporal attention mechanisms, also did not perform optimally. (4) In terms of the predictive accuracy of oxygen uptake at different exercise intensity stages, the five models constructed all showed lower predictive performance at high-oxygen-uptake stages than at moderate and low-oxygen-uptake stages.

4.1. Enhanced VO_2 Prediction Using Accelerometer–Heart Rate Fusion

In this study, we used accelerometer and heart rate signals as dynamic features in the input variables of the VO_2 prediction model. In fact, accelerometer signals reflect the mechanical work generated by the movement itself while the heart rate reflects the body's physiological response to the movement stimulus. The two respectively reflect the internal and external load conditions during exercise.

Research indicates that cumulative triaxial acceleration data is highly correlated with various physiological indicators (such as muscle oxygen content and maximum oxygen uptake) [20]. In this study, the fluctuation characteristics of the accelerometer signals (Figure 6A) and their vector integrals VM (Figure 6C) further corroborated the above correlation. As can be seen from Figure 6, VM fluctuated violently during high-intensity exercise and at the beginning of exercise (when the exercise amplitude changed significantly). However, when the subjects adapted to the running rhythm and performed regular exercises with small amplitude changes, the VM fluctuation frequency decreased significantly. This phenomenon was consistent with Sheridan's limitation that 'slow movements are easily ignored by the system,' revealing the bottleneck in identifying low-dynamic activities through accelerometer signals [21].

The heart rate reflects the body's physiological response to exercise stimuli and is one of the most widely used means of quantifying internal load. This is also consistent with Fick's principle, whereby an increase in cardiac output increases oxygen delivery and uptake, resulting in a positive correlation between the heart rate and VO_2 in a steady state [22]. However, using the heart rate alone also has its limitations. On the one hand, the heart rate is influenced by physiological factors such as the maximum heart rate and resting heart rate. On the other hand, in exercises with rapidly changing rhythms, the heart rate alone cannot accurately reflect sudden changes in intensity, and it is easily affected by factors unrelated to exercise (e.g., the heart rate may increase due to emotional tension) [23].

VO_2 is an output of complex physiological processes and is determined by both external exercise power and internal physiological status. Accelerometer data ensures that the model knows 'what exercise was performed,' while heart rate data lets the model know 'what kind of response the body experienced.'

Previous studies have shown that inputting motion measurement signals such as acceleration and physiological signals such as the heart rate into a non-linear model can significantly reduce VO_2 estimation errors [21]. As shown in Table 4, this study also found that the combined model was able to capture changes in exercise intensity, thus far exceeding single data source models in terms of prediction accuracy and reliability [24].

4.2. The Key Role of CNN in Predicting Oxygen Uptake

In one-dimensional time series applications, CNNs slide over continuous inputs (such as the heart rate or accelerometer signals). This type of local feature learning is well suited for capturing waveform patterns in motion data. This study shows that, compared with the independent LSTM model, introducing a CNN layer can significantly reduce prediction errors and improve the goodness of fit (Table 4). This finding is highly consistent with research conclusions in exercise physiology and related fields. For example, Lee's energy expenditure study based on IMU found that when predicting steady-state energy expenditure, their CNN-LSTM hybrid model demonstrated the best performance among three models (CNN, LSTM, and CNN-LSTM) [25]. Hossain pointed out in energy estimation research that CNN-LSTM models show better performance than simpler networks [26]. Amelard also found that convolutional networks achieved high VO_2 prediction accuracy [27]. The CNN layer effectively captures key action features related to VO_2 changes by extracting local spatial patterns in time series, thereby improving feature extraction capabilities. The subsequent LSTM layers further model the dynamic evolution of these features over time. The combination of the two achieves collaborative modeling of spatial and temporal characteristics, thereby significantly improving the model's ability to characterize VO_2 change trends [28].

4.3. The Impact of the Attention Mechanism on Predicting Oxygen Uptake

As shown in Table 5, compared with the original CNN-LSTM model without attention mechanisms, the introduction of spatial and temporal attention mechanisms resulted in different changes in the model, indicating that the introduction of attention modules does not necessarily improve performance in all cases. Improper or mismatched attention mechanism designs may cause fluctuations in model performance. This phenomenon is consistent with the conclusions of some existing studies: as pointed out by Vaswani, the use of attention mechanisms needs to be combined with task characteristics for targeted design to avoid blindly adding them and causing negative effects [29]. The CLSTA model, which combines temporal and spatial attention, performs worse than the CLSA model, which only includes spatial attention, on the training set. This suggests that simply stacking temporal and spatial attention modules may introduce optimization conflicts or learning redundancy, thereby weakening the actual improvement of the model. Previous studies have also observed similar phenomena: excessive stacking of attention layers does not effectively fuse multiple dependent features [30,31].

The spatial attention mechanism used in this study employs an SE attention module, which is essentially a channel attention mechanism. In the context of the heart rate and acceleration fusion, different channels represent different physiological meanings: the heart rate channel reflects the heart's oxygen supply response, while the three acceleration channels reflect the intensity of movement in different directions of the body. The SE attention module can automatically adjust the weights of these channels based on the motion state, allowing the model to focus on more informative signals at different stages [32]. For example, during steady moderate-intensity exercise, the heart rate is approximately linearly correlated with VO_2 and responds relatively smoothly. At this time, heart rate signals are more indicative of VO_2 predictions, and the SE module may increase the weight of heart-rate-related features. Similarly, during high-intensity interval training, acceleration signals fluctuate dramatically while the heart rate increases with a delay. The model can use channel attention to focus more on features related to instantaneous exercise intensity in the acceleration channel.

In contrast, in time series applications, the temporal attention mechanism is typically viewed as attention to time steps, i.e., assigning weights to the features at each time point. Ideally, temporal attention allows the model to 'focus' on the moments that contribute most to the current VO_2 prediction [33]. However, physiological changes in the VO_2 are smooth and continuous, with a delayed effect. When the intensity of exercise changes, oxygen consumption does not instantly reach a new level but gradually changes through several stages. This means that the VO_2 value at a given moment is the result of the cumulative effect of exercise intensity over a period of time, rather than being determined solely by the current instantaneous heart rate and exercise conditions [34]. After introducing temporal attention, the model may tend to assign excessive weight to certain time points and ignore information from other time periods. For example, the model shown in Figure 6 may overemphasize the heart rate and acceleration peaks at the end of the input sequence, where changes are dramatic. However, due to the lagging characteristics of VO_2, this approach may mislead the model: short-term dramatic changes do not mean that VO_2 will immediately surge proportionally. The improper allocation of time attention may sever the continuous cumulative relationship of the VO_2 signal, causing the model to miss early information that contributes to the current VO_2.

The results indicate that attention mechanisms have great potential for improving model performance, but their effectiveness depends on reasonable module design and integration methods. In subsequent studies, attention modules will be optimized according to task requirements to maximize performance gains and avoid unnecessary performance degradation.

4.4. Increased Error in VO_2 Prediction Model During High-Intensity Exercise Phases

During high-intensity exercise, all models showed significantly increased prediction errors compared to the moderate- and low-intensity phases. In Figure 8, the deviation of the scatter points from the ideal line was significantly larger in each sub-figure. Amelard also pointed out that deep learning models perform well in VO_2 time series prediction, but their performance under different exercise intensity conditions needs further validation [27]. First, this may be related to the fact that as exercise intensity increases, physiological responses (such as the relationship between the heart rate and oxygen consumption) become more complex and non-linear. Some literature indicates that at very low or very high exercise intensities, the relationship between the heart rate and VO_2 becomes significantly non-linear [9]. Secondly, the duration of high-intensity exercise maintained by the subjects was short, resulting in a sample size that was significantly lower than that in the moderate-to-low intensity range. In addition, the attention mechanism had a defect of 'weak local perception,' i.e., limited ability to capture instantaneous rapid changes [35]. Finally, during high-intensity exercise (exceeding the lactate threshold or critical power), human VO_2 kinetics exhibit greater delays and fluctuations [36]. These multiple factors together exacerbated the uncertainty of the model's predictions during high-intensity exercise phases.

Furthermore, research has shown that when continuous targets have a skewed distribution, the lack of observations in certain intervals makes it difficult for a model to 'see' and learn the correct mapping relationships in these intervals, thereby reducing its generalization ability across the entire target range [37]. For the oxygen uptake prediction dataset, high-intensity exercise samples account for only about 36%, which is a relatively small proportion. This imbalance in the target output distribution weakens the model's generalization performance in the high-intensity range. During training, the model primarily optimizes the overall loss, thus paying more attention to medium- and low-intensity samples, which account for a large proportion of the data, and not paying enough attention to high-intensity samples, which account for a relatively small proportion of the data. In addition, high-intensity exercise data itself may have high physiological heterogeneity and noise. Different individuals have large differences in VO_2 responses at extreme intensities, making it more difficult to learn reliable patterns when there are insufficient samples. Therefore, for the model used in this study, the high-intensity portion of the training data was relatively limited, causing the model to make predictions based on limited experience in this range, which naturally led to a decrease in accuracy. In future research, we will further consider appropriate data augmentation, reweighting, or stratified modeling for high-intensity samples to mitigate the impact of sample imbalance on the model.

5. Conclusions

This study used dynamic and static physiological data obtained from resting test and CPET to construct five models based on LSTM, CNN-LSTM, and CNN-LSTM with three attention mechanisms introduced. The models successfully predicted oxygen uptake during exercise. We proposed two innovations: first, we established a multi-source input fusion strategy to optimize feature representation by combining accelerometer dynamic signals with static heart rate data; second, we designed an attention-optimized path to systematically explore the synergistic mechanisms of three attention mechanisms in the CNN-LSTM architecture. The results indicate the following. (1) Combining accelerometer and heart rate data improves the accuracy of oxygen uptake prediction compared to using the heart rate alone. (2) The introduction of the CNN module is beneficial for improving the performance of the oxygen consumption prediction model. (3) Attention mechanisms do not always improve oxygen uptake predictions, and simply stacking attention mechanisms in a prediction model does not necessarily yield the best results. (4) The model's predictive performance is poor at high oxygen uptake levels, and further consideration is needed to resolve this issue. This paper not only provides a new methodological reference for predicting physiological parameters but also offers practical application value for real-time monitoring in the field of sports science. However, this study was still limited by its small sample size and limited data diversity. In future studies, we will expand the cross-group sample size and develop high-intensity error compensation algorithms to achieve more accurate oxygen uptake predictions.

Author Contributions: Z.W., L.P. and Y.S. performed the theoretical analysis. L.P., S.L. and G.S. supervised the writing of the manuscript. Y.S. and Z.W. designed the experimental scheme. Z.W. conducted the experiment. Z.W. and L.P. analyzed the data and wrote the original manuscript. Z.W., S.L., L.P., Y.S. and G.S. provided financial support. All authors have read and agreed to the published version of the manuscript.

Funding: This study was financially supported by Gang Sun (Beijing Science and Technology Plan Project, Grant No. Z221100005222031).

Institutional Review Board Statement: The study adhered to the ethical standards outlined in the Declaration of Helsinki. The ethics committee of the Capital University of Physical Education and Sports approved this study (REC number: 2024A098). The participants signed freely given informed consent to participate in the study and to have the study results anonymously disclosed.

Informed Consent Statement: Informed consent was obtained from all subjects involved in the study.

Data Availability Statement: The data presented in this study are available on request from the corresponding author.

Conflicts of Interest: The authors declare no conflict of interest.

Abbreviations

The following abbreviations have been used in this manuscript:

VO_2	Oxygen Uptake
HR	Heart Rate
ACC	Accelerate
CPET	Cardiopulmonary exercise testing
BMI	Body Mass Index
LSTM	Long Short-Term Memory
CNN	Convolutional Neural Network
SAM	Spatial Attention Module

TAM	Time Attention Mechanism
STAM	Spatio-temporal Attention Module
CLSA	CNN-SAM-LSTM model
CLTA	CNN-TAM-LSTM model
CLSTA	CNN-STAM-LSTM model
RMSE	Root Mean Square Error
MAE	Mean Absolute Error

References

1. Laukkanen, J.A.; Isiozor, N.M.; Kunutsor, S.K. Objectively Assessed Cardiorespiratory Fitness and All-Cause Mortality Risk. *Mayo Clin. Proc.* **2022**, *97*, 1054–1073. [CrossRef]
2. Jones, A.M.; Carter, H. The Effect of Endurance Training on Parameters of Aerobic Fitness. *Sports Med.* **2000**, *29*, 373–386. [CrossRef] [PubMed]
3. Whipp, J.B.; Ward, A.S. Gas Exchange Dynamics and the Tolerance to Muscular Exercise: Effects of Fitness and Training. *Ann. Physiol. Anthropol.* **1992**, *11*, 207–214. [CrossRef]
4. Guazzi, M.; Adams, V.; Conraads, V.; Halle, M.; Mezzani, A.; Vanhees, L.; Arena, R.; Fletcher, G.F.; Forman, D.E.; Kitzman, D.W.; et al. Clinical Recommendations for Cardiopulmonary Exercise Testing Data Assessment in Specific Patient Populations. *Circulation* **2012**, *126*, 2261–2274. [CrossRef] [PubMed]
5. Crouter, S.E.; Antczak, A.; Hudak, J.R.; DellaValle, D.M.; Haas, J.D. Accuracy and Reliability of the ParvoMedics TrueOne 2400 and MedGraphics VO2000 Metabolic Systems. *Eur. J. Appl. Physiol.* **2006**, *98*, 139–151. [CrossRef]
6. Van Hooren, B.; Souren, T.; Bongers, B.C. Accuracy of Respiratory Gas Variables, Substrate, and Energy Use from 15 CPET Systems During Simulated and Human Exercise. *Scand. J. Med. Sci. Sports* **2024**, *34*, e14490. [CrossRef] [PubMed]
7. Wicks, J.R.; Oldridge, N.B.; Nielsen, L.K.; Vickers, C.E. HR Index—A Simple Method for the Prediction of Oxygen Uptake. *Med. Sci. Sports Exerc.* **2011**, *43*, 2005–2012. [CrossRef]
8. Keytel, L.; Goedecke, J.; Noakes, T.; Hiiloskorpi, H.; Laukkanen, R.; Van Der Merwe, L.; Lambert, E. Prediction of Energy Expenditure from Heart Rate Monitoring During Submaximal Exercise. *J. Sports Sci.* **2005**, *23*, 289–297. [CrossRef]
9. Davidson, P.; Trinh, H.; Vekki, S.; Müller, P. Surrogate Modelling for Oxygen Uptake Prediction Using LSTM Neural Network. *Sensors* **2023**, *23*, 2249. [CrossRef]
10. Li, F.; Chang, C.-H.; Chung, Y.-C.; Wu, H.-J.; Kan, N.-W.; ChangChien, W.-S.; Ho, C.-S.; Huang, C.-C. Development and Validation of 3 Min Incremental Step-In-Place Test for Predicting Maximal Oxygen Uptake in Home Settings: A Submaximal Exercise Study to Assess Cardiorespiratory Fitness. *Int. J. Environ. Res. Public Health* **2021**, *18*, 10750. [CrossRef]
11. DiPietro, R.; Hager, G.D. Deep learning: RNNs and LSTM. In *Handbook of Medical Image Computing and Computer Assisted Intervention*; Elsevier: Amsterdam, The Netherlands, 2020; pp. 503–519.
12. Porszasz, J.; Casaburi, R.; Somfay, A.; Woodhouse, L.J.; Whipp, B.J. A Treadmill Ramp Protocol Using Simultaneous Changes in Speed and Grade. *Med. Sci. Sports Exerc.* **2003**, *35*, 1596–1603. [CrossRef] [PubMed]
13. Mei, P.; Li, M.; Zhang, Q.; Li, G.; Song, L. Prediction Model of Drinking Water Source Quality with Potential Industrial-Agricultural Pollution Based on CNN-GRU-Attention. *J. Hydrol.* **2022**, *610*, 127934. [CrossRef]
14. Guo, M.-H.; Xu, T.-X.; Liu, J.-J.; Liu, Z.-N.; Jiang, P.-T.; Mu, T.-J.; Zhang, S.-H.; Martin, R.R.; Cheng, M.-M.; Hu, S.-M. Attention Mechanisms in Computer Vision: A Survey. *Comput. Vis. Media* **2022**, *8*, 331–368. [CrossRef]
15. Hu, J.; Shen, L.; Sun, G. Squeeze-and-Excitation Networks. In Proceedings of the IEEE Conference on Computer Vision and Pattern Recognition, Salt Lake City, UT, USA, 18–22 June 2018; pp. 7132–7141.
16. Woo, S.; Park, J.; Lee, J.-Y.; Kweon, I.S. CBAM: Convolutional Block Attention Module. In *Computer Vision—ECCV 2018*; Ferrari, V., Hebert, M., Sminchisescu, C., Weiss, Y., Eds.; Lecture Notes in Computer Science; Springer International Publishing: Cham, Switzerland, 2018; Volume 11211, pp. 3–19, ISBN 978-3-030-01233-5.
17. American College of Sports Medicine. *ACSM's Guidelines for Exercise Testing and Prescription*, 11th ed.; Wolters Kluwer: Philadelphia, PA, USA, 2021; ISBN 978-1-9751-5326-4.
18. Lu, Z.; Yang, J.; Tao, K.; Li, X.; Xu, H.; Qiu, J. Combined Impact of Heart Rate Sensor Placements with Respiratory Rate and Minute Ventilation on Oxygen Uptake Prediction. *Sensors* **2024**, *24*, 5412. [CrossRef] [PubMed]
19. Bangaru, S.S.; Wang, C.; Aghazadeh, F.; Muley, S.; Willoughby, S. Oxygen Uptake Prediction for Timely Construction Worker Fatigue Monitoring Through Wearable Sensing Data Fusion. *Sensors* **2025**, *25*, 3204. [CrossRef]
20. Gómez-Carmona, C.D.; Bastida-Castillo, A.; Ibáñez, S.J.; Pino-Ortega, J. Accelerometry as a Method for External Workload Monitoring in Invasion Team Sports. A Systematic Review. *PLoS ONE* **2020**, *15*, e0236643. [CrossRef]

21. Sheridan, D.; Jaspers, A.; Viet Cuong, D.; Op De Beéck, T.; Moyna, N.M.; de Beukelaar, T.T.; Roantree, M. Estimating Oxygen Uptake in Simulated Team Sports Using Machine Learning Models and Wearable Sensor Data: A Pilot Study. *PLoS ONE* **2025**, *20*, e0319760. [CrossRef]
22. Nakamura, T.; Kiyono, K.; Wendt, H.; Abry, P.; Yamamoto, Y. Multiscale Analysis of Intensive Longitudinal Biomedical Signals and Its Clinical Applications. *Proc. IEEE* **2016**, *104*, 242–261. [CrossRef]
23. Ernst, G. Heart-Rate Variability—More than Heart Beats? *Front. Public Health* **2017**, *5*, 240. [CrossRef]
24. De Brabandere, A.; Op De Beéck, T.; Schütte, K.H.; Meert, W.; Vanwanseele, B.; Davis, J. Data Fusion of Body-Worn Accelerometers and Heart Rate to Predict VO2max during Submaximal Running. *PLoS ONE* **2018**, *13*, e0199509. [CrossRef]
25. Lee, C.J.; Lee, J.K. IMU-Based Energy Expenditure Estimation for Various Walking Conditions Using a Hybrid CNN–LSTM Model. *Sensors* **2024**, *24*, 414. [CrossRef] [PubMed]
26. Hossain, M.B.; LaMunion, S.R.; Crouter, S.E.; Melanson, E.L.; Sazonov, E. A CNN Model for Physical Activity Recognition and Energy Expenditure Estimation from an Eyeglass-Mounted Wearable Sensor. *Sensors* **2024**, *24*, 3046. [CrossRef] [PubMed]
27. Amelard, R.; Hedge, E.T.; Hughson, R.L. Temporal Convolutional Networks Predict Dynamic Oxygen Uptake Response from Wearable Sensors Across Exercise Intensities. *NPJ Digit. Med.* **2021**, *4*, 156. [CrossRef]
28. Zhu, C.; Liu, Q.; Meng, W.; Ai, Q.; Xie, S.Q. An Attention-Based CNN-LSTM Model with Limb Synergy for Joint Angles Prediction. In Proceedings of the 2021 IEEE/ASME International Conference on Advanced Intelligent Mechatronics (AIM), Delft, The Netherlands, 12–16 July 2021; IEEE: Piscataway, NJ, USA, 2021; pp. 747–752.
29. Vaswani, A.; Shazeer, N.; Parmar, N.; Uszkoreit, J.; Jones, L.; Gomez, A.N.; Kaiser, Ł.; Polosukhin, I. Attention Is All You Need. In *Advances in Neural Information Processing Systems*; MIT Press: Cambridge, MA, USA, 2017; Volume 30.
30. Cao, F.; Yang, S.; Chen, Z.; Liu, Y.; Cui, L. Ister: Inverted Seasonal-Trend Decomposition Transformer for Explainable Multivariate Time Series Forecasting. *arXiv* **2024**, arXiv:2412.18798.
31. Zhou, X.; Sheil, B.; Suryasentana, S.; Shi, P. Multi-Fidelity Fusion for Soil Classification via LSTM and Multi-Head Self-Attention CNN Model. *Adv. Eng. Inform.* **2024**, *62*, 102655. [CrossRef]
32. Zheng, B.; Luo, W.; Zhang, M.; Jin, H. Arrhythmia Classification Based on Multi-Input Convolutional Neural Network with Attention Mechanism. *PLoS ONE* **2025**, *20*, e0326079. [CrossRef]
33. Khan, M.; Hossni, Y. A Comparative Analysis of LSTM Models Aided with Attention and Squeeze and Excitation Blocks for Activity Recognition. *Sci. Rep.* **2025**, *15*, 3858. [CrossRef]
34. Schneider, D.A.; Wing, A.N.; Morris, N.R. Oxygen Uptake and Heart Rate Kinetics During Heavy Exercise: A Comparison Between Arm Cranking and Leg Cycling. *Eur. J. Appl. Physiol.* **2002**, *88*, 100–106. [CrossRef]
35. Zhao, B.; Xing, H.; Wang, X.; Song, F.; Xiao, Z. Rethinking Attention Mechanism in Time Series Classification. *Inf. Sci.* **2023**, *627*, 97–114. [CrossRef]
36. Gløersen, Ø.; Colosio, A.L.; Boone, J.; Dysthe, D.K.; Malthe-Sørenssen, A.; Capelli, C.; Pogliaghi, S. Modeling Vo_2 On-Kinetics Based on Intensity-Dependent Delayed Adjustment and Loss of Efficiency (DALE). *J. Appl. Physiol.* **2022**, *132*, 1480–1488. [CrossRef]
37. Yang, Y.; Zha, K.; Chen, Y.; Wang, H.; Katabi, D. Delving into Deep Imbalanced Regression. In Proceedings of the International Conference on Machine Learning, PMLR, Online, 18–24 July 2021; pp. 11842–11851.

sensors

MDPI

Article

A Comparative Study Between ECG- and PPG-Based Heart Rate Sensors for Heart Rate Variability Measurements: Influence of Body Position, Duration, Sex, and Age

Alexandre Coste [1,*], Geoffrey Millour [1,2] and Christophe Hausswirth [1,3]

1 BeScored Institute, 06560 Valbonne, France
2 Laboratoire Motricité, Interactions, Performance, MIP, UR 4334, Nantes Université, 44109 Nantes, France
3 Inserm CAPS UMR 1093, UFR STAPS, Université Bourgogne Europe, 21078 Dijon, France
* Correspondence: alexandre@bescored.fr

Abstract

This study evaluated the validity of a photoplethysmography (PPG)-based sensor (Polar OH1) for measuring heart rate variability (HRV), compared to an electrocardiography (ECG)-based reference device (Polar H10), considering body position (supine vs. seated), recording duration (2 vs. 5 min), sex, and age (≤40 vs. >40 years). HRV parameters (RMSSD and SDNN) were analyzed in 31 healthy adults using intraclass correlation coefficients (ICCs) and Bland–Altman analyses. Excellent reliability was observed between the devices in the supine position (RMSSD: ICC = 0.955; SDNN: ICC = 0.980), and good to excellent reliability in the seated position (RMSSD: ICC = 0.834; SDNN: ICC = 0.921). Mean biases ranged from −2.1 ms to −8.1 ms, with wider limits of agreement in the seated condition. The change in posture from supine to seated resulted in moderate reliability for both metrics, regardless of the device. Only marginal differences were found between 2- and 5-min recordings. Moreover, agreement was less consistent in older participants and females, suggesting potential effects of age and sex on signal quality. These findings support the use of PPG-based devices for short-term HRV assessment at rest, while highlighting the importance of considering posture, age, and sex when interpreting the results.

Keywords: autonomic nervous system; RMSSD; SDNN; photoplethysmography; electrocardiography; wearable sensors

1. Introduction

In recent years, photoplethysmography (PPG) sensors gained widespread popularity for monitoring heart rate (HR) and heart rate variability (HRV) in wearable devices such as smartwatches and fitness trackers [1]. Unlike electrocardiography (ECG)-based chest straps, which directly measure the heart's electrical activity, PPG relies on optical sensors to estimate HRV by detecting blood volume changes in the peripheral circulation, typically from the wrist or forearm [2]. This approach makes HRV monitoring more accessible and convenient for applications such as lifestyle management, stress assessment, and athletic performance monitoring [1,3–5]. However, despite these advantages, comparative studies evaluating the accuracy and reliability of PPG-based HRV measurements remain limited, particularly when compared to ECG-based measurements, which are considered the gold standard [6].

A fundamental difference between ECG and PPG lies in their measurement mechanisms and recording sites. ECG-based sensors capture the heart's electrical activity directly from the chest, providing precise R–R intervals that enable accurate HRV analysis. In contrast, PPG sensors estimate HRV by detecting peripheral blood volume fluctuations, which are influenced by several factors, such as vascular compliance, pulse arrival time (PAT), pulse transit time (PTT), and microcirculatory regulation [7,8]. As a result, PPG-derived HRV—often referred to as pulse rate variability (PRV)—may differ from ECG-derived HRV due to variations in pulse wave propagation and autonomic regulation at peripheral sites. To such an extent, some authors argue that PRV should be considered a distinct biomarker rather than a surrogate for HRV [9,10].

Several factors may influence the accuracy and comparability of HRV measurements obtained through ECG and PPG. One critical factor is body position. Previous research has shown that autonomic nervous system (ANS) activity varies across postural conditions, with the supine position favoring parasympathetic dominance, while seated or upright positions are associated with increased sympathetic activity [2,6]. PPG has been reported to overestimate parasympathetic activity, particularly in non-supine positions, due to variability in pulse arrival time (PAT) and pulse transit time (PTT) [11,12]. As a result, differences in body position may amplify discrepancies between HRV metrics derived from PPG and those obtained from ECG.

Another important factor influencing HRV measurements is the duration of the recording. Standard HRV assessments typically rely on 5 min recordings, as recommended by the Task Force of the European Society of Cardiology and the North American Society of Pacing and Electrophysiology [13]. However, ultra-short-term recordings (e.g., 2 min) have been proposed as a more practical alternative for use in applied settings [14]. While frequency domain and non-linear HRV metrics can often be reliably estimated from shorter recordings, time domain parameters such as the root mean square of successive differences (RMSSD), and the standard deviation of normal-to-normal intervals (SDNN) generally require longer durations to ensure accuracy [11,13]. Moreover, shorter recordings are more vulnerable to noise and motion artifacts, especially when using PPG-based sensors, as peripheral blood flow is highly sensitive to external disturbances [15,16]. It is therefore recommended to perform HRV measurements at rest.

Individual factors, such as age and sex, also play a key role in HRV variability and measurement accuracy. HRV tends to decline with age due to reduced autonomic flexibility, with time domain metrics such as RMSSD and SDNN showing a gradual decrease [17,18]. For example, [18] analyzed 24 h ECG recordings from 1743 subjects aged 40 to 100 years and observed a linear decline in SDNN. Interestingly, RMSSD followed a U-shaped pattern, decreasing between ages 40 and 60 before increasing again after 70, suggesting complex interactions between aging and autonomic function. Similarly, [19] found that the most significant HRV reductions occur between the second and third decades of life. Sex-related differences in HRV have also been extensively documented. Females generally exhibit greater parasympathetic activity, which influences HRV parameters and results in shorter R–R intervals compared to males [20]. This relative vagal dominance in females has been linked to cardiovascular protective effects but may also lead to differences in HRV measurement reliability across sensor modalities. In contrast, males tend to show greater sympathetic dominance, which can cause more pronounced discrepancies in HRV parameters between ECG and PPG due to their differing sensitivities to autonomic fluctuations [2,19]. Additionally, vascular properties, such as arterial stiffness and endothelial function, which vary between males and females, may further affect PPG-derived HRV measurements by influencing pulse wave propagation and peripheral circulation dynamics [21].

In light of these considerations, the aim of this study is to investigate differences in HRV parameters, specifically RMSSD and SDNN, obtained from ECG and PPG signals. We assess how body position (supine vs. seated), measurement duration (2 min vs. 5 min), and individual factors, such as age and sex, affect the comparability of HRV measures between these two modalities. By accounting for these variables, we aim to improve our understanding of the reliability of PPG-based HRV and its applicability in different populations and settings.

2. Materials and Methods

2.1. Participants

Thirty-one healthy participants were recruited for the study. Their characteristics, including age, height, and body mass, are summarized in Table 1. Inclusion criteria required participants to be between 18 and 70 years old, free of known heart conditions or diseases, and without hypertension. Additionally, due to the influence of skin pigmentation on PPG measurements [22], only individuals with Fitzpatrick skin phototypes I, II, or III were included. Exclusion criteria were regular use of medications affecting the cardiovascular or endocrine systems, current smoking, or pregnancy. All participants received detailed information about the study's purpose, procedures, potential risks, and benefits, and provided written informed consent prior to participation. The study protocol was approved by the National Ethics Committee (ethical approval: IRB00012476-2024-13-11-352) and conducted in accordance with the 2024 Declaration of Helsinki [23].

2.2. Apparatus

Two commercially available devices were used to collect HRV data during the study:

Polar H10 Chest Strap

The Polar H10 (Polar Electro Oy, Kempele, Finland) is a high-precision chest strap heart rate monitor widely used in sports and research for HRV analysis [24]. Equipped with two electrodes embedded in the chest strap, it detects the electrical signals generated by the heart with each beat. These signals are used to calculate the R–R intervals, which represent the time intervals between successive R-wave peaks in the ECG signal. R–R intervals are essential for HRV analysis, as they reflect the autonomic nervous system's regulation of cardiac function. In this study, raw R–R interval data were recorded using the Elite HRV app (Elite HRV, Inc., Asheville, NC, USA) and analyzed with the MATLAB software (R2022a, The MathWorks, Natick, MA, USA).

Polar OH1 PPG Sensor

The Polar OH1 (Polar Electro Oy, Kempele, Finland) is a wearable heart rate sensor that uses PPG technology to measure HR by detecting changes in blood volume. It has been validated in sports settings, demonstrating high accuracy for heart rate measurement, particularly when chest and arm movements are limited [25]. Worn on the upper arm, it employs the same PPG technology found in many modern fitness trackers and smartwatches, utilizing green LEDs. In this study, the peak-to-peak interval (PPI) mode of the Polar OH1 was activated using the official Polar Software Development Kit (SDK, https://github.com/polarofficial/polar-ble-sdk accessed on 4 November 2024), enabling the extraction of pulse rate variability (PRV) data. The sensor was connected via Bluetooth to a custom-built web application developed in JavaScript using the Web Bluetooth API, which enabled real-time acquisition and storage of PPG data. To minimize interference from arm movements, the Polar OH1 was worn on the non-dominant arm (i.e., left forearm for right-handed participants and right forearm for left-handed participants). This placement was chosen to avoid any potential movement-related interference, even though all measurements were taken at rest in a static position.

2.3. Study Design and Procedures

We employed a cross-over design where all participants completed both seated and supine conditions in a randomized order. Data were collected from December 2024 to March 2025, between 11:00 A.M. and 7:00 P.M. Testing was conducted on a massage table for the supine position and a comfortable office chair for the seated position. All measurements took place in a controlled environment (quiet, dark room) to minimize sensory interference. Participants were instructed to relax, breathe normally, and keep their eyes closed throughout the 5 min measurement sessions, each preceded by a 1 min stabilization phase to allow heart rate to return to baseline. The Polar H10 and Polar OH1 sensors were synchronized for simultaneous recording, enabling direct comparison of ECG- and PPG-based HRV measurements.

2.4. Data Analysis

All data were stored in an electronic database, then preprocessed and analyzed using MATLAB and Microsoft Excel (Redmond, Washington, DC, USA). Time domain HRV metrics, including RMSSD and SDNN, were extracted from both the Polar H10 and Polar OH1 devices using the HRVTool MATLAB toolbox [26,27]. Two filters were tested [26,28] to identify the most accurate method for processing R–R intervals. We selected the HRV.RRfilter function, which minimizes fluctuations exceeding 15% of the previous interval, helping to remove artifacts while preserving physiologically relevant HRV variations [26]. To compare HRV parameters between devices and conditions, we used intraclass correlation coefficients (ICCs), mean absolute error (MAE), root mean square error (RMSE), and Bland–Altman analysis. ICCs were interpreted according to [29]: <0.50 = poor, 0.50–0.75 = moderate, 0.75–0.90 = good, and >0.90 = excellent reliability. Bland–Altman analysis calculated mean differences and 95% limits of agreement (LoA). Measurements were analyzed over 2 and 5 min intervals, with primary focus on the 5 min window to enable comparisons by sex (male vs. female) and age group (≤40 years vs. >40 years). The 5 min duration is standard for short-term HRV assessment, providing stable results during normal breathing [6]. The 2 min segment was taken from the middle of the 5 min recording, starting 1 min 30 s after onset and ending 1 min 30 s before completion, to avoid artifacts typically present at the beginning (due to stabilization) and the end (due to anticipatory movements) of measurements [30].

3. Results

3.1. Participant Characteristics

Table 1 shows the general characteristics of our study sample. Descriptive statistics are provided for age, height, and body mass.

Table 1. General participant characteristics and subgroup breakdown by age (≤40 vs. >40) and sex (male vs. female). Values are presented as mean ± standard deviation, with minimum and maximum values in brackets. n: number of participants.

	Overall Participants (n = 31)
Sex (number)	Female: 18—Male: 13
Age (years)	43 ± 12 [21–66]
Height (m)	1.71 ± 0.09 [1.50–1.89]
Body mass (kg)	72 ± 16 [46–115]

Table 1. *Cont.*

	Overall Participants (n = 31)	
	≤40 years old (n = 14)	**>40 years old (n = 17)**
Sex (number)	Female: 8—Male: 6	Female: 10—Male: 7
Age (years)	33 ± 5 [21–40]	52 ± 7 [41–66]
Height (m)	1.73 ± 0.10 [1.59–1.89]	1.69 ± 0.09 [1.50–1.85]
Body mass (kg)	77 ± 19 [50–115]	67 ± 13 [46–89]
	Females (n = 18)	**Males (n = 13)**
Age (years)	44 ± 12 [23–66]	43 ± 12 [21–63]
Height (m)	1.65 ± 0.06 [1.50–1.75]	1.78 ± 0.07 [1.64–1.89]
Body mass (kg)	67 ± 18 [46–115]	78 ± 12 [62–100]

3.2. Impact of Sensor Type on HRV Parameters

The comparison between the two sensors demonstrated good agreement for HRV measurements across both recording durations, particularly in the supine position (see Figure 1 and Table 2). For RMSSD, ICCs (3,1) between the Polar H10 and OH1 were good to excellent in the supine position (ICC = 0.955 for 5 min; 0.869 for 2 min) and remained good in the seated position (ICC = 0.834 for 5 min; 0.868 for 2 min). Mean differences between the H10 and OH1 were relatively small when supine (−3.21 ms for 5 min; −2.91 ms for 2 min), increasing slightly in the seated position (−8.05 ms for 5 min; −6.14 ms for 2 min). A similar pattern was observed for SDNN, with excellent ICCs (3,1) in both supine (ICC = 0.980 for 5 min; 0.929 for 2 min) and seated (ICC = 0.921 for 5 min; 0.916 for 2 min) positions. Mean differences for SDNN were small in the supine position (−2.11 ms for 5 min; −2.63 ms for 2 min) and slightly larger in the seated position (−6.02 ms for 5 min; −5.23 ms for 2 min), accompanied by wider limits of agreement (LoA). MAE and RMSE values mirrored these trends, with lower errors observed in the supine position compared to seated.

3.3. Impact of Body Position on HRV Parameters

When comparing the effect of body position, HRV values remained generally consistent between the supine and seated conditions for both sensors, although reliability decreased and variability increased. ICCs (3,1) for the OH1 were slightly lower than those for the H10 and fell within the moderate range (RMSSD 5 min: 0.560 vs. 0.608; SDNN 5 min: 0.674 vs. 0.728). A similar pattern was observed for 2 min recordings, with ICCs (3,1) dropping into the poor-to-moderate range (RMSSD 2 min: 0.468 vs. 0.482; SDNN 2 min: 0.507 vs. 0.621). Notably, SDNN consistently showed higher reliability than RMSSD across all durations and sensors. Mean differences between body positions were small to moderate for both sensors (−5.32 ms to 1.35 ms for H10; −7.92 ms to −1.89 ms for OH1), but the limits of agreement remained wide across devices, regardless of HRV metric or recording duration. MAE and RMSE values between postures followed a similar trend, with slightly larger errors observed for the OH1, particularly in the 2 min condition for SDNN. Nonetheless, the magnitude of error remained comparable between RMSSD and SDNN.

3.4. Influence of Age on HRV Parameters

When comparing HRV parameters between age groups (≤40 vs. >40 years), a general decline in RMSSD and SDNN values was observed with increasing age (see Figure 2 and Table 3). For RMSSD, ICCs (3,1) between the H10 and OH1 were good to excellent across both age groups and body positions (ranging from 0.812 to 0.981), though slightly lower in the seated position and among older participants. Mean differences between sensors were greater in the seated than in the supine position for both younger

(−3.31 ms vs. −1.94 ms) and older participants (−12.08 ms vs. −4.47 ms), with wider limits of agreement (LoA) in the older group. MAE and RMSE values were also higher among older participants, particularly in the seated condition. For SDNN, ICCs (3,1) remained excellent across positions and age groups (0.912–0.984), yet mean differences and LoA were again larger in the older group. MAE and RMSE followed the same pattern, with higher errors observed in older participants and in the seated position. When comparing body positions, RMSSD values were relatively consistent between supine and seated conditions across age groups and sensors, with moderate to good reliability (ICCs: 0.581–0.623). However, mean differences, LoA, MAE, and RMSE were all higher in the older group. For SDNN, ICCs between positions were lower in the younger group than in the older group (0.598 and 0.624 vs. 0.754 and 0.693 for H10 and OH1, respectively), though younger participants displayed smaller mean differences, narrower LoA, and lower MAE and RMSE values.

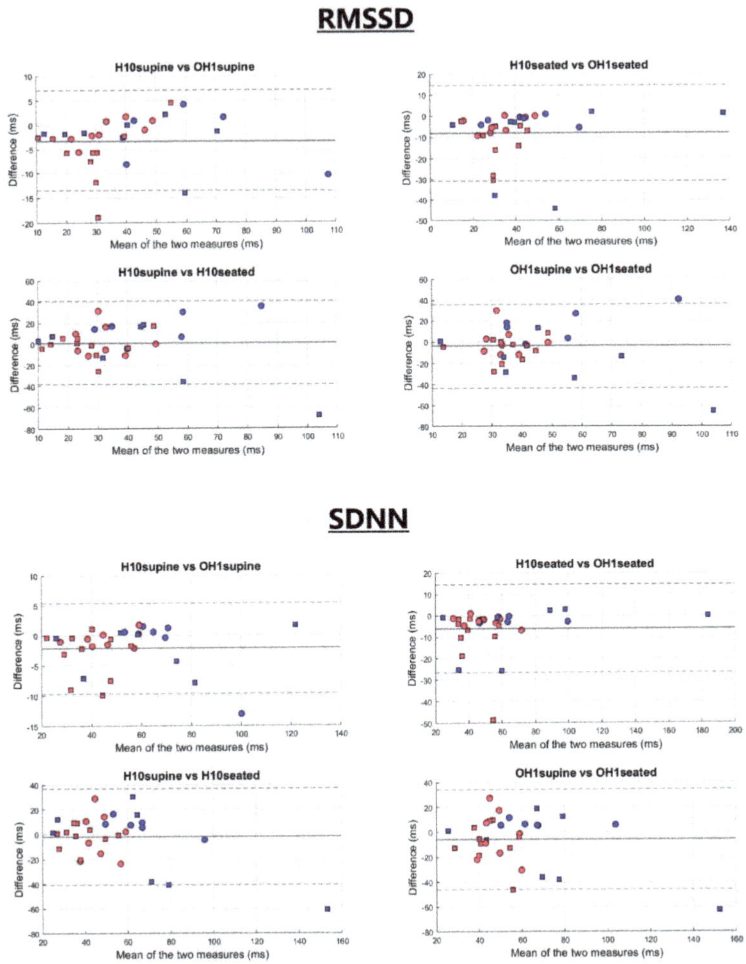

Figure 1. Bland–Altman analysis of RMSSD and SDNN across the different body position conditions (supine and seated) and devices (H10 vs. OH1). The continuous grey line represents the bias, while the dashed grey lines indicate the upper and lower limits of agreement. Markers indicate participant groups: circles for participants aged ≤40 years, squares for participants aged >40 years; blue for men and pink for women.

Table 2. Comparison of RMSSD and SDNN across the different body position conditions (supine and seated) and devices (H10 vs. OH1) using intraclass correlation coefficients (ICC), mean absolute error (MAE), root mean square error (RMSE), and Bland–Altman analysis.

Variables	Conditions (1 vs. 2)	Mean ± SD (1 vs. 2)	ICC (95% CI)	MAE	RMSE	Mean Diff.	Lower LoA	Upper LoA
RMSSD 5 min (ms)	*H10sup.* vs. *OH1sup.*	37 ± 21 vs. 41 ± 20	0.955 (0.911–0.978)	4.32	6.09	−3.21	−13.51	7.09
	H10seat. vs. *OH1seat.*	36 ± 25 vs. 44 ± 23	0.834 (0.699–0.912)	8.33	13.92	−8.05	−30.69	14.59
	H10sup. vs. *H10seat.*	37 ± 21 vs. 36 ± 25	0.608 (0.338–0.786)	13.99	19.85	1.22	−38.25	40.69
	OH1sup. vs. *OH1seat.*	41 ± 20 vs. 44 ± 23	0.560 (0.270–0.756)	14.38	20.23	−3.61	−43.28	36.05
RMSSD 2 min (ms)	*H10sup.* vs. *OH1sup.*	36 ± 18 vs. 39 ± 21	0.869 (0.757–0.931)	5.64	9.98	−2.91	−21.93	16.12
	H10seat. vs. *OH1seat.*	34 ± 22 vs. 41 ± 20	0.868 (0.756–0.931)	6.89	10.72	−6.14	−23.65	11.37
	H10sup. vs. *H10seat.*	36 ± 18 vs. 34 ± 22	0.482 (0.169–0.707)	13.12	19.90	1.35	−38.19	40.88
	OH1sup. vs. *OH1seat.*	39 ± 21 vs. 41 ± 20	0.468 (0.145–0.701)	13.46	20.95	−1.89	−43.47	39.69
SDNN 5 min (ms)	*H10sup.* vs. *OH1sup.*	51 ± 22 vs. 54 ± 22	0.980 (0.959–0.990)	2.72	4.32	−2.11	−9.62	5.40
	H10seat. vs. *OH1seat.*	54 ± 31 vs. 60 ± 29	0.921 (0.848–0.960)	6.43	11.96	−6.02	−26.60	14.57
	H10sup. vs. *H10seat.*	51 ± 22 vs. 54 ± 31	0.728 (0.545–0.845)	14.00	19.54	−2.02	−40.75	36.72
	OH1sup. vs. *OH1seat.*	54 ± 22 vs. 60 ± 29	0.674 (0.454–0.817)	15.44	20.90	−5.92	−45.86	34.02
SDNN 2 min (ms)	*H10sup.* vs. *OH1sup.*	45 ± 21 vs. 48 ± 22	0.929 (0.861–0.964)	4.89	7.96	−2.63	−17.60	12.34
	H10seat. vs. *OH1seat.*	51 ± 31 vs. 56 ± 29	0.916 (0.833–0.957)	6.77	12.28	−5.23	−27.36	16.90
	H10sup. vs. *H10seat.*	45 ± 21 vs. 51 ± 31	0.621 (0.392–0.778)	13.79	22.56	−5.32	−48.99	38.35
	OH1sup. vs. *OH1seat.*	48 ± 22 vs. 56 ± 29	0.507 (0.223–0.712)	17.04	25.92	−7.92	−57.09	41.25

Table 3. Comparison of RMSSD and SDNN between age groups (≤40 vs. >40 years) across the different body position conditions (supine and seated) and devices (H10 vs. OH1) using intraclass correlation coefficients (ICC), mean absolute error (MAE), root mean square error (RMSE), and Bland–Altman analysis.

Variables	Conditions (1 vs. 2)	Mean ± SD (1 vs. 2)	ICC (95% CI)	MAE	RMSE	Mean Diff.	Lower LoA	Upper LoA
RMSSD ≤40 years old (ms)	*H10sup.* vs. *OH1sup.*	42 ± 21 vs. 44 ± 23	0.981 (0.944–0.994)	3.17	4.22	−1.94	−9.89	6.01
	H10seat. vs. *OH1seat.*	35 ± 16 vs. 38 ± 15	0.951 (0.870–0.982)	3.31	4.47	−3.31	−9.91	3.29
	H10sup. vs. *H10seat.*	42 ± 21 vs. 35 ± 16	0.584 (0.207–0.810)	14.11	17.60	7.28	−22.39	36.95
	OH1sup. vs. *OH1seat.*	44 ± 23 vs. 38 ± 15	0.585 (0.228–0.804)	12.93	17.35	5.91	−25.16	36.99

Table 3. *Cont.*

Variables	Conditions (1 vs. 2)	Mean ± SD (1 vs. 2)	ICC (95% CI)	MAE	RMSE	Mean Diff.	Lower LoA	Upper LoA
RMSSD >40 years old (ms)	*H10sup.* vs. *OH1sup.*	31 ± 18 vs. 36 ± 17	0.912 (0.787–0.965)	5.27	7.27	−4.47	−16.06	7.12
	H10seat. vs. *OH1seat.*	36 ± 31 vs. 49 ± 28	0.812 (0.594–0.919)	12.45	18.36	−12.08	−40.01	15.85
	H10sup. vs. *H10seat.*	31 ± 18 vs. 36 ± 31	0.623 (0.335–0.805)	13.89	21.52	−5.11	−47.34	37.13
	OH1sup. vs. *OH1seat.*	36 ± 17 vs. 49 ± 28	0.581 (0.286–0.775)	15.57	22.33	−12.72	−49.80	24.37
SDNN ≤40 years old (ms)	*H10sup.* vs. *OH1sup.*	55 ± 17 vs. 56 ± 19	0.977 (0.941–0.991)	1.89	3.68	−1.08	−8.55	6.39
	H10seat. vs. *OH1seat.*	53 ± 17 vs. 55 ± 18	0.984 (0.957–0.994)	2.46	2.96	−2.46	−6.22	1.30
	H10sup. vs. *H10seat.*	55 ± 17 vs. 53 ± 17	0.598 (0.129–0.849)	12.43	14.57	1.97	−28.46	32.39
	OH1sup. vs. *OH1seat.*	56 ± 19 vs. 55 ± 18	0.624 (0.167–0.860)	12.26	15.08	0.58	−31.17	32.33
SDNN >40 years old (ms)	*H10sup.* vs. *OH1sup.*	48 ± 25 vs. 51 ± 25	0.980 (0.949–0.992)	3.40	4.79	−3.01	−10.53	4.52
	H10seat. vs. *OH1seat.*	53 ± 40 vs. 62 ± 37	0.912 (0.787–0.965)	9.70	15.92	−9.07	−35.50	17.36
	H10sup. vs. *H10seat.*	48 ± 25 vs. 53 ± 40	0.754 (0.542–0.875)	15.31	22.84	−5.50	−50.30	39.30
	OH1sup. vs. *OH1seat.*	51 ± 25 vs. 62 ± 37	0.693 (0.423–0.850)	18.05	24.69	−11.57	−55.63	32.49

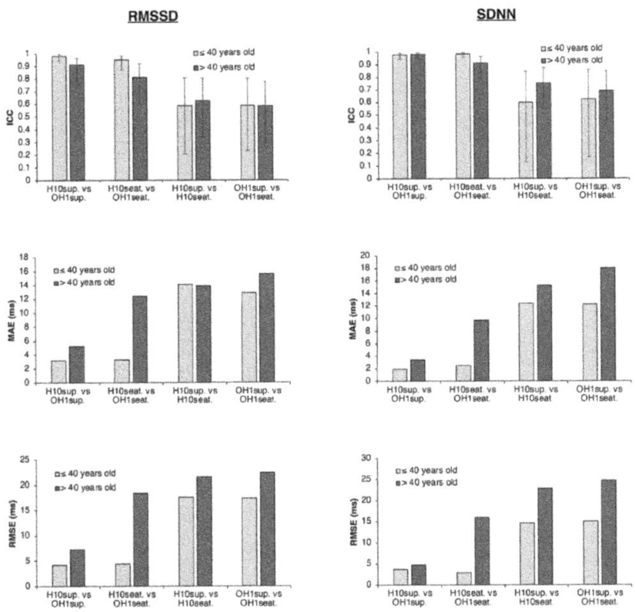

Figure 2. Bar plots of ICC, MAE, and RMSE for RMSSD and SDNN according to age groups (≤40 years vs. >40 years) across different body position conditions (supine and seated) and devices (H10 vs. OH1). Light gray bars represent participants aged ≤40 years and dark gray bars represent participants aged >40 years. Error bars on ICC indicate 95% confidence intervals.

3.5. *Influence of Sex on HRV Parameters*

When comparing HRV parameters between sexes, females exhibited lower absolute RMSSD and SDNN values than males in both supine and seated positions (see Figure 3 and Table 4). For RMSSD, ICCs (3,1) between H10 and OH1 in the supine position were good for females and excellent for males (0.851 vs. 0.974), with mean differences of −3.76 ms and −2.46 ms, respectively. In the seated position, ICCs were lower, particularly among females (0.521 vs. 0.870), and mean differences increased in both groups (−8.27 ms for females vs. −7.74 ms for males). MAE and RMSE values were higher in the seated condition but remained similar between sexes. Comparable patterns were observed for SDNN, with excellent ICCs in the supine position for both females and males (0.939 vs. 0.980). In the seated position, reliability decreased in females (ICC = 0.513) but remained excellent in males (ICC = 0.967). As with RMSSD, MAE and RMSE values were higher in the seated condition, with similar magnitudes of error across sexes. Regarding the effect of body position, RMSSD showed reduced reliability in females, with poor ICCs between supine and seated positions for both sensors (0.450 for H10 and 0.251 for OH1). In contrast, ICCs in males remained moderate (0.555 for H10 and 0.524 for OH1). For SDNN, reliability between positions was higher in males (ICC = 0.702 for H10 and 0.720 for OH1) than in females (ICC = 0.317 for H10 and −0.031 for OH1). Despite relatively small mean differences across positions and sexes (ranging from −8.27 to 2.09 ms), LoA remained wide, occasionally exceeding ±50 ms. MAE and RMSE values confirmed this variability, with consistently larger errors in the seated condition.

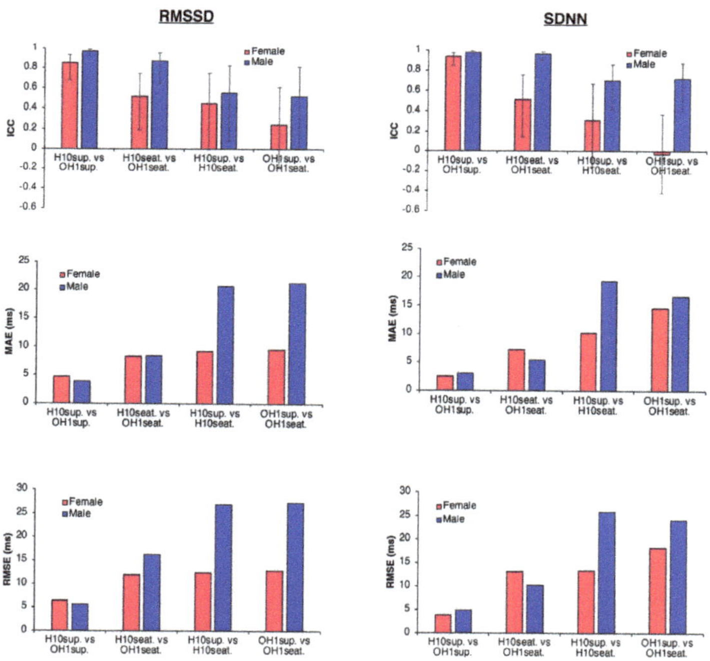

Figure 3. Bar plots of ICC, MAE, and RMSE for RMSSD and SDNN according to sex (male vs. female) across different body position conditions (supine and seated) and devices (H10 vs. OH1). Pink bars represent women and blue bars represent men. Error bars on ICC indicate 95% confidence intervals.

Table 4. Comparison of RMSSD and SDNN between males and females across the different body position conditions (supine and seated) and devices (H10 vs. OH1) using intraclass correlation coefficients (ICC), mean absolute error (MAE), root mean square error (RMSE), and Bland–Altman analysis.

Variables	Conditions (1 vs. 2)	Mean ± SD (1 vs. 2)	ICC (95% CI)	MAE	RMSE	Mean Diff.	Lower LoA	Upper LoA
RMSSD Female (ms)	*H10sup.* vs. *OH1sup.*	29 ± 13 vs. 33 ± 11	0.851 (0.678–0.934)	4.66	6.41	−3.76	−14.24	6.72
	H10seat. vs. *OH1seat.*	29 ± 12 vs. 37 ± 10	0.521 (0.196–0.743)	8.30	11.93	−8.27	−25.62	9.07
	H10sup. vs. *H10seat.*	29 ± 13 vs. 29 ± 12	0.450 (−0.002–0.750)	9.17	12.49	0.59	−24.57	25.75
	OH1sup. vs. *OH1seat.*	33 ± 11 vs. 37 ± 10	0.251 (−0.198–0.613)	9.49	12.90	−3.92	−28.70	20.86
RMSSD Male (ms)	*H10sup.* vs. *OH1sup.*	48 ± 25 vs. 51 ± 26	0.974 (0.921–0.991)	3.86	5.60	−2.46	−12.73	7.82
	H10seat. vs. *OH1seat.*	46 ± 34 vs. 54 ± 32	0.870 (0.646–0.956)	8.36	16.28	−7.74	−36.96	21.49
	H10sup. vs. *H10seat.*	48 ± 25 vs. 46 ± 34	0.555 (0.076–0.826)	20.66	26.89	2.09	−52.61	56.79
	OH1sup. vs. *OH1seat.*	51 ± 26 vs. 54 ± 32	0.524 (0.010–0.819)	21.15	27.31	−3.19	−58.53	52.15
SDNN Female (ms)	*H10sup.* vs. *OH1sup.*	41 ± 11 vs. 43 ± 11	0.939 (0.851–0.976)	2.49	3.86	−2.13	−8.62	4.35
	H10seat. vs. *OH1seat.*	42 ± 12 vs. 50 ± 13	0.513 (0.145–0.757)	7.19	13.09	−7.07	−29.28	15.14
	H10sup. vs. *H10seat.*	41 ± 11 vs. 42 ± 12	0.317 (−0.157–0.672)	10.22	13.28	−1.33	−27.98	25.31
	OH1sup. vs. *OH1seat.*	43 ± 11 vs. 50 ± 13	−0.031 (−0.424–0.373)	14.61	18.28	−6.28	−40.90	28.35
SDNN Male (ms)	*H10sup. vs* *OH1sup.*	66 ± 25 vs. 68 ± 26	0.980 (0.937–0.993)	3.03	4.89	−2.09	−11.11	6.93
	H10seat. vs. *OH1seat.*	69 ± 42 vs. 73 ± 39	0.967 (0.902–0.989)	5.37	10.19	−4.55	−23.15	14.04
	H10sup. vs. *H10seat.*	66 ± 25 vs. 69 ± 42	0.702 (0.419–0.860)	19.26	25.82	−2.96	−55.29	49.36
	OH1sup. vs. *OH1seat.*	68 ± 26 vs. 73 ± 39	0.720 (0.409–0.881)	16.58	24.07	−5.43	−53.26	42.40

4. Discussion

The aim of this study was to assess the validity of PPG-based HRV measurements in comparison with ECG-based measurements, and to examine the influence of recording duration, body position, age, and sex on measurement accuracy.

Our main findings indicate generally good to excellent agreement between the ECG-based Polar H10 and the PPG-based Polar OH1 for the time domain HRV parameters RMSSD and SDNN in healthy individuals. This agreement was consistent across both supine and seated positions, supporting previous research demonstrating the reliability of PPG technology for HRV assessment under controlled conditions [5]. Furthermore, recording duration had a limited impact on measurement accuracy. Although shorter recordings introduced slightly greater variability, our results are consistent with prior studies indicating that 2 min recordings can provide sufficiently accurate RMSSD and SDNN values [14]. This finding is particularly relevant for practical applications, where longer recordings may be impractical. However, ensuring that participants are in a stable physiological state before measurement remains essential to ensure data validity [13].

A more detailed analysis revealed that agreement between sensors varied depending on body position. Specifically, concordance between PPG- and ECG-derived measures was higher in the supine position, but significantly lower in the seated position. These discrepancies were reflected by larger errors, greater mean differences, and wider limits of agreement, particularly for PPG-derived measurements. This suggests that sensor agreement is reduced under certain physiological conditions associated with posture. Furthermore, within-sensor comparisons between supine and seated positions also showed consistently lower agreement, indicating that the observed discrepancies reflect genuine physiological changes rather than sensor inaccuracies alone. The transition from supine to seated posture is known to increase sympathetic activity and reduce parasympathetic tone [11] resulting in distinct autonomic states and, consequently, reduced agreement between positions. Several factors may account for this increased variability. First, PTT introduces fluctuations in PRV that are not directly related to cardiac autonomic modulation [31,32]. These fluctuations—driven by respiration-induced changes in intrathoracic pressure—may be amplified in the seated position due to postural effects on vascular dynamics. Second, the accuracy of beat-to-beat interval extraction from PPG signals is limited, particularly in individuals with increased vascular stiffness or altered pulse wave morphology. For example, reflected waves can distort peak detection in older adults, reducing the reliability of HRV estimates [33]. These limitations primarily affect short-term HRV indices, such as RMSSD and SDNN, although alternative approaches, such as valley-to-valley interval detection, have shown promise in improving accuracy [33]. Together, these findings highlight the importance of considering both sensor type and body position when interpreting HRV data.

When considering the effects of age, our analysis of HRV parameters over a 5 min recording period revealed a general decline in RMSSD and SDNN values with increasing age, which is consistent with previous findings [17,18]. This reduction in HRV among older participants reflects an age-related decrease in autonomic nervous system adaptability [19]. However, prior research suggests that the decline in RMSSD with age does not follow a strictly linear trajectory, but rather a U-shaped pattern, with a slight increase observed beyond the age of 70 [18]. Since our study included only participants aged 18 to 70 years, we were unable to explore this potential non-linear trend. Moreover, the agreement between HRV values derived from the OH1 and H10 was generally lower in participants over 40 years of age, regardless of body position. This may be partially explained by age-related increases in arterial stiffness. In older individuals, the reflected wave in the PPG signal becomes more pronounced, potentially complicating peak detection and reducing the accuracy of HRV estimation [33]. Sex-related differences were also observed, with females displaying lower absolute RMSSD and SDNN values compared to males. These results align with previous literature indicating that women tend to have higher resting heart rates and lower overall HRV, likely due to differences in autonomic regulation [20]. Additionally, the accuracy of PPG-derived HRV measures was slightly reduced in females, particularly in the seated position. This may be attributed to sex-related differences in vascular compliance and endothelial function, which affect pulse wave dynamics and thus the accuracy of PRV estimation [19,21]. Hormonal fluctuations may also contribute to increased intra-individual variability in HRV among females, potentially affecting agreement between ECG- and PPG-based measurements [34]. Nevertheless, given the relatively small sample size, these subgroup-specific observations should be interpreted with caution.

Despite its strengths, this study has several limitations that should be considered when interpreting the findings. First, our sample included only healthy participants aged 18 to 70 years, limiting the generalizability to younger, older, or clinical populations. Additionally, the participants had light skin tones (Fitzpatrick phototypes I–III), which may affect the applicability of results to individuals with darker skin. Indeed, recent research [22] suggests that green-light PPG sensors such as the Polar OH1 may show reduced accuracy in darker skin due to increased light absorption and scattering. Secondly, we focused solely on two time domain HRV metrics, RMSSD and SDNN, commonly used in consumer devices. Although informative, these parameters do not capture the full complexity of autonomic regulation. Future studies should include additional indices, especially frequency domain measures (e.g., LF, HF, and LF/HF ratio), for a more comprehensive evaluation of PPG accuracy. Another limitation is the lack of repeated measurements within each body position. HRV exhibits intra-individual variability even under stable conditions, making it difficult to fully isolate the effect of posture from natural fluctuations. While we randomized the order of recordings and included rest periods to mitigate this, repeated measures would strengthen estimates of measurement reliability and better attribute differences to posture. Future research should address these issues by including more diverse populations, assessing a broader range of HRV parameters, and incorporating repeated recordings. Moreover, applying machine learning techniques to long-term HRV data could reveal health-related trends over time, building upon the foundational validation of PPG-based HRV accuracy provided here.

5. Conclusions

The present findings support the use of PPG-based HRV monitoring for practical assessments in healthy individuals, demonstrating good agreement with ECG-based sensors across conditions. However, as the data were collected exclusively from healthy participants with Fitzpatrick skin phototypes I–III, the results may not be fully generalizable to the wider population. Furthermore, while the observed postural differences likely reflect physiological variations, these findings may not extend to all body positions or PPG sensor types.

Author Contributions: Research design and project management: A.C., G.M. and C.H. Data collection: G.M. Data analysis: A.C. and G.M. Manuscript preparation and editing: A.C., G.M. and C.H. All authors have read and agreed to the published version of the manuscript.

Funding: This research received no external funding.

Institutional Review Board Statement: The study was conducted in accordance with the Declaration of Helsinki, and approved by the National Ethics Committee (ethical approval: IRB00012476-2024-13-11-352).

Informed Consent Statement: Informed consent was obtained from all subjects involved in the study.

Data Availability Statement: The original data and Matlab codes used in the study are openly available in H10_OH1_analysis at https://github.com/GeoffreyMillour/H10_OH1_analysis.git (accessed on 1 September 2025).

Conflicts of Interest: The authors declare no conflicts of interest.

Abbreviations

The following abbreviations are used in this manuscript:

ANS	Autonomic nervous system
ECG	Electrocardiography
HR	Heart rate
HRV	Heart rate variability
LoA	Limits of agreement
PAT	Pulse arrival time
PPG	Photoplethysmography
PPI	Peak-to-peak interval

PTT	Pulse transit time
PRV	Pulse rate variability
RMSSD	Root mean square of successive differences
SDNN	Standard deviation of normal-to-normal intervals

References

1. Rehman, R.Z.U.; Chatterjee, M.; Manyakov, N.V.; Daans, M.; Jackson, A.; O'Brisky, A.; Telesky, T.; Smets, S.; Berghmans, P.-J.; Yang, D.; et al. Assessment of Physiological Signals from Photoplethysmography Sensors Compared to an Electrocardiogram Sensor: A Validation Study in Daily Life. *Sensors* **2024**, *24*, 6826. [CrossRef]
2. Gil, E.; Orini, M.; Bailón, R.; Vergara, J.M.; Mainardi, L.; Laguna, P. Photoplethysmography pulse rate variability as a surrogate measurement of heart rate variability during non-stationary conditions. *Physiol. Meas.* **2010**, *31*, 1271. [CrossRef]
3. Plews, D.J.; Laursen, P.B.; Le Meur, Y.; Hausswirth, C.; Kilding, A.E.; Buchheit, M. Monitoring training with heart-rate variability: How much compliance is needed for valid assessment? *Int. J. Sports Physiol. Perform.* **2014**, *9*, 783–790. [CrossRef]
4. Plews, D.J.; Laursen, P.B.; Stanley, J.; Kilding, A.E.; Buchheit, M. Training adaptation and heart rate variability in elite endurance athletes: Opening the door to effective monitoring. *Sports Med.* **2017**, *47*, 861–880. [CrossRef]
5. Plews, D.J.; Scott, B.; Altini, M.; Wood, M.; Kilding, A.E.; Laursen, P.B. Comparison of heart-rate-variability recording with smartphone photoplethysmography, Polar H7 chest strap, and electrocardiography. *Int. J. Sports Physiol. Perform.* **2017**, *12*, 1324–1328. [CrossRef] [PubMed]
6. Shaffer, F.; Ginsberg, J.P. An overview of heart rate variability metrics and norms. *Front. Public Health* **2017**, *5*, 258. [CrossRef]
7. Armañac-Julián, P.; Kontaxis, S.; Lázaro, J.; Rapalis, A.; Brazaitis, M.; Marozas, V.; Laguna, P.; Bailón, R.; Gil, E. Vascular reactivity characterized by PPG-derived pulse wave velocity. *Biomed. Signal Process. Control* **2025**, *105*, 107641. [CrossRef]
8. Tikhonova, I.V.; Grinevich, A.A.; Tankanag, A.V. Analysis of phase interactions between heart rate variability, respiration and peripheral microhemodynamics oscillations of upper and lower extremities in human. *Biomed. Signal Process. Control* **2022**, *71*, 103091. [CrossRef]
9. Yuda, E.; Shibata, M.; Ogata, Y.; Ueda, N.; Yambe, T.; Yoshizawa, M.; Hayano, J. Pulse rate variability: A new biomarker, not a surrogate for heart rate variability. *J. Physiol. Anthropol.* **2020**, *39*, 21. [CrossRef] [PubMed]
10. Constant, I.; Laude, D.; Murat, I.; Elghozi, J.L. Pulse rate variability is not a surrogate for heart rate variability. *Clin. Sci.* **1999**, *97*, 391–397. [CrossRef]
11. Lu, G.; Yang, F.; Taylor, J.A.; Stein, J.F. A comparison of photoplethysmography and ECG recording to analyze heart rate variability in healthy subjects. *J. Med. Eng. Technol.* **2009**, *33*, 634–641. [CrossRef]
12. Obata, Y.; Ong, Q.J.; Magruder, J.T.; Grichkevitch, H.; Berkowitz, D.E.; Nyhan, D.; Steppan, J.; Barodka, V. Noninvasive assessment of the effect of position and exercise on pulse arrival to peripheral vascular beds in healthy volunteers. *Front. Physiol.* **2017**, *8*, 47. [CrossRef] [PubMed]
13. Task Force of the European Society of Cardiology. Heart rate variability: Standards of measurement, physiological interpretation, and clinical use. *Circulation* **1996**, *93*, 1043–1065. [CrossRef]
14. Munoz, M.L.; Van Roon, A.; Riese, H.; Thio, C.; Oostenbroek, E.; Westrik, I.; de Geus, E.J.C.; Gansevoort, R.; Lefrandt, J.; Nolte, I.M.; et al. Validity of (ultra-) short recordings for heart rate variability measurements. *PLoS ONE* **2015**, *10*, e0138921. [CrossRef]
15. Buchheit, M. Monitoring training status with HRV measures: Do all roads lead to Rome? *Front. Physiol.* **2014**, *5*, 73. [CrossRef] [PubMed]
16. Bent, B.; Goldstein, B.A.; Kibbe, W.A.; Dunn, J.P. Investigating sources of inaccuracy in wearable optical heart rate sensors. *NPJ Digit. Med.* **2020**, *3*, 18. [CrossRef]
17. Nunan, D.; Sandercock, G.R.H.; Brodie, D.A. A quantitative systematic review of normal values for short-term heart rate variability in healthy adults. *Pacing Clin. Electrophysiol.* **2010**, *33*, 1407–1417. [CrossRef]
18. Almeida-Santos, M.A.; Barreto-Filho, J.A.; Oliveira, J.L.M.; Reis, F.P.; da Cunha Oliveira, C.C.; Sousa, A.C.S. Aging, heart rate variability and patterns of autonomic regulation of the heart. *Arch. Gerontol. Geriatr.* **2016**, *63*, 1–8. [CrossRef]
19. Bonnemeier, H.; Wiegand, U.K.; Brandes, A.; Kluge, N.; Katus, H.A.; Richardt, G.; Potratz, J. Circadian profile of cardiac autonomic nervous modulation in healthy subjects: Differing effects of aging and gender on heart rate variability. *J. Cardiovasc. Electrophysiol.* **2003**, *14*, 791–799. [CrossRef] [PubMed]
20. Koenig, J.; Thayer, J.F. Sex differences in healthy human heart rate variability: A meta-analysis. *Neurosci. Biobehav. Rev.* **2016**, *64*, 288–310. [CrossRef]
21. Sista, A.; Ittermann, T.; Gross, S.; Markus, M.R.; Stone, K.; Stoner, L.; Friedrich, N.; Dörr, M.; Bahls, M. Sex and resting heart rate influence the relation between arterial stiffness and cardiac structure and function–insights from the general population. *J. Hum. Hypertens.* **2025**, *39*, 254–261. [CrossRef]
22. Koerber, D.; Khan, S.; Shamsheri, T.; Kirubarajan, A.; Mehta, S. Accuracy of heart rate measurement with wrist-worn wearable devices in various skin tones: A systematic review. *J. Racial Ethn. Health Disparities* **2023**, *10*, 2676–2684. [CrossRef]

23. World Medical Association. World Medical Association Declaration of Helsinki: Ethical principles for medical research involving human participants. *JAMA* **2025**, *333*, 71–74. [CrossRef]
24. Schaffarczyk, M.; Rogers, B.; Reer, R.; Gronwald, T. Validity of the polar H10 sensor for heart rate variability analysis during resting state and incremental exercise in recreational men and women. *Sensors* **2022**, *22*, 6536. [CrossRef] [PubMed]
25. Hermand, E.; Cassirame, J.; Ennequin, G.; Hue, O. Validation of a photoplethysmographic heart rate monitor: Polar OH1. *Int. J. Sports Med.* **2019**, *40*, 462–467. [CrossRef] [PubMed]
26. Vollmer, M. Arrhythmia classification in long-term data using relative RR intervals. In *2017 Computing in Cardiology (CinC)*; IEEE: New York, NY, USA, 2017; pp. 1–4. [CrossRef]
27. Vollmer, M. HRVTool—An open-source MATLAB toolbox for analyzing heart rate variability. In *2019 Computing in Cardiology (CinC)*; IEEE: New York, NY, USA, 2019; pp. 1–4. [CrossRef]
28. Natarajan, A.; Pantelopoulos, A.; Emir-Farinas, H.; Natarajan, P. Heart rate variability with photoplethysmography in 8 million individuals: A cross-sectional study. *Lancet Digit. Health* **2020**, *2*, e650–e657. [CrossRef]
29. Koo, T.K.; Li, M.Y. A guideline of selecting and reporting intraclass correlation coefficients for reliability research. *J. Chiropr. Med.* **2016**, *15*, 155–163. [CrossRef] [PubMed]
30. Lee, E.; Ketelhut, S.; Wiklund, P.; Kostensalo, J.; Kolunsarka, I.; Hägglund, H.; Ahtiainen, J.P. Regular postexercise sauna bathing does not improve heart rate variability: A multi-arm randomized controlled trial. *Physiol. Rep.* **2025**, *13*, e70449. [CrossRef]
31. Yuda, E.; Yamamoto, K.; Yoshida, Y.; Hayano, J. Differences in pulse rate variability with measurement site. *J. Physiol. Anthropol.* **2020**, *39*, 4. [CrossRef]
32. Mejía-Mejía, E.; Kyriacou, P.A. Photoplethysmography-Based Pulse Rate Variability and Haemodynamic Changes in the Absence of Heart Rate Variability: An In-Vitro Study. *Appl. Sci.* **2022**, *12*, 7238. [CrossRef]
33. Chen, X.; Chen, T.; Luo, F.; Li, J. Comparison of valley-to-valley and peak-to-peak intervals from photoplethysmographic signals to obtain heart rate variability in the sitting position. In Proceedings of the 2013 6th International Conference on Biomedical Engineering and Informatics, Hangzhou, China, 16–18 December 2013; IEEE: New York, NY, USA, 2013; pp. 214–218. [CrossRef]
34. Voss, A.; Schroeder, R.; Heitmann, A.; Peters, A.; Perz, S. Short-term heart rate variability—Influence of gender and age in healthy subjects. *PLoS ONE* **2022**, *10*, e0118308. [CrossRef] [PubMed]

MDPI AG
Grosspeteranlage 5
4052 Basel
Switzerland
Tel.: +41 61 683 77 34

Sensors Editorial Office
E-mail: sensors@mdpi.com
www.mdpi.com/journal/sensors

www.ingramcontent.com/pod-product-compliance
Lightning Source LLC
Chambersburg PA
CBHW061442210926
51850CB00008B/1587